Thermoregulation:
The Pathophysiological Basis of Clinical Disorders

8th International Symposium on the Pharmacology of Thermoregulation,
Kananaskis, Alta., August 26–30, 1991

Thermoregulation:
The Pathophysiological Basis of
Clinical Disorders

Editors
P. Lomax, Los Angeles, Calif.
E. Schönbaum, Venhorst

45 figures and 30 tables, 1992

KARGER

Basel · München · Paris · London · New York · New Delhi · Bangkok · Singapore · Tokyo · Sydney

1992

Symposia on the Pharmacology of Thermoregulation

1   The Pharmacology of Thermoregulation. San Francisco, Calif., 1972
    Editors: E. Schönbaum, Toronto, and P. Lomax, Los Angeles, Calif.
    XIV + 586 p., 159 fig., 44 tab., 1973. ISBN 3-8055-1391-7
2   Temperature Regulation and Drug Action. Paris 1974
    Editors: P. Lomax, Los Angeles, Calif.; E. Schönbaum, Oss, and J. Jacob, Paris
    XXII + 405 p., 94 fig., 52 tab., 1975. ISBN 3-8055-1756-4
3   Drugs, Biogenic Amines and Body Temperature. Banff, Alta., 1976
    Editors: K.E. Cooper, Calgary; P. Lomax, Los Angeles, Calif., and E. Schönbaum, Oss
    XX + 284 p., 58 fig., 26 tab., 1977. ISBN 3-8055-2395-5
4   Thermoregulatory Mechanisms and Their Therapeutic Implications. Oxford, 1979
    Editors: B. Cox, Manchester; P. Lomax, Los Angeles, Calif.; A.S. Milton, Aberdeen, and
    E. Schönbaum, Oss
    XVI + 304 p., 68 fig., 38 tab., 1980. ISBN 3-8055-0277-X
5   Environment, Drugs and Thermoregulation. Saint-Paul-de-Vence, 1982
    Editors: P. Lomax, Los Angeles, Calif., and E. Schönbaum, Oss
    XVI + 224 p., 64 fig., 38 tab., 1983. ISBN 3-8055-3654-2
6   Homeostasis and Thermal Stress. Experimental and Therapeutic Advances. Jasper, Alta., 1985
    Editors: K. Cooper, Calgary; P. Lomax, Los Angeles, Calif.; E. Schönbaum, Oss, and
    W.L. Veale, Calgary
    XIV + 210 p., 48 fig., 33 tab., 1986. ISBN 3-8055-4228-3
7   Thermoregulation: Research and Clinical Application. Odense, 1988
    Editors: P. Lomax, Los Angeles, Calif., and E. Schönbaum, Venhorst
    XIV + 250 p., 90 fig., 42 tab., 1989. ISBN 3-8055-4921-0

Library of Congress Cataloging-in-Publication Data
International Symposium on the Pharmacology of Thermoregulation
(8th: 1991: Kananaskis, Alta.
Thermoregulation: the pathophysiological basis of clinical disorders /
8th International Symposium on the Pharmacology of Thermoregulation, Kananaskis, Alta.,
August 26–30, 1991; editors, P. Lomax, E. Schönbaum.
Includes bibliographical references and index.
1. Body temperature – Regulation – Congresses.   2. Hyperthermia – Pathophysiology –
Congresses.   3. Hypothermia – Pathophysiology – Congresses.
I. Lomax, Peter, 1928–.   II. Schönbaum, E.   III. Title.
[DNLM: 1. Body Temperature – drug effects – congresses.   2. Body Temperature Regulation
– congresses.   QT 165 I62t 1991]
RB129.I58   1991
616.9'89 – dc20
ISBN 3-8055-5513-X

©   Copyright 1992 by S. Karger AG, P.O. Box, CH–4009 Basel (Switzerland)
    Printed in Switzerland on acid-free paper by Thür AG Offsetdruck, Pratteln
    ISBN 3-8055-5513-X

CONTENTS

LIST OF PARTICIPANTS

ADLER, MARTIN W.
Philadelphia (USA)

BAKKEVIG, MARTHA KOLO
Trondheim (Norway)

BAUCE, LORENZO
Calgary (Canada)

BELKE, DARRELL
Edmonton (Canada)

BLATTEIS, CLARK M.
Memphis (USA)

CHRISTENSEN, J. DENCKER
Copenhagen (Denmark)

COOPER, KEITH E.
Calgary (Canada)

CUI, YAN
Edmonton (Canada)

DARTANA, SIOE H.
Edmonton (Canada)

DASCOMBE, MICHAEL J.
Manchester (England)

DICKER, ANDREA
Stockholm (Sweden)

DOWNEY, JOHN A.
New York (USA)

FEDERICO, PAOLO
Calgary (Canada)

FEWELL, JAMES
Calgary (Canada)

FREEDMAN, ROBERT
Detroit (USA)

FREGLY, MELVIN J.
Gainesville (USA)

FRENS, JAN
Bokmeer (Netherlands)

GELLER, ELLEN B.
Philadelphia (USA)

GLOSTEN, BETH
Chicago (USA)

GOELST, KATHLEEN
Johannesburg
(South Africa)

GONG, XIAO-WEI
Yamanashi (Japan)

GRANT, Daniel A.
Calgary (Canada)

HALES, J. ROBERT
Kensington (Australia)

HANDLER, CYNTHIA M.
Philadelphia (USA)

HANSEN, E. WIND
Copenhagen (Denmark)

HASSINEN, ESA
Oulu (Finland)

HOOPER, DEBBIE
Calgary (Canada)

HUANG, XIAO-CHEN
Yamanashi (Japan)

IAIZZO, PAUL
Minneapolis (USA)

JACOBS, IRA
North York (Canada)

JONES, DOUG
London (Canada)

JOURDAN, MICHAEL L.
Edmonton (Canada)

KANAMORI, TAKANARI
Kawasaki (Japan)

KATOVICH, MICHAEL
Gainesville (USA)

KONDO, COLLEEN
Calgary (Canada)

LABURN, HELEN
Johannesburg
(South Africa)

LEE, TZE-FUN
Edmonton (Canada)

LIU, BIN
Edmonton (Canada)

LOMAX, PETER
Los Angeles (USA)

MACDONALD, IAN A.
Nottingham (England)

MALKINSON, TERRANCE
Calgary (Canada)

MARSHALL, WILMA
Edmonton (Canada)

MCARTHUR, DAWN
Edmonton (Canada)

MCGUIRE, JOSEPH
San Francisco (USA)

MILTON, ANTHONY S.
Aberdeen (Scotland)

MOAYERI, AZAITA
San Francisco (USA)

NAGAI, MASANORI
Yamanashi (Japan)

NOMOTO, TERUKO
Tokyo (Japan)

OHLSON, KERSTIN
Stockholm (Sweden)

PASSIAS, THANASIS
Burnaby (Canada)

PITTMAN, QUENTIN
Calgary (Canada)

PYORNILA, AHTI
Oulu (Finland)

REINERTSEN, RANDI E.
Trondheim (Norway)

ROTH, JOACHIM
Giessen (Germany)

SAARELA, SEPPO Y.O.
Oulu (Finland)

SACHDEVA, USHA
New Delhi (India)

SCARPACE, PHILIP J.
Gainesville (USA)

SCHÖNBAUM, EDUARD
Venhorst (Netherlands)

SESSLER, DANIEL I.
San Francisco (USA)

SHAPIRO, YAIR
Tel-Aviv (Israel)

SHEFFIELD, CLARK
San Francisco (USA)

SIEMEN, DETLEF
Regensburg (Germany)

SIMROSE, REBECCA
Calgary (Canada)

TALAN, MARK
Baltimore (USA)

UCHIDA, YOKO
Tokyo (Japan)

UCHIDA, YUICHIRO
Tokyo (Japan)

VEALE, WARREN L.
Calgary (Canada)

WANG, LAWRENCE
Edmonton (Canada)

WHITE, MATTHEW
Ste-Foy (Canada)

WILKINSON, MARSHALL
Calgary (Canada)

WILLCOX, BRAD
Calgary (Canada)

WOODWARD, SUZANNE
Detroit (USA)

YOSHIUE, SHOHEI
Kawasaki (Japan)

ZEISBERGER, EUGEN
Giessen (Germany)

ACKNOWLEDGEMENTS

This symposium was supported by the Alberta Heritage Foundation for Medical Research and by the Medical Research Council of Canada.

The symposium was officially sponsored by The University of Calgary, The International Union of Physiological Sciences Commission on Thermal Physiology and The International Union of Pharmacology.

We are grateful for the help and cooperation of The University of Calgary, the University of Alberta and the University of California at Los Angeles. Special thanks are extended to Mrs. Grace Olmstead of the Department of Medical Physiology, The University of Calgary and to Mrs. Margaret-Anne Stroh of the Conference Office, The University of Calgary.

Organizers:

P. Lomax (U.S.A.)
E. Schönbaum (The Netherlands)
W.L. Veale (Canada)
L.C.H. Wang (Canada)

PREFACE

We are pleased to present the Proceedings of the Eighth Symposium on the *Pharmacology of Thermoregulation.* The symposium took place at Kananaskis Village, located in the Canadian Rockies approximately 100 km west of Calgary, Alberta. Kananaskis Village was constructed for the 1988 Winter Olympic Games and the park has been developed since then into a year round recreational facility complete with excellent conference accommodations. This beautiful setting proved to be an outstanding venue for the symposium.

The meeting provided a five day intense forum in which students, postdoctoral fellows and scientists from around the world have had an opportunity to meet to exchange and evaluate scientific ideas in the general field of temperature regulation, encompassing both basic research and clinical applications. Thematic lectures provided a review of the general areas prior to the presentation of related, detailed scientific presentations. The discussions following the oral and poster presentations provided an opportunity to review specific problems and to focus on certain aspects of the subject in which further research is needed. This Proceedings volume makes the scientific findings widely available to all those involved in this field of research, or in the management of patients suffering from disorders related to temperature regulation or exposure to adverse environments. The highlight of the symposium was the mini symposium entitled *Thermoregulation: Past, Present and Future.* Five major topics were discussed by internationally recognized experts in the areas.

As one would expect, considerable help has been received from many different sources and we are most grateful to many colleagues and friends for their cooperation and assistance. We acknowledge the support of the Alberta Heritage Foundation for Medical Research and the Medical Research Council of Canada. Mini-Mitter Corporation of Sunriver, Oregon, U.S.A. contributed generously to the symposium. The collaboration of The University of Calgary, the University of Alberta, the University of California at Los Angeles and the staff of the Conference Office at The University of Calgary was invaluable in arranging the meeting.

Due to political disruptions over the past year several scientists, particularly from the Soviet Union, Eastern Europe and the Middle East, were unable to follow up their plans to attend the symposium. We do hope that in future years these scientists will be able to participate freely in the meetings.

The success of the symposium was in no small way assured by the assistance of Mrs. Grace Olmstead, of the Department of Medical Physiology, and Mrs. Margaret-Anne Stroh, from the Conference Office, of the University of Calgary. Special thanks are extended to Miss Karen Roberts at UCLA for the meticulous preparation of the manuscripts. The cooperation and expertise of the staff of the Karger publishing house has rendered the editors' task a real pleasure. We would like to record our gratitude to Keith Cooper for his outstanding speech, with reminiscences of the earlier symposia, during the banquet. It is our sincere wish that all contributors to these Proceedings will find that their efforts in this scientific endeavor have been most worthwhile.

Kananaskis Village, Alberta, Canada
August, 1991

Peter Lomax
Eduard Schönbaum
Warren L. Veale
Lawrence C.H. Wang

INTRODUCTION

The eighth symposium on the Pharmacology of Thermoregulation was held at The Lodge, Kananaskis, Alberta, Canada from August 26 to 30, 1991. The theme of the meeting was *The Pathophysiological Basis of Clinical Disorders* with the emphasis on the application of fundamental research to the management of thermoregulatory disorders.

There were 80 scientific participants present. The program consisted of a "mini symposium", which opened the proceedings, three thematic review lectures, 21 oral presentations and 25 poster presentations. Communications were scheduled for 7 additional authors who were subsequently unable to attend the meeting. In this Introduction we have included some major points from the talks by those who did not submit manuscripts as well as highlighting specific issues which arose during the lively and extensive discussions.

The mini symposium consisted of five short review lectures, with the general theme *Thermoregulation: Past, Present and Future*. **SCHÖNBAUM** discussed neurotransmitters and the elucidation of their role in temperature control. Current studies of co-transmitters, neuromodulators and neuropeptides render it necessary to reevaluate interdisciplinary research methods, switching from linear analysis to an interactive network approach. The absence of consideration of a possible role of nerve growth factor in the study of cold exposure and acclimation was noted as an example of the need for such reflection. This point was repeated often in ensuing discussions throughout the symposium. **WANG** reviewed his research on the physiology of hibernation, with the focus on the central nervous system. He feels that sleep and hibernation may represent a continuum in which the thermoregulatory set point is progressively lowered. Serotonin can induce sleep and may initiate hibernation. There is increased endogenous opioid function during hibernation and responses to exogenously applied opioids are reduced. The findings that prostaglandin D_2 lowers body temperature and promotes sleep, by an action in the preoptic area of the hypothalamus, whereas prostaglandin E_2 induces fever and wakefulness [see review, Hayaishi, O.: Molecular mechanisms of sleep-wake regulation: roles of prostaglandin D_2 and E_2. FASEB J. **5**:2575-2581 (1991)] are of interest in this respect. The research which has led to the development of the hypothesis that arginine vasopressin (AVP) acts at the ventromedial septal area to promote antipyresis was reviewed by **PITTMAN**. Recent findings indicate that oxytocin enhances the antipyretic effect of AVP in a dose dependent manner. The effects of cold exposure on food and water intake were discussed by **FREGLY**; his research findings are described in his paper in this volume. The question as to whether thermoregulation is impaired with increasing age, particularly in individuals over 65 years, was reevaluated by **LOMAX**. A comprehensive review of the literature reveals little statistical support for the commonly stated view that the incidence of accidental hypothermia and heat stroke (in particular, stress induced heat stroke) is significantly greater in the aged. Additionally, although cardiovascular disease and/or endocrinopathies are considered as major risk factors in the pathogenesis of thermoregulatory disorders, few of these conditions arise characteristically in older patients. Looking to the future, as well as pursuing exciting new avenues of research there is a clear need to reappraise many supposedly established positions in thermoregulatory physiology and pathophysiology.

Temperature regulation during general anesthesia was reviewed by **SESSLER**. The thresholds for the activation of responses to a fall in core temperature are lower during anesthesia while those for activation of heat loss mechanisms are raised. Thus, the interthreshold range is widened and this decreases the sensitivity of the thermoregulatory system. The effects of general anesthesia, with the associated 2-3°C fall in core temperature, on resistance to cutaneous bacterial infection was investigated by **SHEFFIELD**. In guinea pigs, hypothermia during isoflurane anesthesia caused significantly larger dermal lesions from intradermal injection of *E. coli*. Whether the impairment is due to inhibition of the immune response or to vasoconstriction in the skin vessels remains to be determined.

IAIZZO demonstrated that, in the dog, body cooling, and subsequent rewarming by convection, during isoflurane anesthesia regulates the brain temperature and may provide protection from cerebral ischemia in selected patients undergoing neurological or cardiovascular surgery. During epidural anesthesia with lidocaine **GLOSTEN** found that there was a fall in core (tympanic) temperature but this did not correlate with the patient's thermal perception. This may be the result of sympathetic blockade which increases skin temperature due increased perfusion.

In his thematic lecture **MILTON** reviewed the function of cytokines in fever and their role in the immune responses in general. The cover of the Proceedings of the seventh symposium carried a schematic representation of the system and this was updated to encompass most recent research.

That the route of administration of pyrogen significantly affects the fever response in rabbits was demonstrated by **LABURN**. The required dose was 10 times greater by the subcutaneous route compared to an intravenous dose, while intraperitoneal doses are ineffective at less than 100 times the intravenous dose.

Using young lambs, **FEWELL** reported that carotid denervation attenuated the rise in temperature and the increase in metabolic rate following injection of pyrogen. The mechanism of this change was not determined but there was considerable speculation as to its nature in the ensuing discussion.

In his thematic lecture entitled *Hypothalamic Norepinephrine and Body Temperature Control: Another Look* **BLATTEIS** compared his results using slow dialysis of the catecholamine into the rostral hypothalamus, which leads to a dose related fall in core temperature, with the more frequently used microinjection technique, which causes a rise in temperature in several species. It was suggested that microinjection produces tissue damage, possibly with release of prostaglandins, so that the temperature increase is artifactual. Adrenergic antagonists prevented the fall in temperature after dialysis. However, as was pointed out during the discussion, the rise in temperature also is blocked by specific antagonists; furthermore, there are many compounds which lower core temperature following microinjection into the preoptic/anterior hypothalamic nuclei.

Undoubtedly, these interesting and complex questions will continue to be the subjects for ongoing research. In his concluding remarks **LOMAX** raised the question which has concerned the organizers of this series of symposia for some time, namely, whether the pace of research warranted further gatherings, and the appropriate timing. The present symposium has demonstrated clearly that not only are there exciting new avenues to be explored but that earlier conclusions and positions need continuously to be appraised in the light of further knowledge. It is to be expected also that the development of the methodology of molecular biology will stimulate novel approaches to research in the field of thermoregulation. It is within this optimistic context that we look forward to the next symposium in Giessen, Germany in August 1994.

Banff, Alberta, Canada   **Peter Lomax**

August, 1991   **Eduard Schönbaum**

Lomax, Schönbaum (eds.) **Thermoregulation: The Pathophysiological Basis of Clinical Disorders.**
8th International Symposium Pharmacology of Thermoregulation, Kananaskis, Alberta, Canada 1991, pp. 1-5 (Karger, Basel 1992)

EFFECT OF REPEATED EXPOSURES TO COLD ON FOOD AND FLUID INTAKES OF RATS

MELVIN J. FREGLY and JOHN J. BURTON

Department of Physiology, University of Florida, College of Medicine, Gainesville, Florida 32610 (USA)

Exposure of laboratory rats to cold induces a variety of physiological responses that are generally considered to render them better able to survive in a hostile environment. One of the most important of these responses is the ability to increase the production of a sufficient amount of heat to offset increased heat loss. Most studies of heat production in rats show an immediate increase of 35 to 40% upon sudden exposure to cold [6]. One might expect that food intake, which represents an important substrate for the increase in heat production, would also increase immediately by about the same percentage. Surprisingly, most studies reveal that food intake increases gradually on exposure to cold and requires 8 to 10 days to achieve a maximal level [2]. This suggests that the cold exposed rat must make up for the lag in the increase in food intake by calling on body fat to provide the caloric deficit. This fact, among others, affects the gain in body weight of cold exposed rats and the content of white fat in their bodies. The negative caloric balance during the initial phase of exposure to cold is of particular interest since it could affect both performance and survival in the cold.

The primary objective of this study was to: (a) measure the change in food intake of male rats prior to and during a 10 day exposure to cold; and (b) determine whether the mechanisms (hormonal, nervous, etc.) responsible for the increase in food intake would respond more quickly to a second and third exposure to cold; i.e., whether they were adaptable.

METHODS: Twelve male rats of the Sprague Dawley strain, weighing 375-400 g at the start of the experiment, were used. This group was divided randomly into two equal subgroups, one of which served as control and remained at 26 ± 2°C. The second group was exposed to 5 ± 2°C after an initial 5 day control period.

During the control period, rats were kept individually in metabolic cages and provided *ad libitum* access to finely powdered food and tap water. Food containers were spill resistant and have been described elsewhere [1]. Fluid containers were infant nursing bottles with cast bronze spouts [4]. Daily measurements of individual food and fluid intake and urine output, as well as body weight, were made.

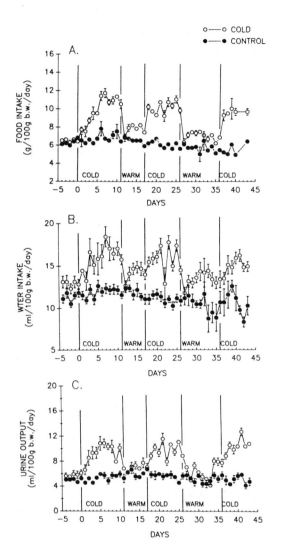

FIGURE 1: Effect of repeated exposure to cold on food intake (A), water intake (B) and urine output (C) of cold treated and control rats. The groups are designated in the figure. $\pm$ 1 SEM is set off at each mean. The vertical lines indicate the day of initiation of exposure to cold (5°C) or warm (26°C) environments.

At the end of the control period, the "cold treated" group was placed in an environmental chamber maintained at 5 $\pm$ 2°C while the control group was kept in an identical chamber maintained at 26 $\pm$ 2°C. Daily intake of food and fluid, and output of urine were measured for 10 days, after which the cold treated group was returned to 26°C. After 6 days at 26°C, the cold treated group was returned to 5°C for 9 days, following which it was removed from cold to 26°C for 10 days. At the end of this time, the cold-treated rats were returned to 5°C for 8 days. Throughout the experiment, daily measurements of food and fluid intake, urine output and body weight of individual rats were made. The experiment ended on the 49th day.

RESULTS: When the rats were exposed to cold for the first time, food intake increased gradually for 6 days at which time it reached a maximal, stable level which was approximately twice that of the control group maintained at 26°C (Fig. 1A). Removal of the rats from cold resulted in a decrease in food intake to control level within 1 day. However, by the second day food intake increased to reach a level significantly ($P < 0.01$) above that of the control group. The food intake was maintained at a level about 20% above that of the control group for the remaining 5 days at 26°C. When the cold treated rats were returned to cold air (i.e., second exposure, days 17 through 26), food intake increased immediately to reach a maximal level within the first day. Food intake remained at this level (approximately twice that of the control group) for the duration of exposure to cold. When the rats were removed from cold to 26°C for the second time, food intake again returned to control level within the first day, but increased above control level (approximately 20%) on the subsequent days of exposure to 26°C. A third cycle of exposure to cold was instituted at the end of the 10 days at 26°C. Again, food intake of the cold treated rats increased to a maximal level within the first day of exposure to cold.

Water intake (Fig. 1B) and urine output (Fig. 1C) followed the pattern of food intake closely, excepting that variability of measurements was greater. While it would appear that water intake reached a maximum more quickly during the second and third cycles of exposure to cold, it is less clear than that of food intake. During the first and second cycles of removal from cold, there were significant ($P < 0.01$) differences between the water intakes of the two groups. In the case of urine output, it is clearer that the maximum was reached more quickly during the second and third cycle than during the first cycle of exposure to cold. During the first and second cycles of removal from cold there were again significant ($P < 0.05$) differences between urine outputs of the two groups.

Exposure to cold resulted in a reduction in the gain of body weight of the cold treated group (Fig. 2). Mean body weight of the cold treated group increased at a greater rate when removed to a warm environment than during the previous or subsequent exposure to cold.

DISCUSSION: It is unclear at present why food intake of rats increases only gradually on first exposure to cold when metabolic rate and energy expenditure increase immediately [2,6]. It seems unlikely that the capacity of the gastrointestinal tract is a limiting factor since food intake reaches a level approximately twice that of controls within 6 days (Fig. 1A). The results suggest that the desire for additional food only slowly manifests itself during the initial exposure to cold. This may occur because hormonal and other mechanisms in the feed-back system controlling food intake respond more slowly than those controlling heat production. This suggests that the two controlling mechanisms are different, with different time constants. Thus, increased secretion of catecholamines, particularly norepinephrine, has been associated with increases in heat production during exposure to cold [3], while increased secretion of insulin, insulin-like growth factors, neuropeptide Y, norepinephrine, opioid peptides, pancreatic polypeptides, growth hormone releasing factor, and gamma-amino butyric acid (GABA) have been associated with increases in food intake [5,7]. It may be that the level of secretion, or interaction among, the hormones required to increase food intake maximally cannot be achieved quickly as is the case for heat production. This remains for further study.

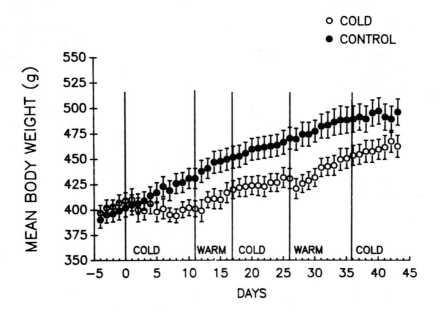

FIGURE 2: Effect of repeated exposures to cold on mean body weight of cold treated and control rats. The groups are designated in the figure. One standard error is set off at each mean. The vertical lines indicate the day of initiation of exposure to cold (5°C) or warm (26°C) environments.

Whatever physiological mechanisms control the intake of food during exposure to cold, the present results suggest that they work more effectively to increase food intake during a second exposure to cold when separated by 6 days from the first exposure to cold. This increased responsiveness was not lost even when the cold exposures were separated by 10 days at 26°C (Fig. 1A). It cannot be stated how long a period of separation between exposure to cold would be required to extinguish this response. It would appear, however, to be an adaptive response; i.e. one that allows the rat exposed to cold for a second time to maintain energy balance more effectively by increasing food intake immediately rather than calling on stores of body fat to maintain energy balance as apparently occurs during the first exposure to cold.

ACKNOWLEDGEMENTS: The authors acknowledge the technical assistance of Mr. T. Connor, Mrs. C. Edelstein, Miss L. Liu and Mr. S. Nayar. Supported by a grant from the Office of Naval Research Grant N00014-88-J-1221.

REFERENCES

1. Fregly, M.J.: A simple and accurate feeding device for rats. J. Appl. Physiol. **15**:539 (1960).
2. Fregly, M.J., Nelson, E.L., Jr. & Tyler, P.E.: Water exchange in rats exposed to cold, hypoxia, and both combined. Aviat. Space Environ. Med. **47**:600-607 (1976).

3. Hsieh, A.C.L., Carlson, L.D. and Gray, G.: Role of the sympathetic nervous system in the control of chemical regulation of heat production. Amer. J. Physiol. **190**:247-251 (1957).

4. Lazarow, A.: Methods for quantitative measurement of water intake. Meth. Med. Res. **6**:225-229 (1954).

5. Leibowitz, S.F.: Brain monoamines and peptides: role in the control of eating behavior. Fed. Proc. **45**:1396-1403 (1986).

6. Sellers, E.A. & You, S.S.: Role of the thyroid in metabolic responses to a cold environment. Am. J. Physiol. **163**:81-91 (1950).

7. Stanley, B.G., Kyrkouli, S.E., Lampert, S. & Leibowitz, S.F.: Neuropeptide Y chronically injected into the hypothalamus: a powerful neurochemical inducer of hyperphagia and obesity. Peptides **7**:1189-1192 (1986).

Lomax, Schönbaum (eds.) **Thermoregulation: The Pathophysiological Basis of Clinical Disorders.**
8th International Symposium Pharmacology of Thermoregulation, Kananaskis, Alberta, Canada 1991, pp. 6-9 (Karger, Basel 1992)

ELEVATED α_2-ADRENERGIC RESPONSIVENESS IN MENOPAUSAL HOT FLUSHES: PHARMACOLOGIC AND BIOCHEMICAL STUDIES

ROBERT R. FREEDMAN and SUZANNE WOODWARD

Department of Psychiatry, Wayne State University School of Medicine, Detroit, Michigan 48202 (USA)

Hot flushes (HFs) are the most common symptom of the climacteric and consist of sensations of internal heat as well as peripheral vasodilation, sweating, and tachycardia. Although HFs accompany the estrogen withdrawal of menopause, their appearance does not correlate with plasma [1], urinary [2], or vaginal [3] estrogen levels. Moreover, LH and LHRH secretion do not appear to be responsible for the initiation of HFs. Gambone *et al.* [4] found that patients with isolated gonadotropin deficiency, who had very low levels of LH, LHRH, and FSH experienced HFs following estrogen withdrawal. In contrast, patients with hypothalamic amenorrhea did not have HFs despite markedly low estrogen levels. The authors reasoned that HFs are not triggered by altered LHRH secretion *per se*, but by altered afferent input to LHRH neurons and suggested norepinephrine (NE) as a likely candidate for this mechanism.

Increased NE turnover in the hypothalamus is one mechanism believed responsible for the activation of central thermoregulatory mechanisms and may be responsible for the peripheral events of the HF that are characteristic of a heat dissipation response [5]. Clonidine, an α_2-adrenergic agonist, acts centrally to reduce NE turnover [6] and has been shown to ameliorate HFs in some clinical studies [7-9]. In a recent study [10] we tested the effects of clonidine vs. placebo during a heating procedure to induce HFs. We also utilized low doses of yohimbine, an α_2-adrenergic antagonist, to provoke HFs.

Subjects were 9 symptomatic menopausal women with frequent HFs documented by 24 h ambulatory monitoring of sternal skin conductance level (SCL, ref. 11). Six asymptomatic menopausal women served as a comparison group. They were prescreened by ambulatory monitoring to have no SCL responses and did not differ from the symptomatic group in age, weight, time since last period, or maturation index. In two blind laboratory sessions, subjects received either clonidine HCl (1 μg/kg iv) or placebo, followed by a 60 min waiting period and then by 45 min of peripheral heating. In two additional blind sessions subjects received yohimbine HCl (.032-.128 μg/kg iv) or placebo. HFs were detected objectively by computer, using the sternal SCL response. Clonidine significantly ($p = 0.01$) increased the amount of heating time needed to provoke a HF compared to placebo (40.6 ± 3.0 min vs 33.6 ± 3.6) and reduced the number of HFs (2 vs 8). A significantly greater number of HFs occurred during yohimbine sessions than in the corresponding placebo sessions (6 vs 0; $p = 0.015$).

The above data support the hypothesis that α_2-adrenoceptors within the central NE system are involved in triggering HFs and suggest that brain NE may be elevated in this process. MHPG is the major metabolite of brain NE [12] and previous studies have shown that plasma MHPG levels are reduced by clonidine [13] and increased by yohimbine [14]. Therefore, in the present study we measured plasma MHPG during spontaneous HFs and during HFs induced by peripheral heating.

METHODS: Thirteen symptomatic and 6 asymptomatic post-menopausal women were prescreened using 24 h ambulatory SCL monitoring [11]. They were supine in a 23°C room and an intravenous line was started for blood drawing. 10 ml blood samples were drawn at the beginning and end of a 60 min period and at the point of an SCL defined HF, if one occurred. Patients were then heated for 45 min as described previously [10]. Blood samples were taken at the beginning and end of this period and during SCL HFs. Blood was drawn from asymptomatic women at time points comparable to those of the symptomatic women. Blood samples were centrifuged and stored at -70°C. Subsequent MHPG determinations were performed by gas chromatography-mass spectrometry. Data were analyzed with repeated measures ANOVAs with simple effects tests.

RESULTS: In the symptomatic women, 6 HFs occurred in the resting period and 7 during the heating period. No HFs occurred in the asymptomatic women during either period. MHPG levels were significantly higher in symptomatic than asymptomatic women at all time points ($p < 0.0001$, Table I). In the symptomatic women, MHPG increased significantly ($p < 0.001$) during resting and heat-induced HFs. There were no significant changes in the asymptomatic women ($p > 0.6$).

TABLE I: Plasma MHPG during resting and heating periods in symptomatic and asymptomatic women (ng/ml)

Symptomatic Women		Asymptomatic Women	
Resting		**Resting**	
Basal	3.5 ± 0.2	Basal	2.6 ± 0.1
HF	4.3 ± 0.2	HF	2.7 ± 0.2
Post	3.8 ± 0.2	Post	2.5 ± 0.2
Heating		**Heating**	
Basal	3.4 ± 0.2	Basal	2.3 ± 0.2
HF	3.9 ± 0.3	HF	2.1 ± 0.1
Post	3.4 ± 0.2	Post	2.2 ± 0.2

DISCUSSION: Using complementary pharmacologic probes, we have shown that HFs can be provoked with an α_2-adrenergic antagonist and reduced with an α_2-adrenergic agonist. These findings suggest that central α_2-adrenergic receptors are involved in the initiation of menopausal HFs. Yohimbine increases NE release by blocking inhibitory presynaptic α_2-adrenoceptors and a reduction in their sensitivity or number would result in elevated NE turnover [15]. Consistent with this mechanism levels of plasma MHPG are significantly higher in symptomatic than asymptomatic women and these levels increase further during HFs. These results agree with previous human studies showing that yohimbine increases [14] and clonidine decreases [13] plasma levels of MHPG.

Investigations of women with menopausal HFs have not found elevations in plasma NE [16,17]. However, this measure derives from peripheral rather than central sympathetic nervous activity [18] whereas plasma MHPG reflects brain NE [12]. Plasma MHPG has not been studied previously with respect to HFs, to our knowledge.

In conclusion, the above data suggest that central α_2-adrenergic receptors are involved in the initiation of menopausal HFs. This mechanism is consistent with the finding of elevated MHPG levels in women with HFs and of further elevations during the HF itself. However the causal relationship, if any, between MHPG levels and α_2-adrenoceptor responsiveness remains to be determined for HFs.

ACKNOWLEDGEMENT: This work was supported by research grant AG-05233 from the National Institute on Aging.

REFERENCES

1. Aksel, S., Schomberg, D.W., Tyrey, L. & Hammond, C.B.: Vasomotor symptoms, serum estrogens, and gonadotropin levels in surgical menopause. Am. J. Obstet. Gynecol. **126:**165-169 (1976).
2. Asch, R.H. & Greenblatt, R.B.: Steroidogenesis in the postmenopausal ovary. Clin. Obstet. Gynaecol. **4:**85-106 (1977).
3. Stone, S.C., Mickal, A. & Rye, P.H.: Postmenopausal symptomatology, maturation index, and plasma estrogen levels. Obstet. Gynecol. **45:**625-627 (1975).
4. Gambone, J., Meldrum, D.R., Laufer, L., Chang, R.J., Lu, J.K.H. & Judd, H.L.: Further delineation of hypothalamic dysfunction responsible for menopausal hot flashes. J. Clin. Endocrinol. Metab. **59:**1097-1102 (1984).
5. Tataryn, I.V., Lomax, P., Bajorek, J.G., Chesarek, W., Meldrum, D.R. & Judd, H.L.: Postmenopausal hot flushes: a disorder of thermoregulation. Maturitas **2:**101-107 (1980).
6. Schmitt, H.: The pharmacology of clonidine and related products. In Gross, *Antihypertensive agents*, pp. 299-396 (Springer-Verlag, New York 1977).
7. Laufer, L.R., Erlik, Y., Meldrum, D.R. & Judd, H.L.: Effect of clonidine on hot flushes in postmenopausal women. Obstet. Gynecol. **60:**583-589 (1982).
8. Clayden, J.R., Bell, J.W. & Pollard, P.: Menopausal flushing: Double blind trial of a non-hormonal medication. Br. Med. J. **1:**409-412 (1974).
9. Schindler, A.E., Muller, D., Keller, E., Goser, R. & Runkel, F.: Studies with clonidine (Dixarit) in menopausal women. Arch. Gynecol. **227:**341-347 (1979).
10. Freedman, R.R., Woodward, S. & Sabharwal, S.C.: α_2-Adrenergic mechanism in menopausal hot flushes. Obstet. Gynecol. **76:**573-578 (1990).
11. Freedman, R.R.: Laboratory and ambulatory monitoring of menopausal hot flushes. Psychophysiology **26:**573-579 (1989).
12. Roth, R.H.: Neuronal activity, impulse flow and MHPG production. In Mass, *MHPG: Basic Mechanisms and Psychopathology*, pp. 19-33 (Academic Press, New York 1983).

13. Leckman, J.F., Maas, J.W., Redmond, D.E. & Heninger, G.E.: Effects of oral clonidine on plasma MHPG in man. Life Sci. **26**:2179-2185 (1980).

14. Charney, D.S., Heninger, G.R. & Sternberg, D.E.: Assessment of α_2 adrenergic autoreceptor function in humans: Effects of oral yohimbine. Life Sci. **30**:2033-2041 (1982).

15. Starke, K., Gothert, M. & Kilbringer, H.: Modulation of neurotransmitter release by presynaptic autoreceptors. Physiol. Rev. **69**:864-989 (1989).

16. Casper, R.F., Yen, S.S.C. & Wilkes, M.M.: Menopausal flushes: A neuroendocrine link with pulsatile luteinizing hormone secretion. Science **205**:823-825 (1979).

17. Kronenberg, F., Carraway, R., Cote, L.J., Crawshaw, L.I. & Downey, J.A.: Changes in thermoregulation, immunoreactive neurotensin, catecholamines and LH during menopausal hot flashes. Maturitas **6**:31-43 (1984).

18. Goldstein, D.S., McCarty, R., Polinsky, R.J. & Kopin, I.J.: Relationship between plasma norepinephrine and sympathetic neural activity. Hypertension **5**:552-559 (1983).

Lomax, Schönbaum (eds.) **Thermoregulation: The Pathophysiological Basis of Clinical Disorders.**
8th International Symposium Pharmacology of Thermoregulation, Kananaskis, Alberta, Canada 1991, pp. 10-13 (Karger, Basel 1992)

THERMOREGULATION AND SLEEP IN POSTMENOPAUSAL WOMEN

SUZANNE WOODWARD and ROBERT R. FREEDMAN

Department of Psychiatry, Wayne State University School of Medicine, Detroit, Michigan 48202 (USA)

Menopause is marked by the cessation of the menses, elevated FSH and LH levels and reduced estrogen production. The most common symptom of the menopause is the hot flush consisting of profuse sweating and vasodilation, followed by a lowering of body temperature [1-3]. The exact etiology of menopausal hot flushes is not clear but the thermoregulatory mechanism is thought to involve altered hypothalamic catecholamines due to estrogen loss as well as altered afferent input to LHRH neurons [1]. In animals, LHRH has been shown to change the firing rate in the preoptic/anterior hypothalamic nuclei, thought to be the major center for thermoregulation [4,5].

Strong evidence exists linking thermoregulation and sleep generation. Blood flow and diathermic warming studies have indicated that the rostral hypothalamus and the preoptic region are the location for slow wave sleep (SWS) generation in animals [5,6]. In humans, a lower level of energy expenditure is maintained during SWS (Stages 3 and 4) and is dependent on stable reductions in body and brain temperatures maintained by active autonomic control mechanisms. Positive thermal loads presented prior to sleep, or following sleep onset, have been shown to alter subsequent SWS, and rapid-eye-movement (REM) sleep [7-9]. Of particular interest are studies showing increases in SWS, particularly Stage 4 sleep, following a warm bath presented approximately 2 hours prior to sleep onset [9,10]. The increases in body temperature shown during heating and the slow decline following heating may act as a stimulus for SWS [11-12]. The thermoregulatory changes of a menopausal hot flush may have the potential for altering SWS in much the same manner. We therefore performed all-night sleep recordings in women with and without menopausal hot flushes to determine if alterations in SWS occurred in the former group.

METHODS: Eight post-menopausal women with hot flushes (mean age 51.63 ± 4.77) and five post-menopausal women without flushes (mean age 53.20 ± 6.68) participated in our study. The women with flushes reported at least 5 hot flushes per day and the non-flushing women reported never having had a flush. All subjects were at least one year post-menopausal, in good health and free from medication including exogenous estrogen. Subjects slept *ad lib* in their own bed and bedroom. All subjects gave informed consent and were paid for their participation.

Twenty-four hour ambulatory monitoring was performed using an 8-channel cassette recorder and playback system. Recorders were attached and started in our laboratory during the afternoon and run continuously until subjects returned the following day. Skin conductance level (SCL) was recorded from the sternum using a 0.5 volt constant voltage circuit and electrocardiogram (ECG) was recorded with Meditrace ambulatory monitoring electrodes in a lead II configuration. The electroencephalogram (EEG) was recorded from C_4-A_1; the electro-oculogram (EOG) was recorded from the outer canthus of each eye, and the electro-myogram (EMG) was recorded from submental muscle beneath the chin. Excess lead lengths were taped to the body to reduce artifacts. In order to detect hot flushes, the Medilog tapes were replayed at 20 X real time into an Analog Devices A/D board and IBM computer and sampled at the real time equivalent of 100 Hz. The computer was programmed to detect any SCL increase of at least 2 μmho within 30 sec and to score the surrounding 4-6 min period before and after the peak of the SCL response. This criterion SCL change has been shown in our laboratory to demarcate menopausal hot flushes with a high degree of reliability [3]. Women reporting hot flushes were excluded from the analysis if they failed to show at least 5 flushes meeting our SCL criterion during the 24 h recording. Women reporting no flushes were excluded if any SCL criterion changes were found.

Sleep portions of the tapes were transferred onto standard chart recordings at real-time speed. These records were scored (blind to flushing or non-flushing status) in 30 sec epochs by conventional criteria [13].

Students' t-tests were used to compare women with flushes to women without flushes on all sleep parameters. All correlations were done using Pearson product-moment correlations.

RESULTS: A summary of the whole night sleep data for both flushing and non-flushing women is presented in Table I. Women with hot flushes had significantly more Stage 4 sleep than women without hot flushes for the entire night (t = 2.87, p < 0.05). In non-rapid-eye-movement sleep period 1 (NREM 1) the amount of SWS was not different between groups, but in the NREM period following the first REM period (NREM 2), the women with hot flushes had significantly more Stage 4 sleep than the non-flushing women (p < 0.05). The total amount of REM sleep was not different between the groups; however the first REM period was significantly shorter in women with flushes (p < 0.05).

The number of flushes that occurred in the 2 h prior to sleep onset showed a significant positive correlation with both the total amount of SWS (r = 0.75, p. < 0.05), as well as Stage 4 sleep (r = 0.70, p < 0.05) in NREM 2.

DISCUSSION: The results show that postmenopausal hot flushes, particularly flushes occurring approximately 2 h prior to sleep onset, are associated with increased Stage 4 sleep and a shortened first REM period. These findings are similar to those of studies showing that a warm bath, presented prior to sleep, is associated with increased SWS and Stage 4 sleep as well as a shortened first REM period [9,10]. These studies also suggest that when the heating is presented temporally closer to the onset of sleep (approximately 2-3 h) the amount of heating required to achieve increases in SWS need not be as intense as that presented approximately 8 h prior to sleep. Our subjects showed no association between flushes experienced in an earlier period 7 h prior to sleep and increases in Stage 4 sleep. Hot flush frequency was not different between the early and late time periods indicating that hot flushes occurring just prior to sleep onset may elicit a compensatory drop in body temperature that continues into sleep affecting the induction and maintenance of SWS. Nighttime hot flush frequency has been shown to increase waking episodes [14,15]. SWS, when thermoregulatory mechanisms are maximally operative, is the only sleep stage where hot flushes are not consistently accompanied by an arousal [16].

Tympanic and rectal temperatures have been shown to increase with passive heating [10,12]. During menopausal hot flushes, no such temperature increases have been noted [2]. It is feasible that altered firing of warm sensitive neurons in the preoptic region may drive brain cooling mechanisms during menopausal hot flushes rather than a physiological thermal load. The resultant episodes of periodic cooling would then be responsible for the alterations of SWS seen during the subsequent night's sleep.

TABLE I: Sleep in postmenopausal flushers and non-flushers

Parameter	Flushers	Non-Flushers
Time in Bed	453.75 ± 69.00	455.90 ± 64.45
Total Sleep Time	412.87 ± 68.73	435.10 ± 59.57
Intermittent Awake	40.06 ± 15.75[1]	20.10 ± 10.12[1]
Sleep Efficiency	90.04 ± 4.18[1]	95.41 ± 2.15[1]
Number of Stage Changes	89.25 ± 29.26[1]	50.36 ± 25.59[1]
Percentage of		
Stage 1 (%)	4.62 ± 02.91	4.34 ± 3.27
Stage 2 (%)	47.09 ± 13.94	48.66 ± 7.36
Stage 3 (%)	11.14 ± 4.11	16.78 ± 6.96
Stage 4 (%)	14.10 ± 7.55[1]	3.28 ± 4.50[1]
SWS (%)	25.26 ± 8.91	20.08 ± 9.24
REM (%)	23.01 ± 8.37	26.94 ± 2.62
REM Latency (Min)	61.31 ± 28.20	72.60 ± 24.66
Number of REM Periods	4.62 ± 0.92	4.60 ± 0.55
Number of NREM Periods	5.62 ± 0.92	5.60 ± 0.55
REM1 Length	13.00 ± 7.77[1]	27.00 ± 14.23[1]
NREM2 Length	96.94 ± 17.50	79.70 ± 25.37
NREM2 Stage 1%	3.87 ± 3.48	2.02 ± 2.13
NREM2 Stage 2%	43.60 ± 24.70	57.14 ± 13.93
NREM2 Stage 3%	16.95 ± 8.53[1]	36.44 ± 15.72
NREM2 Stage 4%	27.34 ± 21.66	0.96 ± 2.15[1]
NREM2 SWS %	44.29 ± 23.53	37.40 ± 16.35
NREM2 Awake (Min)	8.24 ± 5.62	3.46 ± 2.04

Cell entries are mean ± SD.
[1]$p < 0.05$.

ACKNOWLEDGEMENTS: This work was supported by research grant AG-05233 from the National Institute on Aging.

REFERENCES

1.   Tataryn, I.V., Lomax, P., Bajorek, J.G., Chesarek, W., Meldrum, D.R. & Judd, H.L.: Postmenopausal hot flushes: A disorder of thermoregulation. Maturitas **2**:101-107 (1980).
2.   Molnar, G.W.: Body temperatures during menopausal hot flashes. J. Appl. Physiol. **38(3)**:499-503 (1975).
3.   Freedman, R.R.: Laboratory and ambulatory monitoring of menopausal hot flashes. Psychophysiology **26(5)**:573-579 (1989).
4.   McGinty, D., Szymusiak, R.: The basal forebrain and slow wave sleep: Mechanistic and functional aspects. In Wauquier, Dugovic & Radulovacki, *Slow Wave Sleep: Physiological, Pathophysiological, and Functional Aspects*, pp. 61-71 (Raven Press, Ltd., New York 1989).

5. Nikolaishvili, L.S. & Devdariani, M.I.: Dynamics of local blood flow in different regions of the hypothalamus in the sleep-wakefulness cycle. Neurosci. Behav. Physiol. **18(4)**:310-315 (1988).

6. Roberts, W.W. & Robinson, T.C.L.: Relaxation and sleep induced by warming of preoptic region and anterior hypothalamus in cats. Exp. Neurol. **25**:282-294 (1969).

7. Bunnell, D.E. & Horvath, S.M.: Effects of body heating during sleep interruption. Sleep **8(3)**:274-282 (1985).

8. Haskell, E.H., Palca, J.W., Walker, J.M., Berger, R.J. & Heller, H.C.: The effects of high and low ambient temperatures on human sleep stages. Electroencephalogr. Clin. Neurophysiol. **51**:494-501 (1981).

9. Horne, J.A. & Reid, A.J.: Night-time sleep EEG changes following body heating in a warm bath. Electroencephalogr. Clin. Neurophysiol. **60**:154-157 (1985).

10. Horne, J.A. & Shackell, B.S.: Slow wave sleep elevations after body heating: Proximity to sleep and effects of aspirin. Sleep **10(4)**:383-392 (1987).

11. Berger, R.J., Palca, J.W., Walker, J.M. & Phillips, N.H.: Correlations between body temperatures, metabolic rate and slow wave sleep in humans. Neurosci. Lett. **86**:230-234 (1988).

12. Horne, J.A. & Staff, L.H.E.: Exercise and sleep: Body-heating effects. Sleep **6**:36-46 (1983).

13. Rechtschaffen, A. & Kales, A. (eds.): *A Manual of Standardized Terminology, Techniques, and Scoring Systems for Sleep Stages of Human Subjects.* (U.S. Government Printing Office, Washington, D.C. 1968).

14. Erlik, Y., Tataryn, I.V., Meldrum, D.R., Lomax, P., Bajorek, J.G. & Judd, H.L.: Association of waking episodes with menopausal hot flushes. JAMA **245(17)**:1741-1744 (1981).

15. Thomson, J. & Oswald, I.: Effect of oestrogen on the sleep, mood, and anxiety of menopausal women. Br. Med. J. **2**:1317-1319 (1977).

16. Woodward, S. & Freedman, R.R.: Increased menopausal hot flashes in slow wave sleep. Ann. NY Acad. Sci. **592**:479-480 (1990).

Lomax, Schönbaum (eds.) **Thermoregulation: The Pathophysiological Basis of Clinical Disorders.**
8th International Symposium Pharmacology of Thermoregulation, Kananaskis, Alberta, Canada 1991, pp. 14-18 (Karger, Basel 1992)

THE CLIMACTERIC HOT FLUSH: AN UPDATE

E. SCHÖNBAUM[1] and P. LOMAX[2]

[1]Formerly Scientific Development Group, Organon International BV, Oss (The Netherlands) and Department of Pharmacology, University of Toronto (Canada) and [2]Department of Pharmacology, School of Medicine and the Brain Research Institute, University of California at Los Angeles, Los Angeles, California 90024-1735 (USA)

Some ten years ago there was not sufficient information about the postmenopausal hot flush (HF) to include it in the plans for a handbook on thermoregulation [1], but subsequent research justified the publication of a monograph [2], and now this update. For general surveys see [2-4]. The HF is a transient reddening of the face and frequently other areas, including the neck, upper chest and epigastric area which occurs in women passing from the reproductive to the nonreproductive phase of life [2-4]. Objective measurements of the physiological components of the HF [5-10] have shown that it is triggered by a sudden downward shift in the thermoregulatory set point [11] which event causes the prodromal sensations of the HF. When the set temperature is lower than the core temperature (probably that of the hypothalamus), compensatory mechanisms come into play and continue until core and set temperatures are the same, or until the set point has returned to its initial level. This hypothesis is descriptive; it does not explain the link between HF and the endocrine events of the climacteric.

EPIDEMIOLOGY: Cultural and racial factors are of importance in the experience of, and the response to, the HF. In North America and Europe, but not in Japan or Nigeria [12-14], vasomotor symptoms are the most disturbing indicators of hormonal change although, clinically, postmenopausal osteoporosis is far more serious. An Italian study on more than 4,000 women indicated that arthralgia, nervousness, sweating and HFs were the most common complaints [15]. A survey of all women between the ages of 39 and 60 years, resident in the Dutch municipality of Ede (more than 5000 usable replies), showed vasomotor symptoms to be the most frequent complaint [16], followed by joint pain. In Norway tiredness, HFs and pain in the muscles and joints were most prevalent [17]. In the United States, a psychological study of stress and objectively recorded HFs showed that stress increased their incidence [6]. Nevertheless, a study of general practice consultations and menopausal problems in the Oxford (U.K.) area suggested a low overall use of hormone replacement therapy in the general postmenopausal population [18].

MECHANISMS: The rostral hypothalamus is the site for the temporal association between the onset of the HF and pulsatile release of luteinizing hormone releasing hormone (LHRH) [11]. The distribution of fibers containing LHRH suggests close association with, e.g., catecholaminergic and dopaminergic neurons. The involvement of catecholaminergic neurons with thermoregulation and the HF is evidenced also by the loss of facial sweating and flushing in the Holmes-Adie and Ross syndromes [19]. A study of the effects of adrenergic blocking agents in ovariectomized rhesus monkeys showed that the stimulatory effects of catecholamines on pulsatile LHRH release are mediated by α_1-adrenergic receptors but not by α_2- or β- nor by dopaminergic receptors [20]. Target sites for estradiol and dihydrotestosterone were identified in nuclei of many catecholamine cell bodies in the brainstem, and catecholamine nerve terminals were observed near certain steroid hormone target neurons suggesting close interrelations between these agents [21]. LHRH also seems to have a common signal transduction mechanism with endothelin [22]. Endothelin is a potent vasoconstrictor [23] and likely influences cerebral microcirculation and may well interact with catecholamines. Additional evidence for the importance of the sympathetic nervous system in the pathophysiology of hot flushes is offered by clonidine studies (see Medication). In the rostral hypothalamus receptors for estrogen and progesterone have been found [24,25]. The link between the presence of such receptors and the actually demonstrated sites of action of such hormones is tenuous, particularly with respect to the HF. The loss of inhibitory feedback by estrogen in postmenopausal women leads to hypertrophy of neurons expressing the estrogen receptor gene [24], a response most likely secondary to the loss of steroidal inhibitory feedback. Estrogens act on the pituitary: given subcutaneously or intrahypothalamically they suppress LH but not LHRH secretion.

Estrogens also inhibit the LH response to exogenous LHRH [26], but a minimal presence of estrogen is required for an LH surge [27]. Yet, estrogens given in doses sufficient to suppress LH release increase the LHRH content of a discrete region in the median basal hypothalamus [28]. Hypertrophy is seen in certain cells in the hypothalamus of postmenopausal women [24]. A deficiency of certain steroids (estrogens and/or metabolites) could well reduce inhibitory effects on pulsatile release of regulatory peptides [29]. During administration of a potent synthetic agonist of LHRH to normally menstruating women for a period exceeding 2 weeks HFs occurred despite normal serum estradiol levels [30]. The relationships in the hypothalamus, and other areas, between mediators, steroids and catecholamines have been reviewed [11]. Although its role remains controversial [20], dopamine is of interest because, e.g., in postmenopausal Parkinsonian patients some effects of naloxone have been observed. In such patients, normal body temperature is lower than in normal postmenopausal women. Infusing naloxone did not reduce body temperature, although it did so in normal postmenopausal women. This suggested a possible role of opioids in thermoregulation and in HFs [31], at least in the presence of abnormal dopaminergic activity. In physiological doses, estradiol induces hypothalamic opioid activity [32]. This was demonstrated by first suppressing circulating LH levels in postmenopausal women by transdermally administering estradiol and establishing rapidly increasing LH levels by infusing naloxone. Clearly, the opioid system is involved not only in the control of thermoregulation but also in the modulation of LHRH activity; a direct effect on the hypophysis has been ruled out [32]. Treatment of postmenopausal women with a low dose of danazol for 30 days and infusing, on day 30, naloxone did not affect mean plasma LH and FSH levels, but danazol significantly enhanced the thermoregulatory role of endogenous opioids [33]. It is possible also that interleukins influence hypothalamic LHRH release [34].

It is generally noted that HFs occur more often at night. When this happens, the woman awakens first and only thereafter the set point is lowered and the HF triggered [35]. Other studies [6] have shown that "stress" [and therefore the release of corticotropin releasing hormone (CRH)] increases the incidence of HFs. CRH in ovariectomized monkeys acutely inhibits both FSH and LH [36], which will affect the LHRH pulses. Peripheral factors are important in the pathogenesis of the HF. Simple hysterectomy, with preservation of the ovaries, revealed a high prevalence of HFs [37]. The mechanism involved here is not clear.

MEDICATION: Estrogens appear the most logical choice of treatment for those suffering from signs and symptoms of the climacteric [2,4,38]. In spite of their general safety, there are risks since estrogens, particularly if unopposed by progestogens or, sometimes, androgens, can lead to metaplasia in the endometrium or the breast parenchyma [39]. A new synthetic steroid, tibolone, that combines weak estrogenic, progestational and androgenic properties has been introduced and is under intensive study [40]. The search for a suitable non-hormonal treatment is difficult. Clonidine has been studied extensively because it suppresses, primarily, central sympathetic activity. Intravenous clonidine reduced, and intravenous yohimbine increased, the amount of peripheral heating required to provoke a hot flush [41]. Nevertheless, the many contradictions in clinical reports on the therapeutic efficacy of clonidine do not permit a clear conclusion.

A study with a dopamine antagonist, veralipride [42], showed encouraging results. However, suppression by non-hormonal medication of vasomotor complaints still leaves the clinically much more important risk of osteoporosis. One wonders whether there is a set point for parathyroid function that is altered during the climacteric.

Therapeutic progress is hindered by experimental difficulties. Non-human primates are very expensive and the interpretation of data obtained from lower species difficult: oöphorectomy in lower species [20] does not induce signs similar to those in the climacteric.

CONCLUSION: The recently discovered multiple functions of 'regulatory' peptides, e.g. opioids, interleukins and other mediators require a critical review of present knowledge of the HF and make more neuroendocrine research necessary. An inaccurate and oversimplified idea of the integration of various possible mechanisms can actually render further research more difficult [43].

REFERENCES

1. Schönbaum, E. & Lomax, P. (eds): *Thermoregulation. Physiology and Biochemistry. Int. Encycl. Pharmacol. Ther. Section 131* (Pergamon Press, New York 1990); *Thermoregulation. Pathology, Pharmacology and Therapy. Int. Encycl. Pharmacol. Ther. Section 132* (Pergamon Press, New York 1991).
2. Schönbaum, E. (ed). *The Climacteric Hot Flush. Progr. Basic Clin. Pharmacol. vol. 6* (Karger, Basel 1991).
3. Flint, M., Kronenberg, F. & Utian, W. (eds): Multidisciplinary Persectives on Menopause. Ann. N.Y. Acad. Sci. 592 (1990).
4. Studd, J.W.W. & Whitehead, M.I. (eds): *The Menopause* (Blackwell, Oxford 1988).
5. Molnar, G.W.: Body temperatures during menopausal hot flashes. J. Appl. Physiol. **38**:499-503 (1975).
6. Swartzman, L.C., Edelberg, R. & Kemmann, E. Impact of stress on objectively recorded menopausal hot flushes and on flush report bias. Health Psychology **9**:529-545 (1990).
7. Lomax, P. Bajorek, J.G., Chesarek, W. & Tataryn, I.V.: Thermoregulatory effects of luteinizing hormone releasing hormone in the rat. In Cox, Lomax, Milton & Schönbaum *Thermoregulatory Mechanisms and Their Therapeutic Implications*, pp. 208-211 (Karger, Basel 1980).
8. Silverman, R.W., Bajorek, J.G., Lomax, P. & Tataryn, I.V.: Monitoring the pathophysiological correlates of postmenopausal hot flushes. Maturitas **3**:39-46 (1981).
9. Tataryn, I.V. Meldrum, D.R., Frumar, A.M., Lu, K.H., Judd, H.L., Bajorek, J.G., Chesarek, W. & Lomax, P.: The hormonal and thermoregulatory changes in postmenopausal hot flushes. In Cox, Lomax, Milton & Schönbaum *Thermoregulatory Mechanisms and Their Therapeutic Implications*, pp. 202-207 (Karger, Basel 1980).
10. Freedman, R.R.: Laboratory and ambulatory monitoring of menopausal hot flashes. Psychophysiol. **26**:573-578 (1989).
11. Lomax, P.: The pathophysiology of postmenopausal hot flushes. In Schönbaum *The Climacteric Hot Flush. Progr. Basic Clin. Pharmacol. Vol. 6*, pp. 61-82 (Karger, Basel 1991).
12. Lock, M.: Hot flushes in cultural context: The Japanese case as a cautionary tale for the West. In Schönbaum *The Climacteric Hot Flush. Progr. Basic Clin. Pharmacol. Vol. 6*, pp. 40-60 (Karger, Basel 1991).
13. Lock, M., Kaufert, P. & Gilbert, P.: Cultural construction of the menopausal syndrome: the Japanese case. Maturitas **10**:317-332 (1988).

14. Okonofua, F.E., Lawal, A. & Bamgbose, J.K.: Features of menopause and menopausal age in Nigerian women. Int. J. Gynecol. Obstet. **31**:341-345 (1990).
15. De Aloysio, D., Fabiani, A.G., Mauloni & Bottiglioni, F.: Analysis of the climacteric syndrome. Maturitas **11**:43-53 (1989).
16. Oldenhave, A. & Jaszmann, L.J.B.: The climacteric: Absence or presence of hot flushes and their relation to other complaints. In Schönbaum *The Climacteric Hot Flush. Progr. Basic Clin. Pharmacol. Vol. 6*, pp. 6-39 (Karger, Basel 1991).
17. Holte, A. & Mikkelsen, A.: Climacteric complaints as a major health problem in the ageing population year 2000: Prognoses based on the distribution of climacteric complaints in a Scandinavian normal population. In Cortes-Prieto, Alvarez de los Heros, Neves-E-Castro & Vasquez-Benitez *Medicina de la Reproduccion Año 2000. Revista de la universidad de Alcala, No. 1*, pp. 233-243 (1990).
18. Barlow, D.H., Brockie, J.A., Rees, C.M.P. & Oxford General Practitioners Menopause Study Group: Study of general practice consultations and menopausal problems. Br. Med. J. **302**:274-276 (1991).
19. Drummond, P.D. & Edis, R.H.: Loss of facial sweating and flushing in Holmes-Adie syndrome. Neurology **40**:847-849 (1990).
20. Gearing, M. & Terasawa, E.: The α-1-adrenergic neuronal system is involved in the pulsatile release of luteinizing hormone-releasing hormone in the ovariectomized female rhesus monkey. Neuroendocrinology **53**:373-381 (1991).
21. Heritage, A.S., Stumpf, W.E., Sar, M. & Grant, L.D.: Brainstem catecholamine neurons are target sites for sex steroid hormones. Science **207**:1377-1379 (1980).
22. Stojilkovic, S.S., Merell, F., Iida, T., Krsmanovic, L.Z. & Catt, K.J.: Endothelin stimulation of cytosolic calcium and gonadotropin secretion in anterior pituitary cells. Science **248**:1663-1666 (1990).
23. Yanagisawa, M., Inoue, A., Ishikawa, T., Kasuya, Y., Kimura, S., Kumagaye, S., Nakajima, K., Watanabe, T.X., Sakakibara, S., Goto, K. & Masaki, T.: Primary structure, synthesis, and biological activity of rat endothelin, an endothelium-derived vasoconstrictor peptide. Proc. Natl. Acad. Sci. USA **85**:6964-6967 (1988).
24. Rance, N.E., McMullen, N.T., Smialek, J.E., Price, D.L. & Young, III, W.S.: Postmenopausal hypertrophy of neurons expressing the estrogen receptor gene in the human hypothalamus. J. Clin. Endocrinol. Metab. **71**:79-85 (1990).
25. Langub, M.C., Jr., Maley, B.E. & Watson, R.E., Jr.: Ultrastructural evidence for luteinizing hormone-releasing hormone neuronal control of estrogen responsive neurons in the preoptic area. Endocrinology **128**:27-36 (1991).
26. Pau, K-Y.F., Gliessman, P.M., Hess, D.L., Ronnekleiv, O.K., Levine, J.E. & Spies, H.G.: Acute administration of estrogen suppresses LH secretion without altering GnRH release in ovariectomized rhesus macaques. Brain Res. **517**:229-235 (1990).
27. Karande, V.C., Scott, R.T. & Archer, D.F.: The relationship between serum estradiol-17β concentrations and induced pituitary luteinizing hormone surges in postmenopausal women. Fertil. Steril. **54**:217-221 (1990).
28. Roselli, C.E. & Resko, J.A.: Regulation of hypothalamic luteinizing hormone-releasing hormone levels by testosterone and estradiol in male rhesus moneys. Brain Res. **509**:343-346 (1990).
29. Lomax, P. & Schönbaum, E.: Neuroendocrine mechanisms in postmenopausal hot flushes. Submitted to: Life Sci. Adv.
30. Bider, D., Ben-Rafael, Z., Shalev, J., Mashiach, S., Serr, D.M. & Blankstein, J.: Hot flushes during Gn-RH analogue administration despite normal serum oestradiol levels. Maturitas **11**:223-228 (1989).
31. Cagnacci, A., Bonuccelli, U., Melis, G.B., Soldani, R., Piccini, P., Napolitano, A., Muratorio, A. & Fioretti, P.: Effect of naloxone on body temperature in postmenopausal women with Parkinson's disease. Life Sci. **46**:1241-1247 (1990).

32.   D'Amico, J.F., Greendale, G.A., Lu, J.K.H. & Judd, H.L.: Induction of hypothalamic opioid activity with transdermal estradiol administration in postmenopausal women. Fertil. Steril. **55:**754-758 (1991).

33.   Cagnacci, A., Melis, G.B., Paoletti, A.M., Soldani, R. & Fioretti, P.: Thermoregulatory and endocrine effects of a low dose of danazol in postmenopausal women: Interaction with the effect of naloxone. Life Sci. **48:**1051-1058 (1991).

34.   Kalra, P.S., Sahu, A. & Kalra, S.P.: Interleukin-1 inhibits the ovarian steroid-induced luteinizing hormone surge and release of hypothalamic luteinizing hormone-releasing hormone in rats. Endocrinology **126:**2145-2152 (1990).

35.   Parmeggiani, P.L.: Thermoregulation during sleep in mammals. NIPS **5:**208-212 (1990).

36.   Reyes, A., Luckhause, J. & Ferin, M.: Unexpected inhibitory action of N-methyl-D,L-aspartate on luteinizing hormone release in adult ovariectomized rhesus monkeys: A role of the hypothalamic-adrenal axis. Endocrinology **127:**724-729 (1990).

37.   Menon, R.K., Okonofua, F.E., Agnew, J.E., Thomas, M., Bell, J., O'Brien, P.M.S. & Dandona, P.: Endocrine and metabolic effects of simple hysterectomy. Int. J. Gynaecol. Obstet. **25:**459-463 (1987).

38.   L'Hermite, M. (ed.): *Update on Hormonal Treatment in the Menopause. Progr. Reprod. Biol. Med. 13* (Karger, Basel 1989).

39.   Colditz, G.A., Stampfer, M.J., Willett, W.C., Hennekens, C.H., Rosner, B. & Speizer, F.E.: Prospective study of estrogen replacement therapy and risk of breast cancer in postmenopausal women. **264:**2648-2653 (1990).

40.   Tax, L.: Hormone replacement therapy? Livial Ⓡ (Org OD 14), a new possibility. In Schönbaum *The Climacteric Hot Flush. Progr. Basic Clin. Pharmacol. Vol. 6*, pp. 143-159 (Karger, Basel 1991).

41.   Freedman, R.R., Woodward, S. & Sabharwal, S.C.: α_2-Adrenergic mechanisms in menopausal hot flushes. Obstet. Gynecol. **76:**573-578 (1990).

42.   Melis, G.H., Gambacciani, M., Cagnacci, A., Paoletti, A.M., Mais, V. & Fiorett, P.: Effects of the dopamine antagonist veralipride on hot flushes and luteinizing hormone secretion in postmenopausal women. Obstet. Gynecol. **72:**688-692 (1988).

43.   Harris, R.B.S.: Role of set-point theory in regulation of body weight. FASEB J. **4:**33110-33118 (1990).

Lomax, Schönbaum (eds.) **Thermoregulation: The Pathophysiological Basis of Clinical Disorders.**
8th International Symposium Pharmacology of Thermoregulation, Kananaskis, Alberta, Canada 1991, pp. 19-24 (Karger, Basel 1992)

VASOPRESSIN INDUCED ANTIPYRESIS AND CONVULSIVE LIKE ACTIVITY IN THE MEDIAL AMYGDALOID NUCLEUS

P. FEDERICO, B.J. WILLCOX, K.E. COOPER and W.L. VEALE

Neuroscience Research Group, Department of Medical Physiology, University of Calgary, Calgary, Alberta T2N 4N1 (Canada)

Perfusion of the neuropeptide arginine vasopressin (AVP) within the medial amygdaloid nucleus (meA) has recently been shown to evoke antipyresis in the urethane anaesthetized rat [1]. Other studies have demonstrated increased AVP content in amygdalar nerve terminals during fever and during the development of pyrogen tolerance [2-4]. Taken together, these data provide support for the hypothesis that AVP might act within the meA as an endogenous antipyretic.

Currently it is unknown whether AVP is antipyretic when administered exogenously within the meA of the conscious rat. Consequently, experiments were undertaken to determine if AVP, microinjected into the meA, could attenuate fever. Since the amygdala is also a sensitive locus for kindling induced convulsion in the conscious rat [5] and since centrally administered AVP has been reported to evoke motor disturbances, including myotonic/myoclonic convulsions [6], experiments were designed to assess whether AVP could induce convulsive like activity when microinjected into the meA of the conscious rat.

METHODS: Under sodium pentobarbital anaesthesia (Somnotol; 65 mg/kg ip), 57 male Sprague-Dawley rats (weighing 250-300 g) had 23 gauge (thin-wall) stainless steel guide cannulae implanted bilaterally over the meA. In addition, 20 gauge stainless steel guide cannulae were similarly positioned over the lateral cerebral ventricles. Body temperature was measured at 5 min intervals using biotelemetry devices that were implanted intraperitoneally. 10 days after surgery, all animals were subjected to two experimental trials, the order of which was counterbalanced and separated by at least 5 days.

In the first experimental series, 18 animals were subjected to two experimental trials. In both trials, animals were made febrile by an icv injection of PGE_1 (50 ng/5 μl artificial cerebrospinal fluid; aCSF; see [1]). 5 min prior to this, either AVP (40 pmol/1 μl aCSF per side) or aCSF (1 μl) was bilaterally injected into the meA area. Tissue injections were made with a Harvard infusion pump over a period of 60 sec.

In the second experimental series, 17 animals were subjected to two experimental trials. In both trials, each rat received an icv injection of aCSF (5 μl) and 5 min prior to this, either AVP (40 pmol/1 μl per side) or aCSF (1 μl per side) was bilaterally injected into the meA region.

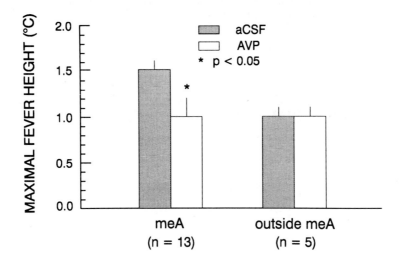

FIGURE 1: Summary of mean ($\pm$ S.E.M.) maximal fever height in response to icv PGE$_1$ (50 ng) with prior bilateral injection of aCSF (1 μl; filled bars) or AVP (40 pmol; open bars) into the meA or sites outside the meA (meA injection: n, 13; *$P < 0.05$, injection outside meA: n, 5; $P > 0.05$).

Upon completion of the experiments, all injection sites were verified using standard histological procedures. Animals were divided into two groups: those receiving tissue injection within the meA on at least one side of the brain, and those receiving tissue injection within sites surrounding, but not impinging upon the meA on both sides of the brain. For each trial, the maximal temperature deviation following icv injection of PGE$_1$ or aCSF was calculated. Baseline temperature recordings were obtained for 1 h prior to tissue injection. Temperature data were subjected to an analysis of variance followed by Newman-Keuls post-hoc comparisons.

In the third experimental series, guide cannulae bilaterally directed toward the meA were implanted into 22 animals, as previously described. 10 days following surgery, each rat received bilateral injections of AVP (100 pmol/1 μl over 60 sec; Day 1). For 10 min immediately following tissue injection, behavioral responses were recorded. 24 h later (Day 2), the animals were again subjected to AVP injection and behavioral assessment as in Day 1.

Animals in this experimental series were divided into two groups based on injection sites as in series I and II. Differences in the frequency of convulsive-like activity between the two groups were analyzed according to Fisher's exact test. Convulsive-like activity was defined as muscular rigidity of the fore- and hindlimbs and/or clonic spasm.

RESULTS: Fig. 1 illustrates the effect of AVP pretreatment on PGE$_1$ fever. Injection of PGE$_1$ (50 ng icv) with aCSF pretreatment resulted in fevers that reached an average maximum 1.5 $\pm$ 0.1°C above baseline within 35 min. However, when the icv injection of PGE$_1$ was preceded by a bilateral injection of AVP (40 pmol) into the meA, the maximal rise in core temperature was attenuated to 1.0 $\pm$ 0.2°C (n, 13; $P < 0.05$; Fig. 1).

When data from animals receiving tissue injections outside the meA were analyzed separately, it was apparent that AVP injection did not reduce fever height. Thus, the maximum rise in core temperature in response to icv PGE_1 was identical ($1.0 \pm 0.1°C$) with either aCSF or AVP (40 pmol) pretreatment (n, 5; $P > 0.05$; Fig. 1).

Injection of AVP into the meA or sites outside the meA did not significantly alter afebrile core temperature compared to control aCSF injection (n, 17; $P > 0.05$; data not shown).

Injection of AVP (100 pmol) into the meA or sites surrounding the meA on Day 1 evoked no convulsive like behaviour (Fig. 2). However, when AVP was injected into the meA on Day 2, convulsive like activity occurred with a significantly greater frequency than in animals who received AVP injection in sites surrounding, but not impinging upon the meA (n, 12; $P = 0.0046$; Fig. 2).

DISCUSSION: An antipyretic agent can be defined as a substance which diminishes febrile body temperature while having no significant effect on afebrile body temperature. In this study, injection of AVP into the meA of the conscious rat was found to reduce the maximal height of PGE_1 fever, while having no significant effect on afebrile core temperature. Thus, AVP is an effective antipyretic when microinjected into the meA of the conscious rat. This finding is consistent with the hypothesis that AVP might normally be released into the meA during fever to function as an endogenous antipyretic, limiting the magnitude of fever. Support for the endogenous release of AVP into the meA comes from previous studies demonstrating an increase in AVP immunoreactivity in amygdalar nerve terminals during fever and during the development of pyrogen tolerance in pregnant and nonpregnant guinea pigs [2-4].

One mechanism through which AVP could act within the meA to evoke antipyresis is through a neurotransmitter/neuromodulatory action on neurons that are part of thermoregulatory pathways which influence the ability of PGE_1 to evoke fever. Consistent with this possibility are studies demonstrating the presence of V_{1a}-like AVP receptors [7,8] and vasopressinergic nerve terminals [9,10] within the meA as well as reciprocal connections between the meA and sites considered to be important in fever and antipyresis such as the rostral hypothalamus, medial preoptic area, ventral septal area, and bed nucleus of the stria terminalis [10-15]. Conclusive support of this possibility, however, awaits further investigation. In addition, future studies should be directed at characterizing the central receptor(s) mediating this antipyretic action and in determining the contribution of the meA to endogenous antipyresis.

The results of the second experimental series demonstrate that AVP, when microinjected into the amygdala, can evoke convulsive-like activity through a sensitization process. Furthermore, this effect appears to be localized to the meA, where AVP-induced antipyretic action is also localized [1]. Thus, it appears that as is the case with the ventral septal area [16], the meA is a site where AVP can evoke antipyresis as well as convulsive like behavior (through a sensitization process). Though the precise neuroanatomical substrate mediating AVP induced convulsive like activity within the meA is unclear, reciprical connections of this site with the bed nucleus of the stria terminalis, basal ganglia, prefrontal cortex and thalamic nuclei provide both direct and indirect connections linking the meA with areas important in motor behavior [17-19].

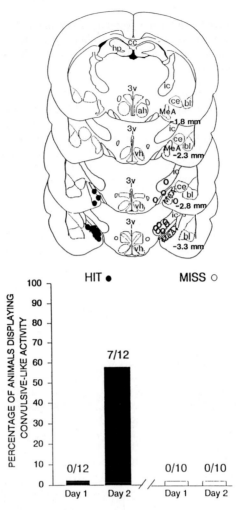

FIGURE 2: Upper panel. Histological representation of coronal sections of the rat forebrain taken at 60 μm indicating sites at which AVP (100 pmol) was effective (filled circles) or ineffective (open circles) at evoking convulsive-like activity. Numbers in the coronal sections indicate distance in mm caudal to bregma. Abbreviations, 3v, third ventricle; ah, anterior hypothalamus; bl, basolateral amygdaloid nucleus; cc, corpus callosum; ce, central amygdaloid nucleus; hp, hippocampal area; ic, internal capsule; MeA, medial amygdaloid nucleus; vh, ventromedial hypothalamus. Lower panel. Summary of behavioral responses to the bilateral injection of AVP (100 pmol) into the meA (filled bars) or sites outside the meA (open bars) on Day 1 and Day 2. Numbers above the bars indicate the proportion of rats displaying convulsive-like behavior.

The present observation that the meA is a sensitive locus for both AVP induced convulsion along with a putative role for this site in endogenous antipyresis raises the possibility that AVP may somehow play a role in the initiation or development of febrile convulsions. While this hypothesis is difficult to test due to the absence of good animal models for febrile convulsions, it has been demonstrated that homozygous Brattleboro rats (which lack AVP) do not convulse until their body temperatures are significantly more elevated than those of control rats [20]. Furthermore, following icv injection of an antiserum specific for AVP into Long-Evans rats, the hyperthermia induced response becomes similar to that displayed by homozygous Brattleboro rats: that is, these animals do not convulse as readily as do control animals (which received preimmune serum) when their body temperatures are elevated. No study to date, however, has localized a central locus where AVP might be involved in the development of febrile convulsions.

Another feature common to febrile convulsion is that an infant which has previously convulsed will be more likely to convulse subsequently. Certain aspects of the response to AVP injection into the meA resemble this phenomenon in that a sensitization process appears to be involved in the development of convulsive-like activity following AVP administration.

In conclusion, the meA appears to be a site where AVP can evoke both antipyretic and convulsive like activity (through a sensitization process). These observations also raise the possibility that the meA might be involved in the initiation or development of febrile convulsions.

ACKNOWLEDGEMENTS: This work was supported by the Medical Research Council of Canada. P. Federico holds a studentship from the Medical Research Council of Canada and the Alberta Heritage Foundation for Medical Research.

REFERENCES

1. Federico, P., Malkinson, T.J., Cooper, K.E., Pittman, Q.J. & Veale, W.L.: Vasopressin-induced antipyresis in the medial amygdaloid nucleus of the urethan-anesthetized rat. Soc. Neurosci. Abstr. **16**:496.8 (1990).
2. Merker, G., Blähser, S. & Zeisberger, E.: Reactivity pattern of vasopressin-containing neurons and its relation to the antipyretic reaction in the pregnant guinea pig. Cell Tissue Res. **212**:47-61 (1980).
3. Cooper, K.E., Blähser, S., Malkinson, T.J., Merker, G., Roth, J. & Zeisberger, E.: Changes in body temperature and vasopressin content of brain neurons, in pregnant and non-pregnant guinea pigs, during fevers produced by Poly I:Poly C. Pflugers Arch. **412**:292-296 (1988).
4. Merker, G., Roth, J. & Zeisberger, E.: Thermoadaptive influence on reactivity pattern of vasopressinergic neurons in the guinea pig. Experientia **45**:722-726 (1989).
5. Gillis, B.J. & Cain, D.P.: Amygdala and pyriform cortex kindling in vasopressin deficient rats (Brattleboro strain). Brain Res. **271**:375-378 (1983).
6. Balaban, C.D., Starcevic, V.P. & Severs, W.B.: Neuropeptide modulation of central vestibular circuits. Pharm. Rev. **41**:53-90 (1989).
7. Dorsa, D.M., Petracca, F.M., Baskin, D.G. & Cornett, L.E.: Localization and characterization of vasopressin-binding sites in the amygdala of the rat brain. J. Neurosci. **4**:1764-1770 (1984).
8. Freund-Mercier, M.J., Stoeckel, M.E., Dietl, M.M., Palacios, J.M. & Richard, P.: Quantitative autoradiographic mapping of neurohypophyseal hormone binding sites in the rat forebrain and pituitary gland-I. Characterization of different binding sites and their distribution in the Long-Evans strain. Neurosci. **26**:261-272 (1988).
9. Buijs, R.M. & Swaab, D.F.: Immuno-electron microscopical demonstration of vasopressin and oxytocin synapses in the limbic system of the rat. Cell Tissue Res. **204**:355-365 (1979).
10. De Vries, G.J., Buijs, R.M., van Leeuwen, F.W., Caffé, A.R. & Swaab, D.F.: The vasopressinergic innervation of the brain in normal and castrated rats. J. Comp. Neurol. **233**:236-254 (1985).

11. Conrad, L.C.A. & Pfaff, D.W.: Efferents from medial basal forebrain and hypothalamus in the rat. I. An autoradiographic study of the medial preoptic area. J. Comp. Neurol. **169:**185-220 (1976).

12. Conrad, L.C.A. & Pfaff, D.W.: Efferents from medial basal forebrain and hypothalamus in the rat. II. An autoradiographic study of the anterior hypothalamus. J. Comp. Neurol. **169:**221-262 (1976).

13. Caffé, A.R., van Leeuwen, F.W. & Luiten, P.G.M.: Vasopressin cells in the medial amygdala of the rat project to the lateral septum and ventral hippocampus. J. Comp. Neurol. **261:**237-252 (1987).

14. Disturnal, J.E., Veale, W.L. & Pittman, Q.J.: Electrophysiological analysis of potential arginine vasopressin projections to the ventral septal area of the rat. Brain Res. **342:**162-167 (1985).

15. Mathieson, W.B., Federico, P., Veale, W.L. & Pittman, Q.J.: Single-unit activity in the bed nucleus of the stria terminalis during fever. Brain Res. **486:**49-55 (1989).

16. Burnard, D.M., Veale, W.L. & Pittman, Q.J.: Arginine vasopressin: its possible involvement in febrile convulsions. In Cooper, Lomax, Schönbaum & Veale, *Homeostasis and Thermal Stress. 6th Int. Symp. Pharmacol. Thermoregulation*, pp. 57-61 (Karger, Basel 1986).

17. de Olmos, J.S., Alheid, G.F. & Beltramino, C.A.: In Paxinos, *The Rat Nervous System (Vol. 1): Forebrain and Midbrain*, pp. 223-334 (Academic Press, Toronto 1985).

18. Russchen, F.T. & Price, J.L.: Amygdalostriatal projections in the rat. Topographical organization and fiber morphology shown using the lectin PHA-L as an anterograde tracer. Neurosci. Lett. **47:**15-22 (1984).

19. Gaykema, R.P.A., Van Weeghel, R., Hersh, L.B. & Luiten, P.G.M.: Prefrontal cortical projections to the cholinergic neurons in the basal forebrain. J. Comp. Neurol. **303:**563-583 (1991).

20. Kasting, N.W., Veale, W.L., Cooper, K.E. & Lederis, K.: Vasopressin may mediate febrile convulsions. Brain Res. **213:**327-333 (1981).

Lomax, Schönbaum (eds.) **Thermoregulation: The Pathophysiological Basis of Clinical Disorders.**
8th International Symposium Pharmacology of Thermoregulation, Kananaskis, Alberta, Canada 1991, pp. 25-27 (Karger, Basel 1992)

THE MODULATORY ROLE OF PERIPHERAL CORTICOTROPHIN-RELEASING FACTOR (CRF) IN THE FEBRILE RESPONSE TO POLYINOSINIC:POLYCYTIDYLIC ACID (POLY-I:C)

A.S. MILTON and N.G.N. MILTON

Division of Pharmacology, University of Aberdeen, Marischal College, Aberdeen, AB9 1AS (Scotland)

The febrile response is thought to be mediated by peripheral production of prostaglandins which in turn activates central thermoregulatory centres in the hypothalamus [1]. Corticotrophin-releasing factor (CRF), a 41-amino acid hypothalamic peptide, has been shown to have wide ranging regulatory properties during responses to stress [2]. It is a potent activator of the hypothalamo-pituitary-adrenocortical (HPA) axis and, in addition, has a regulatory role within the cardiovascular, respiratory, immune and autonomic nervous systems. The proposed link between CRF and the immune system suggests a potential role for CRF in fever. Two contradictory studies have recently been published, one showing that centrally administered CRF has antipyretic effects [3], the other that both centrally administered anti-CRF antibodies and a CRF antagonist inhibit the febrile response [4]. The antipyretic actions of centrally administered CRF have been confirmed in another study which also showed that centrally administered CRF increased body temperature, but did not potentiate IL-1 induced fever [5].

In order to evaluate the thermoregulatory role of peripheral CRF in fever we have studied the effects of peripherally administered monoclonal anti-CRF antibodies [6] and a CRF antagonist (α-helical CRF 9-41; [7]) on the febrile response and on circulating levels of prostaglandins and cortisol in conscious rabbits following the administration of the pyrogenic interferon inducer polyinosinic:polycytidylic acid (Poly-I:C). The effects of peripheral administration of CRF on temperature and prostaglandin responses have also been studied.

METHODS: Male Dutch rabbits (1.7-2.3 kg) were used and core body temperature continuously measured. For studies into the role of peripheral CRF, test substances were administered intravenously (iv). Studies of central CRF antagonism used rabbits which had indwelling third cerebral ventricle cannulae. Purified immunoglobulin (IgG) fractions of mouse monoclonal anti-CRF-41 antibody (KCHMB001, [6]) or control normal mouse serum were used for all studies. A dose of 2.5 μg/kg poly-I:C or saline vehicle was administered at time zero and responses were followed for 5 h. For specific antibody experiments control animals were given a non-specific IgG preparation. Blood was collected into tubes containing EDTA and ketoprofen. Cortisol, PGE_2 and $PGF_{2\alpha}$ were extracted using Sep-Pak Cin columns [8] and assayed by RIA.

RESULTS: Poly-I:C (2.5 μg/kg) caused a biphasic rise in core body temperature with a lag phase of 45-60 min and peak rises of $1.1 \pm 0.2\,^{\circ}$C and $1.4 \pm 0.2\,^{\circ}$C at 90 min and 3.75 h respectively. A 5-fold rise in circulating levels of PGE_2 and a 2.5-fold rise in $PGF_{2\alpha}$ were observed with delays of 1 h and 2 h respectively. The Poly-I:C also caused a 5-fold rise in cortisol, again with a delay of 1 h. Peripherally administered anti-CRF antibody (15 nmol/kg) or CRF receptor antagonist (6.25 nmol/kg), given 5 min prior to poly-I:C, significantly attenuated the febrile responses. Peak rises in core body temperature 3.75 h after poly-I:C being reduced from 1.3 ± 0.1 to $0.7 \pm 0.3°C$ by anti-CRF antibody, and from 1.4 ± 0.2 to $0.5 \pm 0.3°C$ by CRF receptor antagonist. The 5-fold rise in cortisol was abolished by the anti-CRF antibody treatment but not by the low dose of CRF receptor antagonist used. However, the antagonist did significantly reduce the cortisol response at 2.5 h. The increase in circulating PGE_2 was slightly reduced by CRF receptor antagonist treatment whilst the 2.5-fold rise in $PGF_{2\alpha}$ was abolished by both treatments. When antibody was given 1 h following poly-I:C, a significant $0.75°C$ drop in temperature was observed within 5 min followed by a subsequent continuation of the rise in body temperature from a baseline $0.5°C$ below responses observed in control antibody treated animals. Central administration of CRF receptor antagonist (625 pmol/kg) had no effect on the febrile response to peripherally administered poly-I:C. Peripheral administration of CRF (5 nmol/kg) caused a significant stimulation of circulating PGF_2 (3-fold increase) and $PGF_{2\alpha}$ (1-fold increase). This dose of CRF also caused a hypothermic response and inhibited the febrile, but not prostaglandin, responses to poly-I:C. Lower doses of CRF (50 and 500 pmol/kg) had no significant effect on the febrile response.

DISCUSSION: The peripheral immunoneutralisation and CRF receptor antagonist administration studies show that CRF antagonism, as well as reducing the cortisol response, reduced the febrile and $PGF_{2\alpha}$ responses stimulated by poly-I:C. Whilst anti-CRF antibodies abolished the cortisol response, the dose of CRF receptor antagonist used only slightly reduced the cortisol response. These observations suggest that the attenuation of the febrile response is independent of the HPA axis response and suggests a modulatory role for CRF itself. When the CRF receptor antagonist was administered centrally no effect on body temperature was observed. However, when antibodies to CRF were given peripherally during the initial poly-I:C stimulated rise in body temperature a rapid drop in body temperature was observed. The development of a febrile response with a new, lower baseline, after peripheral anti-CRF antibody administration suggests that CRF is not itself the stimulus for fever. From these results it is concluded that peripheral CRF has a modulating role in the development of the febrile response to poly-I:C. The observations that CRF is found in and released by central nervous system tissue suggests that peripheral CRF may come from a central source. Central administration of anti-CRF antibodies, which attenuates the febrile response to centrally administered IL-1 in rats [4], would antagonise actions on central receptors and may also inhibit release of central CRF-41 into the peripheral circulation.

The observations that peripherally administered CRF stimulated rises in circulating PGE_2 and $PGF_{2\alpha}$ and that antagonism of peripheral CRC blocked the poly-I:C stimulated rise in $PGF_{2\alpha}$ suggests that this modulator role of peripheral CRF may involve effects on prostaglandins. The high dose of CRF also caused a significant hypothermic response and reduced the poly-I:C induced rises in body temperature suggesting another action for CRF in modulating the febrile response.

In conclusion, antagonism of peripheral but not central CRF has inhibitory effects on the febrile response to poly-I:C. The mechanism of action is unknown but such antagonism of CRF inhibits increases in $PGF_{2\alpha}$ stimulated by poly-I:C. Peripheral CRF administration in high doses also causes hypothermic responses and stimulates prostaglandin production suggesting that CRF may have more than one modulatory role in temperature regulation, in agreement with the conclusions reached by Opp, Obál and Krueger [5].

ACKNOWLEDGEMENTS: N.G.N. Milton is a Sir Halley Stewart Trust Scholar. This study was supported by a grant from the Nuffield Foundation to Professor A.S. Milton.

REFERENCES

1. Milton, A.S.: Thermoregulatory actions of eicosanoids in the central nervous system with particular regard to the pathogenesis of fever. Ann. N.Y. Acad. Sci. **559**:392-410 (1989).
2. Dunn, A.J. & Berridge, C.W.: Physiological and behavioural responses to corticotropin releasing factor administration: is CRF a mediator of anxiety or stress responses? Brain Res. Rev. **15**:71-100 (1990).
3. Bernardini, G.L., Richards, D.B. & Lipton, J.M. Antipyretic effects of centrally administered CRF. Peptides **5**:57-59 (1984).
4. Rothwell, N.J.: CRF is involved in the pyrogenic and thermogenic effects of interleukin 1β in the rat. Am. J. Physiol. **256**:E111-E115 (1989).
5. Opp, M., Obál Jr., F. & Krueger, J.M.: Corticotropin-releasing factor attenuates interleukin 1-induced sleep and fever in rabbits. Am. J. Physiol. **257**:R528-R535 (1989).
6. Milton, N.G.N., Hillhouse, E.W., Nicholson, S.A., Self, C.H. & McGregor, A.M.: Production and utilisation of monoclonal antibodies to human/rat corticotrophin-releasing factor-41. J. Mol. Endocrinol. **5**:159-166 (1990).
7. Rivier, J., Rivier, C. & Vale, W.: Synthetic competitive antagonists of corticotrophin releasing factor: effects on ACTH secretion in the rat. Science **224**:889-891 (1984).
8. Rotondo, D., Abul, H.T., Milton, A.S. & Davidson, J.: Pyrogenic immunomodulators increase the level of prostaglandin E_2 in the blood simultaneously with the onset of fever. Eur. J. Pharmacol. **154**:145-152 (1988).

Lomax, Schönbaum (eds.) **Thermoregulation: The Pathophysiological Basis of Clinical Disorders.**
8th International Symposium Pharmacology of Thermoregulation, Kananaskis, Alberta, Canada 1991, pp. 28-32 (Karger, Basel 1992)

RELEASE OF INTERLEUKIN-6 AND TUMOR NECROSIS FACTOR DURING LIPOPOLYSACCHARIDE INDUCED FEVER IN GUINEA PIGS

J. ROTH[1], C. CONN[2], M.J. KLUGER[2] and E. ZEISBERGER[1]

[1]Physiologisches Institut, Klinikum der Justus-Liebig-Universität, Aulweg 129, D-6300 Giessen (Germany) and [2]Department of Physiology, University of Michigan, Medical School, Ann Arbor, Michigan 48109 (USA)

The increase in body temperature during fever is regarded as a component of complex host responses to infection accompanying the release of mediators from the immune system, the endogenous pyrogens (EP). The anterior hypothalamus has long been regarded as the site of action of EP [1]. The first immune mediator or cytokine, which was equivalent to EP was interleukin-1 (IL-1) [2]. However, nowadays it is apparent that other cytokines, such as tumor necrosis factor (TNF) [3] or interferon β_2, which is now known as interleukin-6 or IL-6 [4] are also capable of causing fever.

In rats, blood plasma levels of IL-6 and TNF were monitored after application of bacterial lipopolysaccharide (LPS) [5,6] and plasma activity of IL-6 correlated with the fever magnitude [5], while TNF levels in blood plasma peaked before a significant increase in body temperature.

The aims of the present study were to determine if IL-6 and TNF are detectable in blood plasma, and in perfusates of the anterior hypothalamus (the putative site of action), in guinea pigs before and after LPS application; and to investigate if different stages of fever correlate with different IL-6 and TNF levels.

METHODS: The experiments were performed in guinea pigs chronically equipped either with catheters in the left carotid artery or with push-pull cannulae stereotaxically implanted into the rostral hypothalamus.

The febrile response to intramuscular injection of bacterial LPS (*E. coli*, 20 μg/kg) was monitored by measurement of the colonic temperature every 30 min with a thermocouple inserted 6 cm beyond the anus. The sampling of blood plasma or push-pull perfusion of the anterior hypothalamus were performed 60 min before, 60 min after and 180 min after LPS application. The push-pull perfusions lasted 20-25 min with a perfusion speed of 20 μl/min.

Determination of TNF was performed by a bioassay based on the cytotoxic effect of TNF on the mouse fibrosarcoma cell line WEHI 164 subclone 13 [7]. The percent viable cells, incubated either with different concentrations of TNF standard or with biological samples were measured by use of the dimethylthiazol-diphenyltetrazolium bromide (MTT) colorimetric assay [8]. Determination of IL-6 was based on the dose dependent growth stimulation of IL-6 on the B-9 hybridoma cell line [9]. After incubation of B-9 cells with different concentrations of IL-6, or with biological samples, incorporation of ^{3}H-thymidine into the DNA of the cells was measured by a β-scintillation counter. For details on the TNF and IL-6 assays [see 5,6,10].

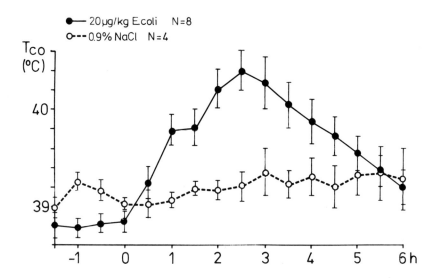

FIGURE 1: Colonic temperature-time curves of guinea pigs before and after intramuscular injection of bacterial lipopolysaccharide (*E. coli*, 20 μg/kg) or of the solvent (0.9% saline).

RESULTS: The effects of intramuscular injection of either LPS (20 μg/kg) or of the solvent (0.9% saline) on colonic temperature of guinea pigs are shown in Fig. 1. LPS injections resulted in fever with the highest colonic temperatures occurring 150 min after injection.

The influence of LPS injection on IL-6 levels in blood plasma and in perfusates of the hypothalamus are summarized in Fig. 2.

The mean level of IL-6 in arterial plasma was 248 units/ml 60 min before LPS application and increased to 24,972 units/ml 60 min after and even to about 1,480,000 units/ml 180 min after injection. The plasma level of IL-6 seemed to correlate with the magnitude of fever. The injection of the solvent did not cause significant changes in plasma level of IL-6. In hypothalamic push-pull perfusates of 3 guinea pigs the basal level of IL-6 (234 units/ml, 60 min before LPS injection) increased in the mean to a 20-fold level 60 min after LPS injection (4,234 units/ml) and declined again to 3,008 units/ml 180 min after LPS application. The IL-6 level in the perfusates of 1 animal injected with the solvent did not alter apparently.

The influence of LPS injection on TNF levels in plasma and hypothalamic perfusates are presented in Fig. 3.

Before the LPS injection, TNF in blood plasma of guinea pigs was hardly detectable (lower than 1 unit/ml). 60 min after injection TNF level in plasma increased strongly to 3,006 units/ml and declined to 1,331 units/ml 180 min after LPS application. In animals injected with 0.9% saline TNF in plasma remained hardly detectable during all stages of the experiment.

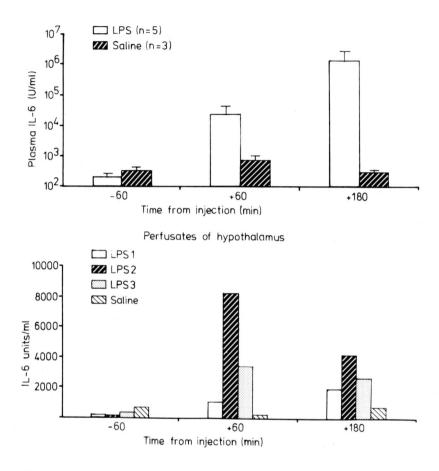

FIGURE 2: IL-6 activity in arterial blood plasma (upper part) and in push-pull perfusates of the anterior hypothalamus (lower part) 60 min before, 60 min after and 180 min after injection of LPS or the solvent.

In hypothalamic push-pull perfusates 2 of the 3 LPS treated animals showed an increase in TNF level 60 min after injection, which continued to rise up to about 6,500 units/ml measured 180 min after injection. In the third animal, LPS treatment seemed to be without effect on the hypothalamic TNF level similar to the control animal injected with 0.9% saline.

DISCUSSION: The data of this study showed that IL-6 and TNF-activity can be monitored not only in blood plasma but also in push-pull perfusates of the anterior hypothalamus in guinea pigs. LPS injections caused strong increases in peripheral and central levels of these two cytokines. The patterns of the IL-6 and TNF levels in blood plasma were similar to those observed in rats [5,6]; the IL-6 level correlated with the change in body temperature during fever, while the TNF level was

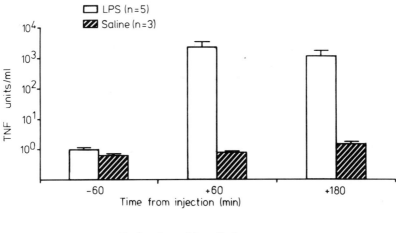

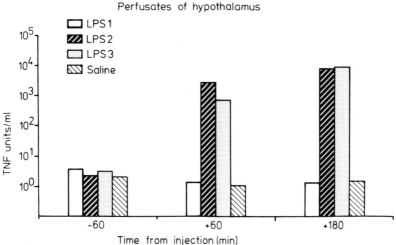

FIGURE 3: TNF activity in arterial blood plasma (upper part) and in push-pull perfusates of the anterior hypothalamus (lower part) 60 min before, 60 min after and 180 min after injection of LPS or the solvent.

higher in the first stage of fever rise than at the fever peak. These results are possibly in agreement with the observation that TNF is a potent inducer of IL-6 [11].

The levels of IL-6 and TNF in hypothalamic perfusates during fever were different from those in blood plasma. The IL-6 level seemed to be higher in the first stage of fever than at the fever maximum, while the hypothalamic TNF level seems to correlate with the magnitude of fever. The data of this pilot study have, of course, to be completed, before we can draw conclusions on the patterns of central increase in IL-6 and TNF levels during the time course of fever. The few data presented here allow, however, some conclusions, which are partly speculative.

The past and present assumptions about the mechanism of EPs are that one or several EPs are released into the circulation, then penetrate the blood-brain barrier in some areas, such as the circum-ventricular organs, and cause an elevation in the thermoregulatory set point [12,13]. If this is the case for IL-6 or TNF, one would expect a correlation between the increase in peripheral and central levels of these cytokines. Another possibility is that IL-6 and TNF are produced in the central nervous system following an induction signal from the periphery. Indeed, it has recently been discovered that ex-planted mediobasal hypothalami of rats can be stimulated by bacterial endotoxin to release IL-6 [14]. It might therefore be likely that the mode of action of EPs will have to be discussed and investigated in a new way in the future.

ACKNOWLEDGEMENTS: This study was supported by the "Deutsche Forschungsgemeins-chaft, project Ze 183. The technical assistance of Miss B. Störr is gratefully acknowledged.

REFERENCES

1. Cooper, K.E., Cranston, W.J. & Snell, E.S.: Observation on the site and mode of action of pyrogens in the rabbit brain. J. Physiol. **191**:325-337 (1967).

2. Dinarello, C.A.: Interleukin-1. Rev. Infect. Dis. **6**:51-95 (1984).

3. Dinarello, C.A., Cannon, S.M., Wolff, H.A., Bernheim, B., Beutler, A., Cerami, I.S., Figari, M.A., Palladino, Jr. & O'Connor, J.V.: Tumor necrosis factor (cachectin) is an endogenous pyrogen and induces production of interleukin 1. J. Exp. Med. **163**:1433-1450 (1986).

4. Nijsten, M.W.N., DeGroot, H.J., Klasen, H.J., Hack, C.E. & Aarden, L.A.: Serum levels of interleukin-6 and acute phase response. Lancet II:921 (1987).

5. Long, N.C., Kunkel, S.L., Vander, A.J. & Kluger, M.J.: Antiserum against tumor necrosis factor enhances lipopolysaccharide fever in rats. Am. J. Physiol. **258**:R332-R337 (1990).

6. LeMay, L.G., Vander, A.J. & Kluger, M.J.: Role of interleukin 6 in fever in rats. Am. J. Physiol. **258**:R798-R803 (1990).

7. Espevic, T. & Nissen-Meyer, J.: A highly sensitive cell line, WEHI 164 clone 13, for measuring cytotoxic factor/tumor necrosis factor from human monocytes. J. Immunol. Meth. **95**:99-105 (1986).

8. Gerlier, D. & Thomasset, N.: Use of MTT colorimetric assay to measure cell activation. J. Immunol. Meth. **94**:57-63 (1986).

9. Aarden, L.A., DeGroot, E.R., Schaap, O.L. & Landsdorp, P.M.: Production of hybridoma growth factors by human monocytes. Eur. J. Immunol. **17**:1411-1416 (1987).

10. LeMay, D.R., LeMay, L.G., Kluger, M.J. & D'Alecy, L.G.: Plasma profiles of IL-6 and TNF with fever-inducing doses of lipopolysaccharide in dogs. Am. J. Physiol. **259**:R126-R132 (1990).

11. Akira, S., Hirando, T., Taga, T. & Kishimoto, T.: Biology of multifunctional cytokines: IL-6 and related molecules (IL 1 and TNF). FASEB J. **4**:2860-2867 (1990).

12. Zeisberger, E.: The role of septal peptides in thermoregulation and fever. In Bligh & Voight, *Thermoreception and Temperature Regulation*, pp. 274-283 (Springer, Berlin, Heidel-berg 1990).

13. Kluger, M.J.: The febrile response. In *Stress Proteins in Biology and Medicine*, pp. 61-78 (Cold Spring Harbor Laboratory Press 1990).

14. Spangelo, B.L., Judd, A.M., MacLeod, R.M., Goodman, D.W. & Isakson, P.C.: Endotoxin induced release of interleukin-6 from rat medial basal hypothalami. Endocrinology **127**:1779-1785 (1990).

Lomax, Schönbaum (eds.) **Thermoregulation: The Pathophysiological Basis of Clinical Disorders.**
8th International Symposium Pharmacology of Thermoregulation, Kananaskis, Alberta, Canada 1991, pp. 33-36 (Karger, Basel 1992)

EFFECTS OF VARIOUS DOSES OF INDOMETHACIN AND DEXAMETHASONE ON RECTAL TEMPERATURE AND HYPOTHALAMIC PROSTANOIDS IN FEBRILE RATS

JACOB KAPLANSKI, HILA HADAS and URIEL SOD-MORIAH

Departments of Clinical Pharmacology and Life Sciences, Ben Gurion University of the Negev, Beer Sheva 84120 (Israel)

In recent studies we have demonstrated that lipopolysaccharides (LPS) cause fever and enhance the synthesis of prostaglandin E_2 (PGE_2) in rat hypothalami [1]. The temperature elevation was inhibited by the nonsteroidal antiinflammatory drug (NSAID) indomethacin (INDO) and dexamethasone (DEXA) which block PG synthesis [2,3]. In this paper we extended the research to some other prostanoids and quantified the dose relationship of the INDO and DEXA to the febrile and prostanoids responses.

METHODS: Male Sprague-Dawley rats 12-15 weeks old weighing 250-350 g were maintained in a room kept at $22 \pm 1°C$ and relative humidity of 35-55% for at least 2 weeks before commencing the experiments. The rats were housed on wood shavings, 2 per cage with water and food *ad libitum*. Rats were injected either with lipopolysaccharide (LPS, E. coli 250 μg ip) or saline (0.5 ml ip). In the first experiment, 22 h post injection, groups of animals were injected with INDO (1, 10 or 50 mg/kg) in 2% $NaHCO_3$ (0.5 ml/100 g ip). In the second experiment 48 h, 24 h, and 2 h before decapitation LPS treated rats were injected with DEXA (1 or 10 mg/kg sc). Rectal temperature (RT) was measured before each treatment with thermistor probe [3] inserted 5 cm into the rectum. Following the final RT measurement 2 h after the INDO or 24 h after the LPS administration, the rats were decapitated and the rostral hypothalami (HT), weighing about 40 mg each, were excised. One or two HT were incubated per vial (6-8 vials per group) for 3 h in Krebs-Henselite buffer containing glucose (0.2%) under an environment of O_2 (95%) and CO_2 (5%) at 37°C. In the third experiment, INDO (1 μM) or DEXA (1 or 100 μM) were added every 30 min to HT slices in the vials. The buffer was replaced every 30 or 60 min. The buffer samples that were recovered were frozen and were assayed at a later time for PGE_2, TXA_2, 6-keto-$PGF_{1\alpha}$ (prostacyclin, PGI) by radioimmunoassay. Statistical evaluation was carried out using student's t test (two-tailed) and factorial analysis.

RESULTS: In rats treated with LPS the RT was significantly higher compared to controls ($p < 0.01$) (Table I, II). The *ex-vivo* experiments show that the output of PGE_2 and PGI_2 were significantly increased ($p < 0.01$) as compared to controls. No such effects were seen for the TXA_2 output (Table I). INDO (50 mg/kg) reversed LPS induced elevations in RT to control values, whereas the decreased RT by INDO (1 or 10 mg/kg) were moderately reduced (Table I). DEXA (1 or 10 mg/kg) decreased significantly ($p < 0.01$) the RT but not to control values (Table 2). INDO (50 mg/kg) decreased the rate of PGE_2, PGI_2 and TXA_2 synthesis at each time point. INDO (1 or 10 mg/kg) reduced the synthesis of the prostanoids only in the first hour of incubation. In the 2nd and 3rd hours of incubation no such effect occurred (Table I). DEXA (1 mg/kg) reduced the synthesis of

PGE_2 to about 80% of the values of LPS treated rats whereas DEXA (10 mg/kg) reduced the synthesis of PGE_2 to about 25% of PGE_2 output of the LPS treated rat HT (Table II). INDO (1 μM) added to HT slices in the medium reduced the PGE_2 output after 30 min to about 40% of the control values and after 120 min it was undetectable. DEXA (1 μM) did not reduce the PGE_2 output at 30 min and later the reduction was minor (70-50% from control; Table III). Larger doses of DEXA (10 or 100 μM) did not change the picture.

TABLE I: **Effects of LPS and various doses of INDO on RT and *in-vivo* prostanoids production in HT of rats**

	RT°C	PGE$_2$			PGI			TXA$_2$
		(pg/mg tissue/h)						
	24 h after LPS	60 min	120 min	180 min	60 min	120 min	180 min	60 min
CON	37.3 ±0.08	8.8 ±0.5	8.2 0.6	8.7 0.9	35.2 2.4	18.0 2.7	28.4 4.1	53.5 1.3
LPS	38.3[1] ±0.06	27[1] ±1.9	29.1[1] 1.3	30.2[1] 3.3	50.7[1] 3.7	28.2[1] 3.2	45.0[1] 2.5	65.7 3.9
LPS + INDO (1 mg)	38.0[1,2] ±0.05	16[1,2] 1.0	34.1[1] 1.8	40.1[1] 3.1	28.0[2] 3.4	34.1[1] 3.4	49.3[1] 3.5	61.7 3.7
LPS + INDO (10 mg)	37.9[1,2] ±0.05	7.0[2] ±0.61	25.2[1] 2.4	31.5[1] 3.2	14.3[1,2] 1.6	28.5[1] 3.0	44.1[1] 3.9	24.5[1,2] 3.6
LPS + INDO (50 mg)	37.4[2] ±0.04	3.8[2] 0.4	6.7[2] 1.0	15.0[1,2] 1.3	5.7[1,2] 1.6	15.2[2] 2.5	29.3[2] 2.4	1.2[1,2] 0.14

Mean ± S.E.M.
[1]Significant difference (p < 0.01) versus control
[2]Significant difference (p < 0.01) versus LPS

TABLE II: **Effects of LPS and various doses of DEXA on RT and *in-vitro* PGE$_2$ production in HT of rats**

	RT°C	PGE$_2$ (pg/mg tissue/h)		
	24 h after LPS	60 min	120 min	180 min
CON	37.3	12.5	13.4	13.8
	0.5	0.9	2.2	1.5
LPS	38.5[1]	40.0[1]	37.2[1]	38.3[1]
	0.5	2.2	2.3	2.9
LPS + DEXA (1)	37.8[1,2]	28.0[1,2]	26.4[1,2]	37.1[1]
	0.18	4.5	2.3	3.2
LPS + DEXA (10)	37.6[1,2]	9.4[2]	8.6[2]	12.3[2]
	0.08	1.1	1.3	1.6

Mean ± S.E.M.
[1]Significant difference (p < 0.01) versus control
[2]Significant difference (p < 0.01) versus LPS

DISCUSSION: In this paper we have shown a correlation between the increased RT due to LPS treatment and the increased synthesis of PGE$_2$ and PGI$_2$ in rat HT. INDO, only in the high dose (50 mg/kg), reversed the RT to control values. Such treatment reduced PGE$_2$, PGI$_2$ and TXA$_2$ output of rat HT in the 3 h samples. The smaller dose (10, 1 mg/kg) reduced the RT to a lesser extent and did not decrease the prostanoid output into the medium in the 2nd and 3rd h. Phenomena like this were reported by Shohami [4] and Danon [5]. DEXA reduced the RT and PGE$_2$ output in the *ex-vivo* experiments in a dose-related manner. On the other hand, it seems that in the *in-vitro* experiments the reduction of the synthesis was not seen in the first measurement (30 min) and later was small. This phenomenon seems to coincide with the fact that DEXA needs to initiate a cascade of events leading to blockade of phospholipase A$_2$ and, later, synthesis of PGE$_2$ [6].

TABLE III: INDO and DEXA added to rats' hypothalamic slices on PGE$_2$ **production**

	PGE$_2$ (pg/mg tissue/30 min)			
	30 min	60 min	90 min	120 min
CON	15.0	9.0	6.0	5.0
	1.8	0.5	0.2	0.3
INDO (1 μM)	4.5[1]	2.7[1]	1.8[1]	0
	0.3	0.3	0.2	
CON	12.9	4.5	3.6	3.6
	0.5	0.2	0.2	0.3
DEXA (1 μM)	12.0	2.4[1]	2.7[1]	3.0[1]
	0.6	0.4	0.1	0.2
DEXA (100 μM)	10.0[1]	2.4[1]	2.1[1]	2.1[1]
	0.5	0.4	0.3	0.2

Mean $\pm$ S.E.M.
[1]Significant difference (p < 0.01) versus control

REFERENCES

1. Hadas, H., Sod-Moriah, U.A. & Kaplanski, J.: The effect of lipopolysaccharide on fever and thermoregulation in rats. In Mercer, *Thermal Physiology*, pp. 395-400 (Elsevier, Amsterdam 1989).
2. Kaplanski, J., Hadas, H. & Sod-Moriah, U.A.: Effect of indomethacin on hyperthermia induced by lipopolysaccharides on high ambient temperature in rats. In Lomax & Schönbaum, *Thermoregulation: Research and Clinical Application*, pp. 176-178 (Karger, Basel 1989).
3. Kaplanski, J., Hadas, H. & Sod-Moriah, U.A.: Effect of dexamethasone on fever and thermoregulation in acutely heat exposed rats. In Mercer, *Thermal Physiology*, pp. 407-412 (Elsevier, Amsterdam 1989).
4. Shohami, E. & Gross, J.: An ex-vivo method for evaluating prostaglandin synthetase activity in cortical slices of mouse brain. J. Neurochem. **45:**132-136 (1985).
5. Danon, A., Leibson, V. & Assouline, J.: Effects of aspirin, indomethacin, flufenamic acid and paracetamol on prostaglandin output from rat stomach and renal papilla in-vitro and ex-vivo. J. Pharm. Pharmacol. **35:**576-579 (1983).
6. Nakamura, H., Mizushima, Y., Seto, Y., Motoyoshi, S. & Kadokawa, T.: Dexamethasone fails to produce antipyretic and analgesic actions in experimental animals. Agents & Actions **16:**542-547 (1985).

Lomax, Schönbaum (eds.) **Thermoregulation: The Pathophysiological Basis of Clinical Disorders.**
8th International Symposium Pharmacology of Thermoregulation, Kananaskis, Alberta, Canada 1991, pp. 37-41 (Karger, Basel 1992)

FEVER AND AGING: RELATIONSHIP TO BROWN ADIPOSE TISSUE THERMOGENESIS

PHILIP J. SCARPACE

Geriatric Research, Education and Clinical Center, VA Medical Center and Department of Pharmacology, University of Florida, Gainesville, Florida 32610 (USA)

Fever is a highly complex physiological response to infection that appears to serve as an important non-specific, host defense mechanism [1]. Elevated body temperature during bacteremia is directly correlated with survival since mortality rates are lower in patients who develop a high fever during bacteremia compared to those who develop a low grade fever or are afebrile [1]. The elderly, in particular, have an impaired febrile response to infection, but the mechanism underlying this remains obscure.

The febrile response to acute bacteremia involves interaction between bacterial endotoxin and macrophages and is mediated by endogenously released pyrogens, most likely interleukin-1 [1]. The pyrogenic effects of interleukin-1 are mediated centrally and may involve activation of the sympathetic nervous system and stimulation of thermogenesis in the periphery [2]. The peripheral mechanisms responsible for the increase in heat production following infection are controversial. Administration of interleukin-1β to rats increases blood flow and oxygen consumption in brown adipose tissue (BAT), suggesting thermogenesis in BAT is an important source of heat production for the febrile response to interleukins [2].

Thermogenesis in BAT is stimulated by catecholamine activation of adenylate cyclase through a sympathetically innervated β-adrenergic receptor. This receptor is pharmacologically distinct from the conventional β_1- or β_2-adrenergic receptors [3,4]. Thermogenesis can be stimulated preferentially by β-agonists directed towards this distinct receptor [3]. For example, the β-adrenergic antagonist, CGP-12177A uniquely binds to the β-adrenergic receptor in BAT and stimulates thermogenesis [4,5].

The ability to regulate body temperature, including the febrile response, diminishes with age [1] and may involve impaired thermogenic mechanisms in BAT. This is a review of our studies initiated to investigate the mechanisms of the reduced febrile response in aged rodents and will be discussed in three parts. In the first series of experiments, we demonstrated that the febrile response to infection was diminished with age in rats [6]. In a second series of experiments, we established that the source of heat production in response to infection with *E. coli* is from BAT [7]. In the third series of experiments, we determined that the β-adrenergic receptor in BAT is unique and that β-adrenergic signal transduction and β-adrenergic stimulation of thermogenesis is diminished with age in BAT [4,8,9].

TABLE I: Adenylate cyclase activity with age in BAT

Adenylate Cyclase Activity (pmol cAMP/min/mg protein)

Age (month)	Basal	NaF	Forskolin	GTP	ISO
3	17.6 ± 1.6	197 ± 21	197 ± 36	30.6 ± 2.5	182 ± 28
18	11.6 ± 3.6	67 ± 29[1]	40 ± 16[1]	19.2 ± 5.7	64 ± 23[1]
24	11.9 ± 1.9	118 ± 11[2]	48 ± 08[1]	24.4 ± 2.0	97 ± 10[2]

NaF (10 mM) and forskolin (33 μM) represent activity above basal.
Isoproterenol (ISO, 0.1 mM) represents activity above GTP (0.1 mM).
Data represent the mean ± SE of 5 rats. Adapted from [10].
[1]$p < 0.01$ or [2]$p < 0.05$ by one way ANOVA and Dunnett's t-test for differences from 3 month.

RESULTS: *Decreased Febrile Response with Age.* Core temperatures were determined remotely by surgically implanting biotelemetry devices into the peritoneal cavity [7]. This allowed repeated noninvasive measurement of temperature without handling the rats. In 3-, 12-, and 24-month-old rats, the body temperature of control rats was the same for each age group, varying from 38.2 ± 0.2°C at 07:30 h following sham injection to 36.9 ± 0.3°C at 16:00 h [6]. In response to ip injection of 1 x 10[8] colony forming units (CFU) of *E. coli*, the 3- and 12-month-old rats experienced a transient hypothermia followed by a fever at 2.5 h after injection. The peak fever in the 3- and 12-month-old rats at 6.5 h post-injection was 1.3 ± 0.1°C above controls ($p < 0.001$). The 24-month-old rats experienced a greater transient hypothermia of -1.4 ± 0.2°C and did not develop a fever until 6 h post-injection. The peak fever at 7.15 h post-injection (0.9 ± 0.2°C above controls; $p < 0.05$) was less than in the 3- or 12-month-old rats [6].

Role of BAT Thermogenesis in the Febrile Response. To investigate the possible relationship between the increase in body temperature and thermogenesis in BAT following infection with *E. coli*, body temperature and whole body oxygen consumption were assessed simultaneously [7]. Six pairs of animals were either infected with 1 x 10[8] CFU of *E. coli* or sham injected. In control animals, there was a slight downward trend in body temperature throughout the day that was paralleled by a slight decrease in oxygen consumption. In rats infected with *E. coli*, there was a transient hypothermia followed by a fever that was sustained throughout the day. Oxygen consumption increased almost immediately, preceded the development of the fever, and was sustained throughout the fever. There was a significant increase in the average cumulative 4 h body temperature (36.6 ± 0.1°C vs 38.2 ± 0.2, $p < 0.001$) and a 48% increase in the average cumulative 4 h oxygen consumption (18.2 ± 1.7 vs 26.9 ± 3.0 ml/min/kg$^{0.67}$; $p < 0.05$). The increase in oxygen consumption was associated with neither an increase in physical activity nor shivering. There was highly significant correlation (R = 0.736, $p < 0.01$) between oxygen consumption and the body temperature for both controls and infected animals [7].

To investigate the relationship between the increase in body temperature and thermogenesis in BAT, we assessed GDP binding to the uncoupling protein in BAT mitochondria during the development of fever in response to *E. coli* infection. GDP binding was assessed by multi-point Scatchard analysis of ^{3}H-GDP binding to isolated mitochondria. In control rats there were 226 $\pm$ 30 pmol GDP binding sites per mg protein with a dissociation constant of 390 $\pm$ 70 nM [7]. Paired rats were either sham injected or infected with 1 x 10^8 CFU of *E. coli* and sacrificed at 0.5, 1.75, and 3.5 h post injection. At 0.5 h post injection there was neither a fever nor a change in GDP binding. At 1.75 h, during the rising phase of the fever, there was an increase in body temperature of 0.7 $\pm$ 0.2°C with a corresponding 45.4 $\pm$ 7.3% ($p < 0.01$) increase in GDP binding sites. By 3.5 h the fever had reached a peak (1.05 $\pm$ 0.13°C above controls); however, the 31.9 $\pm$ 9.0% increase in GDP binding sites was less than during the rising phase of the fever [7].

Impaired Signal Transudction with Age. The amount of interscapular brown adipose tissue recovered from senescent animals was 30% less than that recovered from the 3- or 12-month-old animals (224 $\pm$ 12 mg, 3 month; 214 $\pm$ 10, 12 month; 152 $\pm$ 14, 24 month) [8]. Cytochrome *c* oxidase activity, when expressed as activity per mg mitochondrial protein, was unchanged with age [8]. However, total cytochrome *c* oxidase activity per tissue, a measure of mitochondrial mass, progressively decreased with age (642 $\pm$ 5 nmol/min, 3 month; 455 $\pm$ 58, 12 month; 267 $\pm$ 57, 24 month) [8]. In addition, both the density and the total number of β-adrenergic receptors in BAT membranes decreased with age [8]. In senescent rats, the density (fmol/mg protein) of receptors in BAT membranes was twofold less than that in the 3-month-old rats (20.1 $\pm$ 2.1, 3 month; 11.1 $\pm$ 1.6, 24 month, $p < 0.005$). When the concentration of β-adrenergic receptors was expressed as the total number per tissue (fmol/tissue), there was a similar twofold decrease between the 3- and the 24-month-old rats (20.3 $\pm$ 2.1 and 9.2 $\pm$ 1.3, respectively).

Basal as well as GTP-, isoproterenol-, NaF-, and forskolin-stimulated adenylate cyclase activity was assessed in BAT membranes [8]. Basal and GTP-stimulated activity was not significantly changed with age (Table I). There was a threefold decrease in NaF-stimulated activity between 3 and 18 months of age and a slight increase between 18 and 24 months of age (Table I). Forskolin stimulated activity, which primarily reflects activation of the catalytic unit of adenylate cyclase, was fourfold greater in the 3-month than in the 18- or 24-month-old rats (Table I). Maximal isoproterenol stimulated adenylate cyclase activity displayed the same pattern of age-related loss of activity as NaF and forskolin [8]. There was a threefold decrease in activity between 3 and 18 months of age and a twofold decrease between 3 and 24 months of age (Table I). Isoproterenol dose-response curves indicated that the dose of isoproterenol that half-maximally activated adenylate cyclase was similar for 3- and 24-month-old rats (3.7 x 10^{-6} M vs. 3.9 x 10^{-6} M) and slightly less for 12-month-old rats (1.7 x 10^{-6} M).

CGP-12177A Uniquely Activates the BAT β-Adrenergic Receptor. CGF-12177A is generally considered to be a hydrophilic β-adrenergic antagonist. However, we recently demonstrated that in BAT, this compound has agonist properties [4]. Agonists can be distinguished from antagonists by their ability to interact with both the high- and low-affinity forms of the β-adrenergic receptor [10]. In the presence of guanyl nucleotides, receptors have a lower affinity for the agonist, whereas there is no effect on the affinity of antagonists [10]. We observed a one- to two-log shift to lower affinity in the presence of Gpp(NH)p [4]. These data indicate that CGP-12177A has agonist properties with respect to the β-adrenergic binding site [4].

Furthermore, CGP-12177A activated adenylate cyclase with two components of activation [4]. The first, stimulated by concentrations between 1 and 100 μM, activates to a level of ~20% of the maximum isoproterenol stimulation. The second, at concentrations > 1 mM, activates to a level equal to 63% of the maximum isoproterenol stimulation (83 $\pm$ 15 pmol cAMP/min/mg vs 132 $\pm$ 10). The high-affinity component of CGP-12177A-stimulated adenylate cyclase activity was completely inhibited by propranolol, whereas the low-affinity component was only weakly blocked. However, pindolol inhibited the low affinity component in a manner similar to the inhibition of isoproterenol-stimulated activity. In contrast, CGP-12177A did not activate adenylate cyclase in heart. Thus the CGP-12177A activation of adenylate cyclase, although occurring at high concentrations, appears to be receptor mediated and does not occur in heart tissue, indicating the β-adrenergic receptor in BAT is atypical [4].

Impaired Thermogenesis with Age. CGP-12177A stimulates oxygen consumption in rats [5,9]. When administered to male F-344 rats of 6, 18, and 24 months of age, CGP-12177A (0.75 mg/kg, ip) rapidly induced an elevation in oxygen consumption that peaked at 15 min post-injection followed by a biphasic decline over 4 h [9]. The peak increase in oxygen consumption over baseline (8.1 $\pm$ 0.9 Δml/min/kg$^{0.67}$, 6 month; 7.1 $\pm$ 1.0, 18 month; 3.8 $\pm$ 0.6, 24 month) and the average cumulative 4 h increase (7.6 $\pm$ 1.1, 6 month; 4.6 $\pm$ 0.7, 18 month; 3.7 $\pm$ 0.7, 24 month) were decreased with age ($p < 0.01$, ANOVA). CGP-12177A induced an increase in body temperature that paralleled but appropriately lagged behind the increase in oxygen consumption [9]. The peak increase in body temperature over baseline at 45 min post-injection (0.76 Δ°C, 6 month; 0.63, 18 month; 0.51, 24 month) and the 4 h cumulative increase (127 $\pm$ 10, 6 month; 94 $\pm$ 16, 18 month; 66 $\pm$ 12, 24 month) were decreased with age ($p < 0.05$, ANOVA).

DISCUSSION: Fever has long been recognized as a host defense mechanism against infection. It has an evolutionary history that dates back hundreds of millions of years to lower animals [1]. In classic studies by Kluger *et al.* [11], lizards infected with bacteria had higher temperatures. Clinical studies have demonstrated a correlation between fever and decreased morbidity and mortality rates with a variety of infections. This is particularly true in the elderly, who are often afebrile during bacteremia [1].

The mechanism of the impaired febrile response with senescence is unknown but may involve inadequate BAT thermogenesis. The present report summarizes the evidence that the sympathetic nervous system is implicated in the genesis of fever and that the mechanism involves β-adrenergic-stimulated thermogenesis in BAT [2,7,9]. Specifically, *E. coli* infection results in increased oxygen consumption and increased GDP binding to BAT mitochondria, culminating in a rise in body temperature [7].

With age, the febrile response to *E. coli* infection is decreased as is the increase in oxygen consumption to the specific BAT β-agonist, CGP-12177A [6,9]. This reduced responsiveness may be a consequence of both diminished mitochondrial mass and decreased β-adrenergic signal transduction [8]. Both the density and total number of receptors are reduced with age as is β-agonist-stimulated adenylate cyclase activity [8].

Collectively, these data suggest that bacterial infection induces thermogenesis in BAT and that this may be contributing to the development of fever. In aging rats, the impaired ability to develop a fever in response to infection appears to be a consequence of inadequate BAT thermogenesis due to the diminished responsiveness to β-adrenergic stimulation. This β-agonist stimulation in BAT is unusual in that it is mediated by a β-adrenergic receptor that is pharmacologically distinct from either the β_1 or β_2 subtype. Our evidence that CGP-12177A uniquely activates this receptor, with no activation in other tissues such as the heart, provides an important pharmacological tool [4]. It may be possible to specifically restore lost thermogenic responsiveness with age by pharmacological manipulation with this compound.

ACKNOWLEDGEMENT: The author greatly acknowledges the contributions of S.E. Borst, B.S. Bender, M. Matheny, and J.E. Morley to the original studies. Supported by the Medical Research Service of the Department of Veterans Affairs.

REFERENCES

1. Norman, D.C., Grahn, D. & Yoshikawa, T.T.: Fever and aging. J. Am. Geriatr. Soc. **33**:859-863 (1985).
2. Jepson, M.M., Millward, D.J., Rothwell, N.J. & Stock, M.J.: Involvement of sympathetic nervous system and brown fat in endotoxin-induced fever in rats. Am. J. Physiol. **255**:E617-E620 (1988).
3. Arch, J.R.S.: The brown adipocyte β-adrenoceptor. Proc. Nutr. Soc. **48**:215-223 (1989).
4. Scarpace, P.J. & Matheny, M.: Adenylate cyclase agonist properties of CGP-12177A in brown fat: Evidence for atypical β-adrenergic receptors. Am. J. Physiol. **260**:E226-E231 (1991).
5. Mohell, N. & Dicker, A.: The β-adrenergic radioligand [^{3}H]CGP-12177, generally classified as an antagonist, is a thermogenic agonist in brown adipose tissue. Biochem. J. **261**:401-405 (1989).
6. Scarpace, P.J., Bender, B.S. & Borst, S.E.: The febrile response to E. coli peritonitis is impaired in senescent rats. Gerontologist **30(special issue)**:215A (1990).
7. Scarpace, P.J., Bender, B.S. & Borst, S.E.: E. coli peritonitis activates thermogenesis in brown adipose tissue: Relationship to fever. Can. J. Physiol. Pharmacol. (June 1991).
8. Scarpace, P.J., Mooradian, A.D. & Morley, J.E.: Age-associated decrease in beta-adrenergic receptors and adenylate cyclase activity in rat brown adipose tissue. J. Gerontol. **43**:B65-B70 (1988).
9. Scarpace, P.J., Matheny, M. & Borst, S.E.: Thermogenesis induced by a unique brown adipose tissue agonist is decreased with age. FASEB J. **5**:A1654 (1991).
10. Sibley, D.R. & Lefkowitz, R.J.: Molecular mechanism of receptor desensitization using the β-adrenergic receptor coupled adenylate cyclase system as a model. Nature Lond. **317**:124-129 (1985).
11. Kluger, M.J., Ringler, D.H. & Anver, M.R.: Fever and survival. Science **188**:166-168 (1975).

Lomax, Schönbaum (eds.) **Thermoregulation: The Pathophysiological Basis of Clinical Disorders.**
8th International Symposium Pharmacology of Thermoregulation, Kananaskis, Alberta, Canada 1991, pp. 42-45 (Karger, Basel 1992)

A SPECIFIC INHIBITORY EFFECT OF HALOTHANE ON BROWN ADIPOSE TISSUE THERMOGENESIS

KERSTIN OHLSON[1,3], ANDREA DICKER[1], NINA MOHELL[1], STEN LINDAHL[2], BARBARA CANNON[1] and JAN NEDERGAARD[1]

[1]The Wenner-Gren Institute, The Arrhenius Laboratories F3, Stockholm University, S-106 91, Stockholm (Sweden), [2]Department of Anesthesiology and Intensive Care, Karolinska Hospital and Institute, S-104 01, Stockholm (Sweden) and [3]Department of Anesthesiology and Intensive Care, University Hospital and University of Lund, S-221 85, Lund (Sweden)

The inability of patients to remain euthermic during anesthesia and surgery is a general clinical problem but has presumably its most important implications during anesthesia of newborn infants and small children. Many factors have been considered to contribute to the fact that the baby is more susceptible to heat loss than an adult, e.g., a large surface area relative to body mass and a smaller amount of insulating subcutaneous fat. However, due to the specific thermoregulatory properties of babies and small infants, a further and more specific explanation may be found.

In newborn children exposed to cold no visible shivering occurs and heat production is provided by nonshivering thermogenesis [1]. The location of nonshivering thermogenesis to brown adipose tissue and the observation that the inhalation anesthetic halothane inhibits lipolysis in white adipose tissue cells [2] initiated the present investigation of the effects of halothane on brown fat thermogenesis. The studies were performed *in vivo* and *in vitro* in golden hamsters.

The results indicate that halothane has a specific inhibitory effect on brown fat thermogenesis and this may aggravate the situation for babies and small infants during anesthesia and surgery.

METHODS: I. *In vivo* studies. Cold acclimated Syrian hamsters were placed in an open circuit metabolic chamber (principally as described in [3,4]) with an air flow of 650 ml/min. Halothane from a conventional vaporizer was carried with the air into the chamber. The halothane concentrations were monitored at the outlet with a gas monitor. Oxygen concentration in the effluent air was measured paramagnetically and corrected for halothane concentration. Oxygen consumption was measured before anesthesia, during undisturbed anesthesia, after intraperitoneal injection of norepinephrine (1 mg/kg) and when the animal was awake again. Control animals were anesthetised with pentobarbital (120 mg/kg). Oxygen consumption was calculated as ml $O_2/(min\text{-}kg^{0.75})$.

II. *In vitro* studies. Brown adipocytes were isolated with a collagenase digestion method from adult hamsters living at 21°C [5]. The rate of oxygen consumption (thermogenesis) was measured polarographically with a Clark-type oxygen electrode. A 15 min preincubation of the cells was performed in a plastic tube with a double needle technique for continuously bubbling with 3% halothane in air with 5% CO_2 (control cells were preincubated without the halothane). Respiratory rate was measured under basal conditions and after addition of increasing concentrations of norepinephrine (0.1 nM - 10 μM). Oxygen consumption was calculated as fmol O/(min•cell).

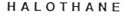

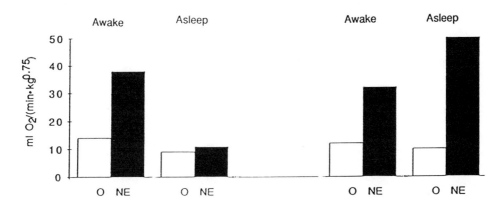

FIGURE 1: Oxygen consumption in hamsters anesthetised with either halothane or pentobarbital. NE: norepinephrine injection.

RESULTS: As seen in Fig. 1 (left panels), an unanesthetised hamster had a low metabolic rate when examined at 24°C. When the hamster was injected with norepinephrine, a high thermogenic response was elicited [6]. However, when the hamster was anesthetised with halothane, the basal metabolism was somewhat diminished, and, very remarkably, the response to norepinephrine was completely abolished.

In a control hamster which was anesthetised with pentobarbital, an increase in oxygen consumption was still found after injection of norepinephrine (Fig. 1, right panels).

As seen in Fig. 2, brown fat cells responded to increasing concentrations of norepinephrine with an increased respiration, as earlier observed [5]. In cells preincubated with halothane, the basal respiratory rate was unaffected. When norepinephrine was added there was practically no increase in oxygen consumption in the halothane incubated cells. Control experiments indicated that the halothane effect was reversible (not shown).

DISCUSSION: In these experiments, we have used cold acclimated hamsters as experimental *in vivo* models for examining a possible brown fat related effect of halothane on thermoregulatory effectors in babies and small infants. This model was chosen because cold acclimated hamsters, just like infants, have a recruited and metabolically active brown adipose tissue.

We found a specific inhibitory effect of halothane on norepinephrine induced thermogenesis in these hamsters, as shown in Fig. 1. As norepinephrine induced thermogenesis is a measure of the capacity for nonshivering thermogenesis [7], these experiments implicate that thermoregulatory nonshivering thermogenesis in the halothane anesthetised infant may be inhibited.

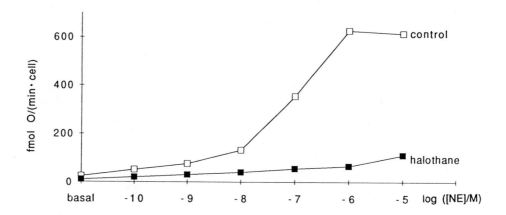

FIGURE 2: Dose-response curves for norepinephrine stimulation of respiration in control and halothane-incubated hamster brown adipocytes.

As nonshivering thermogenesis is located to brown adipose tissue [8] it was likely that the halothane inhibition was a direct effect on the brown fat cells themselves. As shown in Fig. 2, this was apparently the case. The reduced calorigenic activity of the brown adipose tissue may result from an impairment of the norepinephrine induced lipolytic activity, as found in white adipose tissue [2].

The small baby is dependent on nonshivering thermogenesis, i.e., on the adrenergic stimulation of its brown adipose tissue, for thermoregulation during cold stress. The demonstrated inhibitory effect of halothane on heat production in brown adipose tissue suggests that nonshivering thermogenesis during halothane anesthesia is less efficient than during awake conditions and this may contribute to the small child's thermoregulatory problems during anesthesia and surgery.

ACKNOWLEDGEMENTS: These studies were supported by grants from Jeanssons stiftelse and from the Swedish Science Research Council.

REFERENCES

1.   Cannon, B. & Johansson, B.W.: Nonshivering thermogenesis in the newborn. Mol. Aspects Med. **3:**119-223 (1980).
2.   Prokocimer, P.G., Maze, M., Vickery, R.G., Kraemer, F.B., Gandjei, R. & Hoffman, B.B.: Mechanism of halothane-induced inhibition of isoproterenol-stimulated lipolysis in isolated rat adipocytes. Mol. Pharmacol. **33:**338-343 (1988).
3.   Heldmaier, G. & Steinlechner, S.: Seasonal control of energy requirements for thermoregulation in the Djungarian hamster (Phodopus sungorus), living in natural photoperiod. J. Comp. Physiol. **142:**429-437 (1981).
4.   Dicker, A., Raasmaja, A., Cannon, B. & Nedergaard, J.: Effects of hypothyroidism on adrenergic receptors in brown adipose tissue. (Submitted 1991).

5. Mohell, N., Nedergaard, J. & Cannon, B.: Quantitative differentiation of α- and β-adrenergic respiratory responses in isolated hamster brown fat cells: evidence for the presence of an α_1-adrenergic component. Eur. J. Pharmacol. **93:**183-193 (1983).

6. Hissa, R. & Hirsimäki, P.: Calorigenic effects of noradrenaline and inderal in the temperature-acclimated golden hamster. Comp. Gen. Pharmac. **2:**217-224 (1971).

7. Janský, L., Bartunkova, R., Kockova, J., Mejsnar, J. & Zeisberger, E.: Interspecies differences in cold adaptation and nonshivering thermogenesis. Fed. Proc. **28:**1053-1058 (1969).

8. Foster, D.O. & Frydman, M.L.: Nonshivering thermogenesis in the rat. II. Measurements of blood flow with microspheres point to brown adipose tissue as the dominant site of the calorigenesis induced by noradrenaline. Can. J. Physiol. Pharmacol. **56:**110-122 (1978).

Lomax, Schönbaum (eds.) **Thermoregulation: The Pathophysiological Basis of Clinical Disorders.**
8th International Symposium Pharmacology of Thermoregulation, Kananaskis, Alberta, Canada 1991, pp. 46-49 (Karger, Basel 1992)

HYPOTHALAMIC NOREPINEPHRINE AND BODY TEMPERATURE CONTROL: ANOTHER LOOK

NING QUAN, LI XIN, WILLIAM S. HUNTER and CLARK M. BLATTEIS[1]

Department of Physiology and Biophysics, University of Tennessee College of Medicine, Memphis, Tennessee (USA)

Studies on the role of central norepinephrine (NE) in the regulation of body temperature (T_{bo}) conducted to date have yielded inconsistent results. When NE was microinjected into the cerebral ventricles or directly into the preoptic/anterior hypothalamic nuclei (PO/AH), increases, decreases, or no change in T_{bo} were observed [1]. These discrepant findings have generally been ascribed to differences in experimental conditions, e.g., the dose of NE, the animal species, the ambient temperature (T_a), the time of day when the injection was made, and the degree of restraint imposed on the animal during the experiments [2]. Indeed, varying one or another of these factors changes the response to microinjected NE. Unfortunately, these latter responses have, themselves, been inconsistent. For instance, NE given icv induced a rise in T_{bo} at warm T_a's, but T_{bo} falls in cold T_a's in sheep, goats, and rabbits [2], whereas in cats these treatments induced only decreases in T_{bo} at all T_a's [1]. Similarly, conflicting responses were obtained when NE was microinjected directly into the PO/AH.

We found recently that microinjection of NE into the PO/AH of conscious guinea pigs, in confirmation of other studies [3], caused a T_{bo} rise. However, microinjection of pyrogen-free saline (PFS), the control solution and vehicle for NE, similarly caused a gradual elevation of T_{bo}'s. This rise was obviated when PFS was microdialyzed [4]. Additionally, the T_{bo} rise induced by microinjected PFS was prevented by pretreatment with a PGE-synthase blocker, indomethacin [4]. This blocker also converted the T_{bo} rise caused by microinjected NE into a fall [3]. Taken together, these results suggested that non-specific traumatic injury, and the consequent release of PGE, a hyperthermogenic mediator, may attend microinjection but not microdialysis and account for the hyperthermogenic response to NE. We, therefore, re-examined the thermal effect of centrally administered NE, using microdialysis.

METHODS: Adult, male Hartley guinea pigs, weighing 300-350 g, were prepared surgically as described previously [3]. Briefly, guide cannulas were implanted in different animals into the medial PO (MPO), lateral PO (LPO), AH, and lateral septal area (LS). One week later, a microdialysis probe was inserted into each guide such that its membrane tip (10 kDa molecular weight cutoff) protruded 1 mm beyond the guide. The animals were allowed to recover for 2 days before the experiments were begun. PFS containing 0.1% ascorbic acid was the control solution and vehicle for NE. L-NE bitartrate was dissolved freshly to various concentrations (0.05-60 $\mu l/\mu l$) in PFS immediately before use. Adrenergic α-(phentolamine, PHE) or β-(propranolol, PRO) receptor antagonists were dissolved to 1 $\mu g/\mu l$ in PFS, alone or with NE (10 $\mu g/\mu l$), respectively. After a 90 min stabilization period, a drug was microdialyzed through the pre-implanted probe at 2 $\mu l/min$ for another

2 h. Most experiments were conducted by day (09:00 h), and some at night (21:00 h). The animals, fully conscious, were exposed to T_a 24 ± 1, 31 ± 1, or 15 ± 2°C, and their T_{bo}, skin temperature (T_{sk}), and oxygen consumption (V_{O2}) monitored, using previously described methods [3,5].

RESULTS & DISCUSSION: At 24°C, NE microdialyzed into the MPO induced dose-related T_{bo} falls (Table I). PFS and 0.05 $\mu g/\mu l$ of NE had no thermal effect (not illustrated), but NE (5, 10, 20, 40, or 60 $\mu g/\mu l$) caused statistically significant decreases in T_{bo}. The T_{bo} returned towards pretreatment levels immediately after an NE perfusion was ended. The onset latencies tended to grow shorter and the magnitudes of the responses larger with increasing NE doses; viz., the latencies after 5 and 10 $\mu g/\mu l$ were significantly longer than after the higher doses, and the T_{bo} fall evoked by 5 $\mu g/\mu l$ was significantly smaller than that by any of the higher concentrations of NE. Thus, these results show that the thermal action of NE microdialyzed into the MPO of guinea pigs causes hypothermia, in contrast to its hyperthermic effect after microinjection. Since the latter was blocked by pretreatment with indomethacin [3], it is probable that it is an injury related artifact peculiar to the technique. The T_{bo} fall induced by microdialyzed NE in 24 ± 1°C was also site-specific, the MPO being most sensitive (-0.7 ± 0.2°C), the LS (-0.5 ± 0.1°C) and AH (-0.4 ± 0.2°C) less sensitive, and the LPO (-0.2 ± 0.2°C) insensitive. These results correlate with the known distribution of thermosensitive neurons [6] and noradrenergic terminals in these hypothalamic regions [7].

The NE induced T_{bo} fall also occurred in the cold, but not in the warm environment (Table I). The latter was expected, since at 31°C there should be little capacity for the already activated body heat dissipation system to be enhanced further by the hypothermic effect of NE. The T_{bo} fall in the cold, however, was smaller than that at 24°C. A priori, this was perplexing because the heat dissipation system should be functioning at its lowest limit in a cold environment and, hence, be available for maximal activation by NE. It is possible, however, that NE did not cause a larger T_{bo} fall because systemic autonomic mechanisms that counteract the effect of cold exosure may already have been operating to prevent a further decrease of T_{bo} under these conditions.

NE dialyzed directly into the PO (iPO) of these guinea pigs during the night also produced a T_{bo} fall (Table I). The response was different from that obtained during the daytime in that recovery from the lowered T_{bo} was slower. Since the NE turnover rate and the expression of adrenoceptors display a circadian rhythm [8], it is possible that this slower recovery of T_{bo} reflected the greater production and density of NE receptors during the active, food-foraging period of these crepuscular animals.

The T_{bo} fall induced by NE was blocked by co-microdialyzed PHE, but not PRO (Table I), suggesting α-, but not β-, adrenoceptor mediation of the effect. Furthermore, the iPO microdialysis of PHE, but not of PRO, alone induced a T_{bo} rise, indicating that α-receptors may be tonically active in maintaining the homeostatic level of T_{bo}. The T_{bo} fall induced by NE was associated with a decrease in V_{O2} (-15 ± 7%); T_{sk} was not changed. Hence, the T_{bo} fall was effected by reduction in the metabolic rate, without attendant cutaneous vasodilation.

TABLE I: Changes in T_{bo} of conscious guinea pigs in response to microdialyzed NE, PHE, and PRO

Drug	N	Dose, $\mu g/\mu l$	T_a °C	Latency, min	Max ΔT_{bo} °C	ΔT_{bo} 5 h, °C
NE	4	5*	24 ± 1	72 ± 10	-0.30 ± 0.08	-0.12 ± 0.10
	6	10*	24 ± 1	72 ± 8	-0.82 ± 0.11	-0.37 ± 0.17
	3	60*	24 ± 1	36 ± 7	-1.23 ± 0.22	-0.45 ± 0.15
NE	5	10	31 ± 1	N/A	-0.00 ± 0.20	-0.14 ± 0.30
	4	10*	15 ± 2	36 ± 5	-0.40 ± 0.20	-0.30 ± 0.22
NE‡	5	10*	24 ± 1	72 ± 8	-0.70 ± 0.20	-0.67 ± 0.26
PHE	5	1*	24 ± 1	47 ± 1	-0.75 ± 0.20	-1.67 ± 0.22
PRO	5	1	24 ± 1	N/A	-0.02 ± 0.02	-0.02 ± 0.03
PHE + NE	5	1 + 10	24 ± 1	N/A	-0.03 ± 0.13	-0.06 ± 0.05
PRO + NE	5	1* + 10	24 ± 1	70 ± 9	-0.76 ± 0.14	-0.35 ± 0.20

Abbreviations and symbols: NE: norepinephrine. PHE: phentolamine. PRO: propranolol. Max ΔT_{bo}: Maximal T_{bo} changes from basal values (the T_{bo} at 6-min intervals averaged voer the last 30 min of a 90 min stabilization period) during the 3 h dialysis period. ΔT_{bo} 5 h: T_{bo} changes from basal values 5 h after the beginning of drug dialysis, i.e., 2 h after the end of dialysis. ‡: experiments conducted during the night in the dark. *: changes in T_{bo} significantly different ($P < 0.05$) from the response to PFS (not illustrated). N/A: not applicable.

CONCLUSION: It would appear that, in conscious guinea pigs, NE acts in the MPO to depress the metabolic rate through an α-adrenoceptor-mediated mechanism, thereby causing the T_{bo} to fall. This response is dose-dependent, site-specific, and consistent under all the ambient conditions examined in this study.

ACKNOWLEDGEMENTS: This research was supported by NIH grant NS 22716 to Clark M. Blatteis.

REFERENCES

1. Clark, W.G. & Lipton, J.M.: Changes in body temperature after administration of adrenergic agents and related drugs including antidepressants. Neurosci. Behav. **10:**153-220 (1986).
2. Blight, J. & Cottle, W.H.: The influence of ambient temperature on thermoregulatory responses to 5-hydroxytryptamine, noradrenaline and acetylcholine injected into the lateral cerebral ventricles of sheep, goats and rabbits. J. Physiol. Lond. **212:**377-392 (1969).

3. Quan, N. & Blatteis, C.M.: Intrapreoptically microdialyzed and microinjected norepinephrine evoke different thermal responses. Am. J. Physiol. **257**:R816-R821 (1989).

4. Quan, N. & Blatteis, C.M.: Microdialysis: a system for localized drug delivery into the brain. Brain Res. Bull. **22**:621-625 (1989).

5. Collins, M.G., Hunter, W.S. & Blatteis, C.M.: Factors producing elevated core temperature in spontaneously hypertensive rats. J. Appl. Physiol. **63**:740-745 (1987).

6. Blatteis, C.M.: Functional anatomy of the hypothalamus from the point of view of temperature regulation. In Szelenyi & Szekely *Advances in Physiological Science*, Vol. 32, Contributions to Thermal Physiology, pp. 3-12 (Pergamon, Oxford 1981).

7. Nieuwenhuys, R.: *Chemoarchitecture of the Brain*. (Springer-Verlag, Berlin 1985).

8. Kafka, M.S., Benedito, M.A., Roth, R.H., Steele, L.K., Wolfe, W.W. & Castravas, G.N.: Circadian rhythms in catecholamine metabolites and cyclic nucleotide production. Chronobiol. Int. **3**:101-115 (1986).

Lomax, Schönbaum (eds.) **Thermoregulation: The Pathophysiological Basis of Clinical Disorders.**
8th International Symposium Pharmacology of Thermoregulation, Kananaskis, Alberta, Canada 1991, pp. 50-53 (Karger, Basel 1992)

COMPARISON OF PERIPHERAL VASCULAR RESPONSES TO HYPOGLYCAEMIA AND TO ADRENALINE INFUSION

D.G. MAGGS and I.A. MACDONALD

Department of Physiology & Pharmacology, University of Nottingham Medical School, Nottingham (UK)

Acute hypoglycaemia is recognised as a common [1] and unpleasant side effect of insulin therapy and its physical characteristics are well described. Changes in heart rate and blood pressure during hypoglycaemia closely parallel cardiovascular changes during an adrenomedullary response. It is therefore not surprising that plasma adrenaline concentrations are found to be elevated during hypoglycaemia [2]. Although many of the physical features of hypoglycaemia are attributed to raised circulating adrenaline [3], our understanding of peripheral blood flow responses are not so well defined. Early work has shown an increase in limb blood flow [4] and this has since been a consistent finding. However, changes in acral and skin blood flow have not been fully established.

The purpose of our work was to determine more accurately peripheral vascular responses in healthy subjects during a period of hypoglycaemia and to separately establish the vascular responses to infused adrenaline.

METHODS: Healthy nondiabetic subjects (see physical characteristics Table I) were recruited for the two following studies which were approved by the Nottingham Medical School Ethics Committee. In both studies subjects were seen in a post-absorptive state, resting supine and lightly clad in thermoneutral conditions (30°C). Measurements of peripheral blood flow were made at 10 min intervals; firstly measured by venous occlusion plethysmography at two sites (forearm and great toe), and secondly, skin blood flow measured by laser doppler flowmetry [Moor instruments, UK] at two sites (dorsum of the foot and great toe pulp).

In the first study responses were observed during a 60 min period of hypoglycaemia (blood glucose 2.5 mmol/l). Hypoglycaemia was induced using a hyperinsulinaemic (Human Actrapid insulin 60 $mU/m^2/min$) clamp [5]. As a means of control, subjects were similarly studied on another occasion during an infusion of saline (placebo).

In the second study responses were observed during a graded adrenaline infusion at 3 consecutive 20 min steps (10, 25 and 50 ng adrenaline/kg/min). As a means of control subjects were similarly studied on another occasion during an infusion of saline (placebo).

Arterialised venous blood was sampled at intervals for adrenaline [6] from a retrograde intravenous cannula inserted into a vein of the dorsum of the hand which was in a hot air box maintained at 50°C.

Data were analysed by analysis of variance with repeated measures.

TABLE I: **Physical characteristics (ranges) of subjects**

	Hypoglycaemia Study	Adrenaline Infusion Study
Number	10	10
Sex	10 male	5 male
Age (years)	20-26	20-27
BMI (kg/m^2)	20.7-26.6	20.4-29.1

RESULTS: The results are summarized in Table II. During hypoglycaemia plasma adrenaline had increased significantly at 20 min and was still rising at the end of the 60 min period. During adrenaline infusion there was an expected rise in plasma adrenaline concentration.

Forearm blood flow increased after 20 min of hypoglycaemia but a return towards baseline measurements was noted at 60 min. During adrenaline infusion there was a stepwise increase in forearm blood flow, the greatest increment being with the highest infusion rate. There was also a smaller, yet nevertheless significant, rise in forearm blood flow during saline infusion.

Toe blood flow fell significantly after 60 min of hypoglycaemia with a fall noted during adrenaline infusion at the highest plasma adrenaline concentration.

After 20 min of hypoglycaemia skin blood flow of the toe pulp fell, this change was sustained at 60 min. Similarly, during adrenaline infusion, skin blood flow of the toe pulp fell at the highest adrenaline concentration. Skin blood flow of the dorsum of the foot fell after 60 min of hypoglycaemia and during the final adrenaline infusion rate.

DISCUSSION: We have demonstrated similar peripheral vascular responses to hypoglycaemia to those observed during adrenaline infusion at comparable plasma adrenaline concentrations. Although described before [4,7], in both studies there were similar increases in forearm blood flow indicating a probable common mechanism, assumedly β-adrenoceptor mediated vasodilatation in muscle. However, a waning of this effect seems an unlikely explanation for the late fall in forearm blood flow noted during hypoglycaemia, especially in the light of a progressively rising plasma adrenaline concentration at this time. It seems probable this reflects accompanying skin vasoconstriction as skin blood flow is a significant component of forearm blood flow, especially with the high starting values observed in these subjects.

The decreases in distal skin blood flow (laser doppler flowmetry) and toe blood flow (strain gauge plethysmography) during adrenaline infusion are in strong accordance wth previous work [8], where skin vasoconstriction was described using much higher doses of adrenaline, using different techniques (this response is mediated through α-adrenoceptors). We have demonstrated similar skin vasoconstriction during hypoglycaemia which, to some extent, contradicts current views. Flushing of the skin is a common symptom of hypoglycaemic subjects, has been described by observers [9] and is consistent with the demonstration of cutaneous hyperaemia of the forearm and face [10]. We observed transient hyperaemia in the skin over the dorsum of the foot at an early stage of hypoglycaemia. Such hyperaemia could be due to the withdrawal of α-adrenergic mediated vasoconstrictor tone [11].

TABLE II: Plasma adrenaline and blood flow responses to hypoglycaemia and adrenaline infusion

	Hypoglycaemia Study			Adrenaline Infusion Study	
	Hypoglycaemia	Control		Adrenaline	Control
Plasma Adrenaline (nmol/l)					
Baseline	0.38 (.06)	0.36 (.04)	Baseline	0.22 (.03)	0.21 (.03)
0 min	0.44 (.08)	0.35 (.04)	Step 1	$1.01\ (.10)^2$	0.23 (.04)
20 min	$2.68\ (.36)^2$	0.38 (.04)	Step 2	$1.86\ (.10)^2$	0.22 (.03)
60 min	$3.73\ (.64)^2$	0.34 (.05)	Step 3	$3.05\ (.20)^2$	0.25 (.04)
Forearm Blood Flow (ml/100 ml/min)					
Baseline	9.1 (1.5)	8.2 (1.8)	Baseline	3.9 (0.5)	4.3 (0.5)
0 min	9.1 (1.4)	7.7 (1.3)	Step 1	5.5 (1.1)	5.5 (0.6)
20 min	$12.0\ (1.6)^1$	7.6 (0.9)	Step 2	$6.6\ (0.7)^1$	5.9 (0.6)
60 min	$10.9\ (1.6)^1$	8.1 (0.8)	Step 3	$8.9\ (1.4)^2$	$6.2\ (0.7)^1$
Toe Blood Flow (ml/100 ml/min)					
Baseline	13.3 (2.3)	13.2 (2.6)	Baseline	11.7 (1.6)	10.2 (1.3)
0 min	14.0 (2.4)	15.4 (2.4)	Step 1	12.0 (1.6)	10.4 (1.2)
20 min	11.2 (2.4)	16.2 (1.7)	Step 2	$10.4\ (1.3)^1$	10.4 (1.2)
60 min	$9.9\ (1.7)^1$	$17.2\ (2.3)^1$	Step 3	$8.9\ (1.2)^2$	10.2 (1.5)
Toe Pulp Blood Flow (relative Change From Baseline)					
0 min	1.13 (.13)	1.13 (.15)	Step 1	0.90 (.06)	$1.67\ (.48)^1$
20 min	$0.62\ (.10)^2$	1.28 (.17)	Step 2	0.87 (.21)	1.48 (.48)
60 min	$0.70\ (.11)^2$	$1.35\ (.18)^1$	Step 3	$0.61\ (.09)^2$	1.68 (.44)
Foot Dorsum Blood Flow (Relative Change From Baseline)					
0 min	$1.92\ (.42)^1$	$1.58\ (.21)^2$	Step 1	$1.59\ (.40)^1$	1.24 (.15)
20 min	1.58 (.15)	1.58 (.21)	Step 2	1.30 (.19)	1.21 (.18)
60 min	$0.86\ (.09)^1$	1.48 (.15)	Step 3	$1.01\ (.13)^1$	1.29 (.25)

Values are means with standard errors (significance: $^1p < .05$; $^2p < .01$).

However, the present study shows vasoconstriction in the skin of the foot and toe, indicating either a marked regional variation in skin vascular responses or, possibly, an effect of duration. We imposed rather sustained hypoglycaemia and saw vasoconstriction consistent with the pallor which is a characteristic of hypoglycaemia in diabetic patients. The other studies may have observed changes occurring at an earlier stage of hypoglycaemia. Toe blood flow during hypoglycaemia had a greater relative decrement when compared with the decrement noted during adrenaline infusion. This may simply be due to slight differences in adrenaline concentration but may indicate an additional vasoconstrictor action during hypoglycaemia, e.g. vasopressin [12] and angiotensin II [13]. The release of adrenaline during hypoglycaemia would explain most, if not all, of the observed peripheral vascular responses.

REFERENCES

1. The DCCT Research Group: Diabetes Control and Complications Trial (DCCT): results of feasibility study. Diabetes Care **10:**1-19 (1987).
2. Holzbauer, T.R. & Vogt, M.: The concentration of adrenaline in the peripheral blood during insulin hypoglycaemia. Brit. J. Pharmacol. **9:**249 (1954).
3. Wallace, J.M. & Harlan, W.R.: Significance of epinephrine in insulin hypoglycaemia in man. Am. J. Med. **38:**531-539 (1965).
4. Lauter, S. & Baumann, H.: Kreislauf und Atmung im hypoglykamischen Zustand. Dtsch. Arch. klin. Med. **163:**161-175 (1929).
5. DeFronzo, R.A., Jordan, D., Tobin, J.D. & Andres, R.: Glucose clamp technique: a method for quantifying insulin secretion and resistance. Am. J. Physiol. **237:**E214-223 (1979).
6. Macdonald, I.A. & Lake, D.M.: An improved technique for extracting catecholamines from body fluids. J. Neurosci. Methods **13:**239-248 (1985).
7. Macdonald, I.A., Bennett, T., Gale, E.A.M., Green, J.H. & Walford, S.: The effect of propranolol on thermoregulation during insulin-induced hypoglycaemia in man. Clin. Sci. **63:**301-310 (1982).
8. Barcroft, H. & Swan, H.J.C.: *Sympathetic Control of Human Blood Vessels* (Edward Arnold, London 1953).
9. French, E.B. & Kilpatrick, R.: The role of adrenaline in hypoglycaemic reactions in man. Clin. Sci. **14:**639-651 (1955).
10. Aman, J., Berne, C., Ewald, U. & Tuvemo, T.: Lack of cutaneous hyperaemia in response to insulin-induced hypoglycaemia in IDDM. Diabetes Care **13:**1029-1033 (1990).
11. Berne, C. & Fagius, J.: Skin nerve sympathetic activity during insulin-induced hypoglycaemia. Diabetologia **29:**855-860 (1986).
12. Thompson, C.J., Thow, J., Jones, I.R. & Baylis, P.H.: Vasopressin secretion during insulin-induced hypoglycaemia: exaggerated response in people with type I diabetes. Diab. Med. **6:**158-163 (1989).
13. Trovati, M., Massucco, P., Mularoni, E., Cavalot, F., Anfossi, G., Mattiello, L. & Emanuelli, G.: Insulin-induced hypoglycaemia increases plasma concentrations of angiotensin II and does not modify atrial natriuretic polypeptide secretion in man. Diabetologia **31:**816-820 (1988).

Lomax, Schönbaum (eds.) **Thermoregulation: The Pathophysiological Basis of Clinical Disorders.**
8th International Symposium Pharmacology of Thermoregulation, Kananaskis, Alberta, Canada, 1991, pp. 54-59 (Karger, Basel, 1992)

EFFECT OF REPEATED ADMINISTRATION OF SUBLETHAL DOSE OF DIVICINE ON BODY TEMPERATURE, SOME BLOOD AND URINE CONSTITUENTS OF RATS

M.S. ARBID and M.A. BASHANDY

Pharmacology Department, National Research Centre and Zoology Department, Faculty of Science, Al-azhar University, Cairo (Egypt)

Favism is an acute haemolytic disease associated with glucose-6-phosphate dehydrogenase deficiency and ingestion of faba beans [1-3]. In the presence of oxygen divicine and isouramil produce free radicals [4] which cause a fall in blood or liver glutathione concentration [1,5-7] leading to peroxidative reactions [8]. Yannai and Marquardt [9], Arbid and Marquardt [10] and Arbid and Bashandy [7] have recently demonstrated that the rat can be sensitised to the effect of vicine, convicine, divicine or isouramil following intraperitoneal injections or intravenous injections of the latter two compounds. The induced signs are similar in many respects to those observed in favism of humans. They noticed an increased respiration rate, generalised cyanosis, and, after several hours, death apparently caused by asphyxiation. The weight of splenic tissue and percent haematocrit decreased 24 h after divicine administration indicating that the damaged erythrocytes were being removed by the reticuloendothelial system.

Cenarruzabitia *et al.* [11] found that the effects of vicia faba diet on urinary nitrogenous compounds and on enzyme activities of pathways directly associated with amino acid metabolism.

MATERIALS & METHODS: ANIMALS: Male albino rats of the Sprague-Dawley strain were used in the present experiments. The animals were of about the same age, size and of average weight about 100-120 g and each rat was kept in a special metabolic cage.

MATERIALS: Divicine was prepared by acid hydrolysis according to the method of Arbid and Marquardt [10].

EXPERIMENTAL DESIGN: Two groups were used each of 15 rats. The first group represents the control and the rats wre intraperitoneally injected with saline solution. The second group was intraperitoneally injected daily with sublethal dose of divicine (1.4 mg/100 g body weight) for two weeks. Daily collection of urine was carried out for each rat.

METHODS & TECHNIQUES: 1. Rectal, Skin, Ear and Tail Temperature: They were measured by using digital thermistor from Cole-Parmer Instrument Company, USA. With two types of electrodes, one with long probe which is inserted in the rectum for three min, the other with a disc probe for measuring the skin, ear and tail temperature, the disc is placed in direct contact with skin, ear or tail for three min.

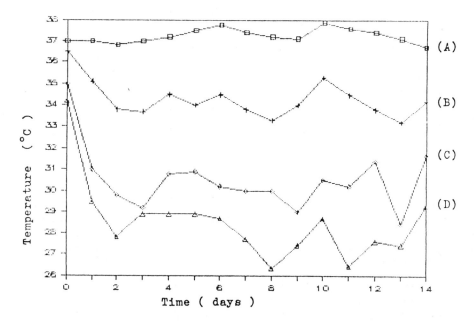

FIGURE 1: Effect of daily injected sublethal dose of divicine on rectal, skin, ear and tail temperature of rats. (A) Rectal temperature, (B) Skin temperature, (C) Ear temperature, (D) Tail temperature.

2. Haematological Investigations: Blood samples were obtained from the retro-orbital venous plexes of rats [12] and examined for erythrocytic count [13], haemoglobin percentage by using kits prepared by Boehringer Mannheim Company and haematocrit value was determined by using heparinized microhaematocrit tubes.

3. Urine Analysis: Urine samples were collected daily from each rat and examined for haemoglobin percentage and creatinine content using kits prepared by Boehringer Mannheim Company. Uric acid content was estimated by Folin's method [14].

4. Statistical Analysis of the Results: They were done according to Snedecor and Gochran [15].

RESULTS & DISCUSSION: The thermoregulatory effect of daily intraperitoneally injected doses of divicine (1.4 mg/100 g B.W.) on the rat is shown in Fig. 1.

There were insignificant changes in rectal temperatures. While significant and highly significant decreases in skin, ear and tail temperature of rats were recorded in most days but at few days the decrease was insignificant. The insignificant change in rectal temperature may be due to that the thermoregulaory centre in the brain was not affected by the injection of sublethal dose of divicine, while the skin, ear and tail temperature indicated decreasing in temperature which may be attributed to the effect of divicine on the peripheral blood vessels which are found in the body surface. The effect of daily administration (1.4 mg/100 g B.W. ip) of divicine on some blood constituents was indicated in Table I. There were insignificant decreases in erythrocytes after the first week of injection. On the other hand, highly significant decrease in erythrocytes was found after second week of injection. Muduuli *et al.* [16] found increasing in fragility of erythrocytes of the laying hen and the growing chick fed vicine which was isolated from faba beans. Spontaneous haemolysis of erythrocytes was recorded in the vicine or convicine fed rats or hens [4,16,17,19]. Leucocytes showed, as in Table I, insignificant increase after first and second week of injection. Arbid and Marquardt [10] reported increases in blood monocytes and neutrophil counts in rats which were injected daily with vicine or convicine, suggesting that vicine and convicine stimulated adrenal corticoid steroid production, but they found decreasing in lymphocytes count. Insignificant increase was indicated in haemoglobin content [Table I]. Hegazy and Marquardt [19]; Arbid and Marquardt [10] and Arbid and Bashandy [7] found that the haemoglobin concentration of rats were not affected.

These results are somewhat different from those obtained with the laying hen [16,18,20], where it was observed that dietary vicine or faba beans caused a marked decrease in haemoglobin concentration. The same results were indicated in injected rats with divicine [21]. The haemoglobinurea [Table II] increased significantly until the third day of administration, while decreasing appeared at the 6th day of administration until the end of administration (2 weeks). Vicine causes mild haemoglobinuria in juvenile dogs [22]. Also, haemoglobinuria was reported in rats, injected with single lethal dose of divicine [7]. Haematocrit value was highly significantly increased (Table I) after both the first and second week of administration. Arbid and Marquardt [10] indicated that haematocrit values of rats increased for blood collected one hour after DV administration, which may be attributed to haemoconcentration caused by the movement of body fluids into the gastrointestinal tract. On the contrary, when a smaller dose of divicine was injected into rats, haematocrit either increased or not affected within 1.5 h of divicine. After 24 h there was dramatic decrease in haematocrit concentration which corresponded with the increase in the weight of the spleen [9,10].

TABLE I: **Effect of daily injected 1/10 LD_{50} of divicine (1.4 mg/100 g body weight) intraperitoneally on some blood constituents (Mean $\pm$ SE)**

Week	R.B.C.$_s$ $10^6/\mu l$	W.B.C.$_s$ $10^3/\mu$	Hb. %	PCV %
		Analysis		
Control	7.06 ± 0.37	12.07 ± 0.42	86.20 ± 2.24	41.30 ± 1.36
After first week	6.35 ± 0.30	14.58 ± 1.63	92.00 ± 2.54	56.03 ± 3.26[1]
After second	5.62 ± 0.27[1]	15.03 ± 1.74	87.11 ± 3.22	51.90 ± 1.55[1]

[1]$P < 0.01$

TABLE II: Effect of daily injected 1/lo LD_{50} of divicine (1.4 mg/100 g body weight) intraperitoneally on creatinine, uric acid and haemoglobinurea in the urine of rats (Mean $\pm$ SE)

Days	Creatinine (mg/100 ml urine)	Analysis Uric Acid (mg/100 ml urine)	Haemoglobinurea %
0	40.04 ± 2.86	31.9 ± 2.83	1.90 ± 0.09
1	73.12 ± 3.33^2	31.0 ± 2.92	5.50 ± 0.93^2
3	59.44 ± 10.55	35.0 ± 2.62	6.22 ± 0.39^2
6	61.12 ± 3.73^2	30.9 ± 2.96	3.66 ± 0.57^1
9	59.96 ± 8.32	33.1 ± 1.80	3.86 ± 0.50^2
12	62.82 ± 2.67^2	27.3 ± 3.38	2.98 ± 0.22^2
15	68.54 ± 2.86^2	31.8 ± 4.49	3.16 ± 0.47

$^1 P < 0.05$
$^2 P < 0.01$

In Table II creatinine excretion was highly significantly increased in most days of administration. Cenarruzabeitia et al. [11] found that the urea and creatinine excretion of rats fed on vicia faba was approximately 90% more than that of control rats. The vicia faba fed rats had increased the activities of liver arginase, arginosuccinate synthetase and alanine aminotransferase. On the other hand, uric acid excretion (Table II) was not affected in all times of experiment. This result is in agreement with that reported by Arbid and Marquardt [21]. They injected the rats with isouramil and divicine.

Body weight was decreased with the control rats. This is due to the effect of divicine on amino acid metabolism [11]. Water consumption and urine volume were not affected during the days of experiment (Table III).

TABLE III: Results of the analysis of variance performed on body weight (%), water consumption (%), and urine volume of rats, injected intraperitoneally with 1/10 LD$_{50}$ of divicine

Source of Variation	Body Weight (%)		Water Consumption (%)		Urine Volume
	D.F.	MS	D.F.	MS	MS
Total	64	--	69	--	--
Weeks	01	630.24[1]	01	01.79	10.03
Days	12	144.79[1]	13	28.00	04.02
Error	51	029.79	55	34.66	03.11

[1]$P < 0.01$

REFERENCES

1. Mager, J., Chevion, M. & Glaser, G.: In Liener *Toxic Constituents of Plant Foods*, p. 266 (Academic Press, New York 1980).
2. Arese, P., Bosia, A., Naitana, A., Gaetani, S., D'Aquino,M. & Gaetan, G.P.: In Brewer *The Red Cell*, p. 725 (Alan R. Liss, New York 1981).
3. Arese, P.: Rev. Pure Appl. Pharmacol. Sci. **3:**123 (1982).
4. Albano, E., Tomasi, A., Mannuzzu, L. & Arese, P.: Detection of a free radical intermediate from divicine of Vicia faba. Biochem. Pharmacol. **33:**1701-1704 (1984).
5. Mager, J., Glaser, G., Razin, A., Izak, G., Bien, S. & Noam, M.: Metabolic effects of pyrimidines derived from faba bean glycosides on human erythrocytes deficient in glucose-6-phosphate dehydrogenase. Biochem. Biophys. Res. Comm. **20:**235-240 (1965).
6. Chevion, M., Navok, T., Glaser, G. & Mager, J.: The chemistry of favism-inducing compounds. The properties of isouramil and divicine and their reaction with glutathione. Eur. J. Biochem. **12:**405-409 (1982).
7. Arbid, M.S. & Bashandy, M.A.: A study of the antimetabolites (Divicine) isolated from faba beans (Vicia faba L.) on some physiological responses with special references to its thermoregulatory effects. 7th International Symposium on the Pharmacology of Thermoregulation, Odense, pp. 149-152, 1988 (Karger, Basel 1989).
8. D'Aquino, M., Gaetani, S. & Spadoni, M.A.: Effect of factors of favism on the protein and lipid components of rat erythrocyte membrane. Biochem. Biophys. Acta **731:**161-167 (1983).
9. Yannai, S. & Marquardt, R.R.: Induction of favism-like symptoms in the rat: effects of vicine and divicine in normal and buthionine sulfoximine-treated rats. J. Sci. Food Agric. **36:**1161-1168 (1985).
10. Arbid, M.S.S. & Marquardt, R.R.: Effect of intraperitoneally injected vicine and convicine on the rats: induction of favism-like signs. J. Sci. Food Agric. **37:**539-547 (1986).

11. Cenarruzabeitia, M.N., Santidrian, S., Bello, J. & Larralde, J.: Effect of raw field bean (vicia faba) on amino-acid-degrading enzymes in rats and chicks. Nutr. Metb. **23(3):**203-210 (1979).

12. Helperin, B.N., Beezi, G., Mene, G. & Benaceroff, B.: Etude quantitative de l'activate granulo plexyue Due systeme reteculo-ends lial por l'injection intraveneus d'encre de chin chez les diverses especes animals. Anr. Inst. Pasteur **80:**582-604 (1951).

13. Harris *et al.* (1951): (Cited from Hawk's physiological chemistry, 14th edition, 1965).

14. Folin (1950): (Cited from Hawk's physiological chemistry, 14th edition, 1965).

15. Snedecor, G.W. & Cochran, W.G.: Statistical methods. Iowa State University Press, Ames 7th Edition (1980).

16. Muduuli, D.S., Marquardt, R.R. & Guenter, W.: Effect of dietary vicine and vitamine E supplementation on the productive performance of growing and laying chickens. Br. J. Nutr. 47-53 (1982).

17. Winterbourn, C.C., Benatti, U. & DeFlora, A.: Contributions of superoxide, hydrogen peroxide, and transition metal ions to auto-oxidation of the favism-inducing pyrimidine aglycone, divicine, and its reactions with haemoglobin. Biochem. Pharmacolgoy **23(12):**2009-2015 (1986).

18. Arbid, M.S., Marquardt, R.R. & El-Habbak, M.M.: A study of the toxic effects of high levels of dehulled faba beans (Vicia faba L.) in the diets of laying hens. Egyptian Poultry Science, Faculty of Agriculture, 5 (1985).

19. Hagazy, M.I. & Marquardt, R.R.: Metabolism of vicine and convicine in rat tissues: Absorption and excretion patterns and sites of hydrolysis. J. Sci. Food Agric. **35:**139-146 (1984).

20. Muduuli, D., Marquardt, R. & Guenter, W.: Effect of dietary vicine on the productive performance of laying chickens. Can. J. Anim. Sci. **61:**757-761 (1981).

21. Arbid, M.S.S. & Marquardt, R.R.: Favism-like effects of divicine and isouramil in the rat: Acute and chronic effects on animal health, mortalities, blood parameters and ability to exchange respiratory gases. J. Sci. Food Agric. **43:**75-90 (1988).

22. Lin, J.Y. & Ling, K.H.: Favism 2. Studies on physiological activities of vicine in vivo. J. Formosan Med. Assoc. **62:**490-494 (1962).

Lomax, Schönbaum (eds.) **Thermoregulation: The Pathophysiological Basis of Clinical Disorders.**
8th International Symposium Pharmacology of Thermoregulation, Kananaskis, Alberta, Canada 1991, pp. 60-64 (Karger, Basel 1992)

NMDA ANTAGONISTS ATTENUATE COCAINE-INDUCED HYPOTHERMIA

M. BANSINATH, H. TURNDORF and V.K. SHUKLA[1]

Department of Anesthesiology, School of Medicine, New York University Medical Center, 550 First Avenue, New York, N.Y. 10016 (USA)

Body temperature is an important factor affecting the dose requirement of the anesthetics [1]. Both non-competitive and competitive NMDA antagonists have anesthetic effects [2,3]. The dissociative anesthetic, ketamine is a non-competitive antagonist at the NMDA receptor. Ketamine is believed to act primarily through binding at a phencyclidine site located within the NMDA receptor complex. Due to its distinct advantages, ketamine has an important place in the practice of anesthesia [3]. With the recent increase in cocaine abuse, the pharmacodynamic interactions of cocaine with drugs used in anesthesia have assumed clinical importance [4]. Body temperature is affected by both cocaine [5] and the NMDA-antagonist-anesthetic, ketamine [6]. The objective of the present investigation was to assess the thermoregulatory interaction between cocaine and NMDA antagonists.

METHODS: Male Swiss Webster [(SW)fBR] mice weighing 25-30 g were housed five per cage in a room with controlled temperture (22 $\pm$ 2°C), humidity and artificial light (06:30-19:00 h). The animals had free access to food and water and were used after minimum of four days acclimation to housing conditions. All experiments were conducted between 09:00-17:00 h in March-May.

The following drugs were prepared by dissolving them in sterile water just before use; cocaine hydrochloride, ketamine hydrochloride, MK-801 (Dizocilpine, (+)-5-methyl-10,11-dihydro-5H-dibenzo[a,d]cyclohepten-5,10-iminehydrogen maleate, Merck Sharp and Dohme, West Point, PA). All the drugs were injected in a volume of 10 ml/kg. The doses used were: cocaine 25, 50, 100 and 150 mg/kg sc. In the combination experiments, cocaine (100 mg/kg sc) injection was followed by either ketamine (30 mg/kg ip) or MK-801 (1 mg/kg ip) injection. Animals in the control group were injected with sterile saline. A minimum of 10 animals were used per group.

The temperature measurements were done at an ambient temperature of 22 $\pm$ 0.2°C. Colonic temperatures of mice were measured using a telethermometer and thermistor probe. The probe was inserted 3.5 cm into the rectum and the temperature was recorded when a constant reading was obtained [7]. While the temperaure measurements were made, the animals were gently restrained (45-60 sec) in chux. The pre-drug temperaure for each mouse was measured twice, 15 min apart and the readings were averaged to obtain the basal temperature of the respective animal. Post drug measurements were taken 0.5, 1, 1.5 and 2 h after the drug injections. Each animal was used only once.

[1]Visiting Assistant Professor, Department of Biophysics, Panjab University, Chandigarh - 160014, India

TABLE I: **Time course of the changes in colonic temperature in cocaine treated animals**

Change in the colonic temperature °C Mean ± SEM

Cocaine (mg/kg sc)	Time (h)			
	0.5	1	1.5	2
Saline	-0.19 ± 0.09	-0.40 ± 0.09	-0.33 ± 0.07	-0.44 ± 0.07
025	-0.04 ± 0.24	-0.87 ± 0.15	-0.24 ± 0.11	-0.16 ± 0.14
050	-1.81 ± 0.12	-0.35 ± 0.15	-0.05 ± 0.08	-0.22 ± 0.07
100	-1.56 ± 0.49	-1.10 ± 0.64	-1.78 ± 0.47	-1.87 ± 0.35
150	-1.00 ± 0.37	-2.02 ± 0.26	-1.55 ± 0.76	-1.74 ± 0.39

RANOVA indicated that the interaction of dose x time was significant ($F_{12,213} = 11.4$, $p < 0.00001$).

For each animal, the change in body temperature compared to preinjection control was calculated and the data are presented graphically as mean changes *versus* time. The thermic response was integrated by the addition of the net temperature change at each consecutive interval after the drug injection [7]. The group mean of the net changes in temperature (temperature index) are presented in bar diagrams. The statistical significance was determined by analysis of variance (ANOVA), repeated measure ANOVA (RANOVA) and Newman-Keuls test where appropriate using a computer program. A $p < 0.05$ was considered as significant.

RESULTS: The time course data of the changes in colonic temperature in cocaine treated mice are shown in Table I. Depending on the dose, cocaine induced hyper- or hypothermia. Repeated measure ANOVA indicated that the interaction of dose x time was significant ($F_{12,213} = 11.4$, $p < 0.00001$). The temperature index (0-120 min) after cocaine treatment is shown in Fig. 1. ANOVA indicated that dose had a significant effect ($F_{4,71} = 21.78$, $p < 0.00001$). The effect of simultaneous administration of NMDA antagonists on the hypothermic response of cocaine (100 mg/kg) is shown in Fig. 2. For these combination studies, based on the results from the pilot experiments, doses of ketamine (30 mg/kg ip) and MK-801 (1 mg/kg ip) were selected such that, when compared to saline treated animals, these drugs by themselves did not significantly alter the temperature index. When ketamine or MK-801 was administered simultaneously with cocaine, cocaine induced hypothermia was attenuated (Fig. 2). ANOVA indicated that the main factors of combination ($F_{1,65} = 18.46$, $p < 0.0001$) and the interaction of drug x combination had significant effect ($F_{2,65} = 3.47$, $p < 0.05$).

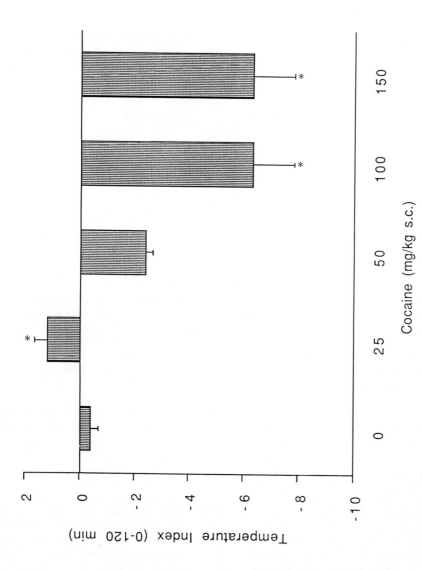

FIGURE 1: The mean (+ SEM) temperature index (0-120 min) after saline (O) or cocaine (25, 50, 100 and 150 mg/kg sc) administration. ANOVA indicated dose had a significant effect ($F_{4,71}$ = 21.78, $p < 0.00001$). *$p < 0.05$ when compared with saline treated group (Newman-Keuls test).

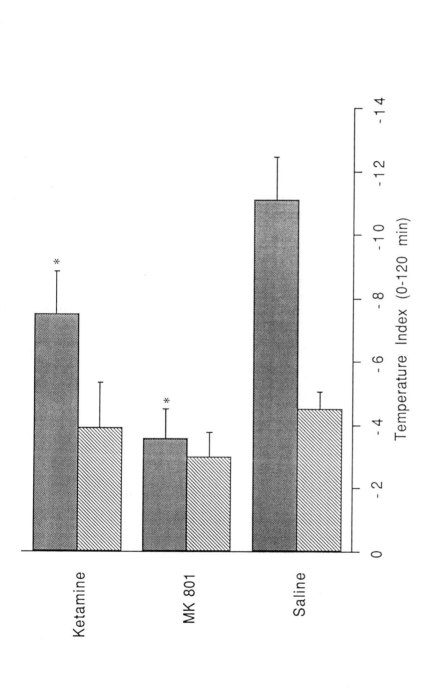

FIGURE 2: The mean (+ SEM) temperature index (0-120 min) after ketamine (30 mg/kg ip), MK-801 (1 mg/kg ip) or saline (10 ml/kg ip) in control (cross hatched bar) and in tests groups (shaded bar) which were treated with above drugs in combination with cocaine (100 mg/kg). ANOVA indicated that the main factors of combination ($F_{1,65} = 18.46$, $p < 0.0001$) and the interaction of drug x combination had significant effect ($F_{2,65} = 3.47$, $p < 0.05$). *$p < 0.05$ when compared to cocaine + saline treated group (Newman-Keuls test).

DISCUSSION: These results demonstrate that, depending on the dose administered, cocaine induces hyper or hypothermic responses in mice. However, hypothermia appears to be the principal effect of cocaine, since it was the response observed at higher doses of cocaine. Thus, these results are in agreement with earlier studies in rats [5]. Among mechanisms by which cocaine affects the body temperature, modulation of central dopaminergic system appears to be important [5]. The non-competitive NMDA antagonist, MK-801, has no effect on body temperature [8]. However, MK-801 potentiates the hypothermic effect of the inhalation anesthetic, halothane [9]. In the present study, the dissociative anesthetic, ketamine and MK-801, in the doses used, did not affect the body temperature. Hence, attenuation of cocaine induced hypothermia cannot be explained on the basis of physiological antagonism. The mechanism of attenuation of hypothermic response, may directly or indirectly involve the NMDA receptor mediated neurotransmission at the thermoregulatory centers.

Modulation of the central dopaminergic system appears to be the mechanism by which cocaine potentiates the ketamine-induced sleeping time in mice [10]. Therefore, the status of the dopaminergic system should also be considered as an important factor affecting the thermoregulatory interaction between NMDA antagonists and cocaine.

REFERENCES

1. Bansinath, M., Turndorf, H. & Puig, M.M.: Influence of hypo- and hyperthermia on disposition of morphine. J. Clin. Pharmacol. **28:**860-864 (1988).
2. France, C.P., Winger, G.D. & Woods, J.H.: Analgesic, anesthetic and respiratory effects of the competitive N-methyl-D-aspartate (NMDA) antagonist CGS 19755 in rhesus monkeys. Brain Res. **526:**355-358 (1990).
3. Zsigmond, E.K. & Domino, E.F.: Clinical pharmacology of ketamine. In Domino *Status of Ketamine in Anesthesiology*, pp. 27-67 (NPP Books, Ann Arbor 1990).
4. Fleming, J.A., Byck, R. & Barash, P.G.: Pharmacology and therapeutic applications of cocaine. Anesthesiology **73:**518-531 (1990).
5. Lomax, P. & Daniel, K.A.: Cocaine and body temperature in the rat: effects of ambient temperature. Pharmacology **40:**103-109 (1990).
6. Ramabadran, K., Bansinath, M., Turndorf, H. & Puig, M.M.: A pharmacological analysis of the interaction of ketamine with kappa opiates. In Domino *Status of Ketamine in Anesthesiology*, pp. 211-227 (NPP Books, Ann Arbor 1990).
7. Bansinath, M., Ramabadran, K., Turndorf, H. & Puig, M.M.: Effect of κ and μ selective agonists on colonic temperature in normoglycemic and streptozotocin-treated hyperglycemic mice. Pharmacol. Toxicol. **66:**324-328 (1990).
8. Nehls, D.G., Park, C.K., MacCormack, A.G. & McCulloch, J.: The effects of N-methyl-D-aspartate receptor blockade with MK-801 upon the relationship between cerebral blood flow and glucose utilization. Brain Res. **511:**271-279 (1990).
9. Corbett, D., Evans, S., Thomas, C., Wang, D. & Jonas, R.A.: MK-801 reduced cerebral ischemic injury by inducing hypothermia. Brain Res. **514:**300-304 (1990).
10. Vanderwende, C., Spoerlein, M.T. & Lapollo, J.: Cocaine potentiates ketamine-induced loss of the righting reflex and sleeping time in mice. Role of catecholamines. J. Pharmacol. Exp. Ther. **222:**122-125 (1982).

Lomax, Schönbaum (eds.) **Thermoregulation: The Pathophysiological Basis of Clinical Disorders.**
8th International Symposium Pharmacology of Thermoregulation, Kananaskis, Alberta, Canada 1991, pp. 65-69 (Karger, Basel 1992)

INFLUENCE OF GABA AGONISTS AND CCK-8 ON AMPHETAMINE INDUCED HYPOTHERMIA IN MICE

GABRIELLE BOSCHI[1], NICOLE LAUNAY and RICHARD RIPS

Faculté de Pharmacie, Pharmacologie-INSERM, 5 rue J.B. Clément, 92296 Châtenay-Malabry Cédex (France)

Central dopaminergic (DA) and serotonergic (5-HT) mechanisms are involved in amphetamine induced hypothermia in mice and these two systems display a functional antagonism [1,2]. However, this hypothermia seems more complex. As the nucleus accumbens appears to be the most responsive area [1], we have examined the possible contributions of other neurotransmitter or neuromodulator systems which are involved in this brain area. The effects of pretreatment with GABA related agent, cholecystokinin (CCK-8), and drugs acting on opioid systems, such as naloxone, on the hypothermia elicited by intracerebroventricular (icv) amphetamine have been investigated in mice. In an attempt to evaluate the contribution of the major metabolites of amphetamine to the induction of hypothermia, the mice were also treated with iprindole and desipramine, which has been reported to inhibit amphetamine metabolism [3,4].

METHODS: Male OF1 mice, 6 weeks old and weighing 26-28 g, were implanted with a guide cannula into the right lateral ventricle. They were maintained at $22 \pm 1°C$ for 1 week. Central injections were made in a volume of 0.5 μl over a period of 50 sec. Rectal temperature was measured with a thermocouple.

RESULTS: The effects of pretreatment with GABA related drugs are shown in Fig. 1. Amphetamine induced hypothermia was not abolished by the GABA antagonists, bicuculine (2 mg/kg ip) or picrotoxin (0.5 mg/kg ip). The $GABA_A$ agonist, muscimol (0.5 mg/kg ip) did not potentiate this hypothermia, whereas the $GABA_B$ agonist, baclofen (2.5 mg/kg ip) did. The GABA analogue, γ-butyrolactone (GBL) (40 mg/kg ip) also induced potentiation.

CCK-8 (0.04 mg/kg ip) caused potentiation, whereas naloxone (2 mg/kg ip) was without effect (Fig. 2a). Iprindole (15 mg/kg ip) did not modify the hypothermia. In contrast, desipramine (20 mg/kg ip) markedly reduced it (Fig. 2b).

---

[1]Author for correspondence. Address for reprint requests: 7, rue Jules Breton, 75013 Paris, France

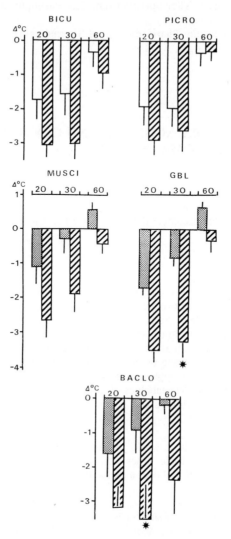

FIGURE 1: Time course of the change in rectal temperature (Δ°C, ordinate scales) in mice produced by a combination of: amphetamine (9 μg icv) and vehicle (open columns); amphetamine (3 μg icv) and vehicle (stippled columns); amphetamine (9 or 3 μg icv) and GABA drugs (hatched columns). Amphetamine (9 or 3 μg) was used to investigate any antagonism or potentiation, respectively. GABA related drugs or vehicle were given before amphetamine. BICU: bicuculline (2 mg/kg ip, 15 min), time zero values: 36.11 ± 0.14°C (vehicle), 36.11 ± 0.19°C (BICU); PICRO: picrotoxin (0.5 mg/kg ip, 15 min), time zero values: 36.31 ± 0.14°C (vehicle), 36.40 ± 0.24°C (PICRO); MUSCI: muscimol (0.5 mg/kg ip, 15 min), time zero values: 36.25 ± 0.19°C (vehicle), 36.40 ± 0.17°C (MUSCI); GBL: γ-butyrolactone (40 mg/kg ip, simultaneously), time zero values: 36.37 ± 0.34°C (vehicle), 36.67 ± 0.28°C (GBL); BACLO: baclofen (2.5 mg/kg ip, 15 min), time zero values: 36.44 ± 0.23°C (controls), 36.68 ± 0.18°C (BACLO). Each column represents the mean of 7 to 12 mice. Vertical bars indicate S.E.M. *p < 0.05, comparison with the appropriate controls (amphetamine + vehicle), Mann-Whitney U test. Abscissa scales: time in min.

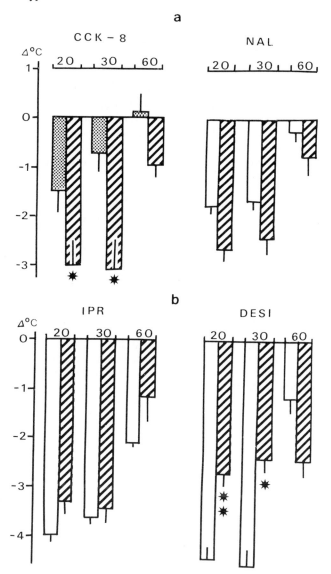

FIGURE 2: Time course of the change in rectal temperature (Δ°C, ordinate scales) in mice produced by a combination of: amphetamine (3 μg icv) and vehicle (stippled columns); amphetamine (9 μg icv) and vehicle (open columns); amphetamine (3 or 9 μg icv) and drugs (hatched columns). Amphetamine (3 μg) was used to investigate any potentiation and 9 μg to investigate any antagonism. Drugs or vehicle were given before amphetamine. (a): CCK-8: cholecystokinin (0.04 mg/kg ip, simultaneously), time zero values: 36.27 ± 0.22°C (vehicle), 36.0.2 ± 0.25°C (CCK-8); NAL: naloxone (2 mg/kg ip, simultaneously), time zero values: 37.20 ± 0.23°C (vehicle), 36.72 ± 0.22°C (NAL); (b): IPR: iprindole (15 mg/kg ip, 30 min), time zero values: 37.00 ± 0.14°C (vehicle), 36.59 ± 0.37°C (IPR); DESI: desipramine (20 mg/kg ip, 1 h), time zero values: 37.42 ± 0.17°C (vehicle), 36.50 ± 0.40°C (DESI). Each column represents the mean of 6 to 11 mice. Vertical bars indicate S.E.M. *p < 0.05; **p < 0.01, comparison with the appropriate controls (amphetamine + vehicle), Mann-Whitney U test. Abscissa scales: time in min.

DISCUSSION: The facilitation of the action of amphetamine by baclofen may result from GABA release induced by baclofen [5]. Studies have shown that GABA exerts an inhibitory control on DA systems. Attenuation of the activity of DA neurons by GABA would result in a decrease in dopamine release and intraneuronal catabolism which would, in turn, increase the neuronal concentration of dopamine. More endogenous dopamine could then be available at the presynaptic nerve endings for release by amphetamine. Baclofen has been reported to increase dopamine in the mesolimbic DA terminals [6] and to inhibit the firing rate of DA nerves [7]. All these mechanisms may be implicated in the potentiation of hypothermia by baclofen, based on the above explanation. In the same way, GBL facilitated hypothermia may result from an increase in dopamine synthesis caused by the blockade of impulse flow [8].

CCK-8 is present in high concentration in a subpopulation of dopamine containing neurons [9]. There is considerable controversy as to whether CCK-8 potentiates or decreases DA transmission. In our study, CCK-8 clearly potentiated the hypothermia induced by amphetamine. This potentiation may depend, at least partially, on DA mechanisms, since it has been suggested that CCK-8 potentiates the effect of dopamine on DA receptors [10]. Consequently, the activity of amphetamine would be enhanced.

Taken together, these results seem to indicate that endogenous dopamine modulates the hypothermia produced by amphetamine via GABA and CCK-8 interactions.

It has recently been reported that the hydroxylated metabolites of amphetamine are capable of influencing DA and 5-HT transmission [11]. If these metabolites are involved in the hypothermic response to amphetamine, their effects may help to explain the complex mechanism of this hypothermia. Iprindole did not modify the hypothermia, whereas desipramine prevented it. This result must be treated with caution since desipramine also influences noradrenaline metabolism.

REFERENCES

1. Boschi, G. & Rips, R.: Forebrain sites for the hypothermic effect of dexamphetamine in mice. Neurosci. Lett. **31:**153-158 (1982).
2. Boschi, G. & Launay, N.: Differential effects of neuroleptic and serotonergic drugs on amphetamine-induced hypothermia in mice. Neuropharmacology **24:**117-122 (1985).
3. Freeman, J.J. & Sulser, F.: Iprindole-amphetamine interactions in the rat: the role of aromatic hydroxylation of amphetamine in its mode of action. J. Pharmacol. Exp. Ther. **183:**307-315 (1972).
4. Consolo, S., Dolfini, E., Garattini, S. & Valzelli, L.: Desipramine and amphetamine metabolism. J. Pharm. Pharmacol. **19:**253-256 (1967).
5. Roberts, P.J., Gupta, H.K. & Shargill, N.S.: The interaction of baclofen (β-(4-chlorophenyl) GABA) with GABA systems in the rat brain: evidence for a releasing action. Brain Res. **155:**209-212 (1978).
6. Kelly, P.H. & Moore, K.E.: Dopamine concentrations in the rat brain following injections into the substantia nigra of baclofen, γ-aminobutyric acid, γ-hydroxybutyric acid, apomorphine and amphetamine. Neuropharmacology **17:**169-174 (1978).
7. Fuxe, K., Hökfelt, T., Ljungdahl, A., Agnati, L., Johansson, O. & Perez de la Mora, M.: Evidence for an inhibitory gabaergic control of the mesolimbic dopamine neurons: Possibility of improving treatment of schizophrenia by combined treatment with neuroleptics and gabaergic drugs. Med. Biol. **53:**177-183 (1975).
8. Roth, R.H., Walters, J.R. & Aghajanian, G.K.: Effect of impulse flow on the release and synthesis of dopamine in the rat striatum. In Snyder and Costa *Frontiers in Catecholamine Research*, pp. 567-574 (Pergamon Press, New York 1973).

9.   Hökfelt, T., Skirboll, L., Rehfeld, J.F., Goldstein, H., Markey, K. & Dann, O.: A sub-population of mesencephalic dopamine neurons projecting to limbic areas containing a cholecystokinin-like peptide: evidence from immunohistochemistry combined with retrograde tracing. Neuroscience **5:**2093-2124 (1980).

10.   Studler, J.M., Reibaud, M., Tramu, G., Blanc, G., Glowinski, J. & Tassin, J.P.: Distinct properties of cholecystokinin-8 and mixed dopamine-cholecystokinin-8 neurons innervating the nucleus accumbens. In Vanderkalghen and Crawley *Cholecystokinin*, pp. 306-314 (Academic Science, New York 1985).

11.   Matsuda, L.A., Hanson, G.R. & Gibb, J.W.: Neurochemical effects of amphetamine metabolites on central dopaminergic and serotonergic systems. J. Pharmacol. Exp. Ther. **251:**901-908 (1989).

Lomax, Schönbaum (eds.) **Thermoregulation: The Pathophysiological Basis of Clinical Disorders.**
8th International Symposium Pharmacology of Thermoregulation, Kananaskis, Alberta, Canada 1991, pp. 70-73 (Karger, Basel 1992)

EXOGENOUS AND ENDOGENOUS PYROGENS: EFFECTS ON CYCLIC AMP EFFLUX FROM RAT BRAIN SLICES *IN VITRO*

M.J. DASCOMBE, G.M. HORWICH and D. PRICE

Neuroscience Research Group, Department of Physiological Sciences, Stopford Building, University of Manchester, Oxford Road, Manchester M13 9PT (England)

The febrile response to an infection or an inflammatory stimulus is mediated initially by the synthesis and release of endogenous pyrogenic cytokines, such as interleukin-1 (IL-1), then the elevation of prostaglandin E_2-like eicosanoid levels in the brain, although the identity of the pyrogenic mediator, if any, actually crossing from the periphery into the brain has yet to be clearly established [1-3].

In contrast to this knowledge of extracellular mediators, the intracellular or second messengers involved in fever, especially those in the brain, are poorly understood. The hypothesis that the cyclic nucleotides, adenosine $3',5'$-monophosphate (cyclic AMP) and guanosine $3',5'$-monophosphate (cyclic GMP) could be intracellular mediators of pyrogens in the brain has resulted in a number of studies being conducted in several species *in vivo*. These reports have been reviewed elsewhere [1,4], but any conclusion from them concerning an involvement of either cyclic AMP or cyclic GMP is debatable, due in part to the difficulties associated with studying a central response such as fever *in vivo* over several hours.

In this report the possible involvement of cyclic AMP in the central action of pyrogens has been studied by determining the effects of the exogenous pyrogen, bacterial lipopolysaccharide (LPS) and its putative endogenous mediators, IL-1 and prostaglandin E_2 (PGE_2), on the release of cyclic AMP from brain tissue incubated *in vitro*, thereby eliminating some of the factors confusing interpretation of data gathered *in vivo* from intact animals.

METHODS: Male Sprague-Dawley rats (150-350 g) were killed humanely. Each brain was removed from the cranium within 2 min and placed in 10 ml Krebs-Henseleit solution [composition (mM): NaCl (118), KCl (4.75), $CaCl_2.6H_2O$ (2.55), $MgSO_4.7H_2O$ (1.2), KH_2PO_4 (1.19), $NaHCO_3$ (25), glucose (11)] at $4°C$. The cerebellum was removed and one hemisphere cross chopped (250 μm x 250 μm) using a McIlwain tissue chopper. Brain slices were suspended in 50 ml sterile, filtered (pore size 22 μm, Millipore) Krebs-Henseleit solution gassed with 95% O_2, 5% CO_2. Slices were incubated for 20 min at $37°C$ with continuous agitation, the incubation medium being renewed after 10 min. The supernatant was then decanted and the brain slices resuspended in 7.5 ml Krebs-Henseleit solution containing the phosphodiesterase inhibitor, 3-isobutyl-1-methylxanthine (IBMX, 5 μM). Incubation volumes (200 μl) of tissue suspension were dispensed into capped reaction tubes gassed with 95% O_2, 5% CO_2 with continuous shaking at $37°C$. Drugs and pyrogens, dissolved in Krebs-Henseleit solution (100 μl) containing IBMX (5 μM), were added to duplicate incubation tubes to give the final incubation concentrations indicated in Results. Following a contact time of 10, 30 or 60 min with the drugs or pyrogens, incubation tubes were placed in a boiling water bath for 10 min to terminate the adenylate cyclase reaction then centrifuged at 720 RCF for 10 min at 4°C. Samples of supernatant fluid (200 μl) were removed and stored at -20°C until the cyclic AMP content was determined by the competitive protein binding assay described by Tovey and co-workers [5] with assay reagents supplied by Amersham International. The protein content of each incubation tube was determined using a Coomassie Blue G-250 based assay reagent (Pierce). Absorbance was read at 595 nm using bovine serum albumin (50-400 μg/ml) as standard. Procedures minimizing contamination of solutions and glassware by extraneous pyrogens were used throughout the incubation period [6].

Results are expressed as the amount of cyclic AMP (pmol) released into the incubation medium by brain tissue (mg protein) during an incubation period of 10, 30 or 60 min as indicated in Results. Values are the mean $\pm$ 1 S.E.M. for n brains. The probability (P) of the significance of the difference between means was evaluated by 2-tailed Student's t and Wilcoxon's Matched Pairs Signed Ranks tests.

The following compounds were studied: dopamine hydrochloride, cholera toxin, phenol extracts of LPS from *Salmonella abortus equi* and *Escherichia coli* serotype 026:B6, PGE$_2$, PGF$_{2\alpha}$, recombinant human IL-1α (specific activity 5 x 10^7U/mg), human IL-1β (specific activity 2 x 10^7 U/mg) and murine IL-1β (specific activity 1 x 10^8U/mg). The endotoxin content of the recombinant cytokines, determined by the Limulus Amoebocyte Lysis assay, was 10 ng/mg protein or less.

RESULTS: Cyclic AMP efflux from rat brain slices was increased by dopamine (1 mM), from 19.3 $\pm$ 4.0 pmol/mg protein/10 min to 25.2 $\pm$ 3.5 pmol/mg protein/10 min (P < 0.05; n, 8), and by forskolin (10 μM), from 21.5 $\pm$ 2.0 pmol/mg protein/10 min to 37.9 $\pm$ 6.1 pmol/mg protein/10 min (P < 0.05; n, 4). Cholera toxin (1 and 10 μg/ml; n, 4) had no effect on cyclic AMP release from brain slices during incubation periods of either 10 min or 30 min.

LPS from *Salmonella abortus equi* (10 μg/ml) did not have a significant effect on cyclic AMP release following contact with brain tissue for either 10 or 30 min when compared to values for time matched control slices from the same rats (Table I). In a few studies (n, 2 or 3), other combinations of concentration and contact time for this LPS (1 μg/ml for 10 min, 10 μg/ml for 60 min, 100 μg/ml for 30 min) were also without effect, as was LPS from *Escherichia coli* (10 μg/ml for 60 min).

Recombinant human IL-1β (1, 10 and 100 ng/ml) had no effect on cyclic AMP release from rat brain slices after a contact time of either 10 min or 30 min (Table I). Human IL-1α (100 ng/ml; n, 8) and murine IL-1β (10 and 100 ng/ml; n, 6) were also without effect on cyclic AMP efflux over 10 min. PGE$_2$ (0.1, 1 and 10 μg/ml) produced a dose related increase in cyclic AMP release over 10 min, but not 30 min (Table I), which was unaffected by flurbiprofen (10 μM). PGF$_{2\alpha}$ (10 μg/ml for 10 min; n, 8) had no effect.

The basal efflux of cyclic AMP from rat brain slices (pmol/mg protein/10 min) was found to decrease with increase in body weight (n, 21) in the range used (150-350 g), but the responses to forskolin (10 μM) and PGE$_2$ (10 μg/ml) were unchanged when assessed as percentage changes in basal release. Slices of rat cerebellum (n, 4) gave similar results to those from forebrain (Table I) over 10 min. PGE$_2$ (10 μg/ml) caused an increase in cyclic AMP (P < 0.05), but LPS (*Salmonella abortus equi* 10 μg/ml) and human IL-1β (100 ng/ml) had no effect.

DISCUSSION: If the hypothesis that cyclic AMP mediates the central action of pyrogens is correct then endogenous levels of the nucleotide should vary with body temperature in a manner commensurate with the purported role of cyclic AMP. The concentration of cyclic AMP in cerebrospinal fluid (CSF) is raised during fever in rabbits [7] and cats [8], however, CSF levels may not represent nucleotide biosynthesis in the brain [4]. Assay of cyclic AMP in pyrogen sensitive parts of the brain would provide more relevant data concerning the involvement of the nucleotide in fever. However, brain levels of cyclic AMP increase rapidly after death and methods developed to minimise these changes are difficult to apply successfully to large species such as the cat and the rabbit commonly used in fever studies. Using microwave irradiation to rapidly inactivate nucleotide metabolism, no change in the cyclic AMP content of the preoptica/anterior hypothalamus was found in rats made febrile by treatment with yeast [9]. This apparent lack of an effect on cyclic AMP *in vivo* could represent the limits of the methods employed and may indicate that changes in brain levels of cyclic AMP *in vivo* are small and/or transient rather than absent.

TABLE I: Effect of *Salmonella abortus equi* lipopolysaccharide (LPS), recombinant interleukin-1β (IL-1β) and prostaglandin E_2 (PGE$_2$) on adenosine 3´,5´-monophosphate (cyclic AMP) release from rat brain slices *in vitro*

Pyrogen	Dose μg/ml	Contact Time (min)	pmol/mg/ incubation	Control Value	n
LPS	10	10	11.5 ± 2.0	9.6 ± 1.2	8
LPS	10	30	5.2 ± 0.7	5.7 ± 1.3	6
Human IL-1β	0.1	10	11.5 ± 2.2	8.8 ± 1.1	8
Human IL-1β	0.1	30	5.2 ± 0.6	5.7 ± 1.3	6
PGE$_2$	10	10	13.3 ± 1.9[1]	9.1 ± 1.0	8
PGE$_2$	10	30	7.10 ± 0.6	5.7 ± 1.3	6

Amount of cyclic AMP (pmol) released into the incubation medium by brain tissue (mg protein) during an incubation period of 10 or 30 min. Values are the mean ± 1 S.E.M. for n brains.

[1]P < 0.05 compared to paired control value.

In this study, brain tissue and pyrogens were incubated together *in vitro* and the effects on cyclic AMP release into the incubation medium determined. The tissue content of cyclic AMP is a balance between its synthesis by adenylate cyclase and its hydrolysis by phosphodiesterases. The cell content of cyclic AMP can also be reduced by active extrusion of the nucleotide into the extracellular fluid [10], a process presumably enhanced if phosphodiesterases are inhibited. In the presence of IBMX, agents known to stimulate adenylate cyclase (dopamine, forskolin, PGE$_2$) increased the efflux of cyclic AMP from rat brain slices during 10 min incubation periods, but not 30 min. The absence of an effect in this study by cholera toxin, an activator of adenylate cyclase, is consistent with the characteristic lag period of several hours before a response is evident in various other tissues [11].

As stated earlier, the identity of the pyrogenic mediator, if any, actually crossing from the periphery into the brain has yet to be clearly established [1-3], therefore the effects of LPS, IL-1 and PGE$_2$ on cyclic AMP release have all been determined in this study. LPS from *Salmonella abortus equi* and *Escherichia coli* had no effect on the amount of cyclic AMP released into the incubation medium by rat brain slices during periods up to 60 min. IL-1 is an endogenous mediator of the febrile response to LPS [1-3] and receptors for this cytokine are distributed throughout the rat brain [12]. Two distinct molecules of IL-1, termed IL-1α and IL-1β have been cloned and sequenced [13]. Both human IL-1α and human IL-1β induce fever in rats after intracerebroventricular injection but apparently by different mechanisms [14]. However, neither human IL-1α nor human IL-1β had an effect on cyclic AMP release. Murine IL-1β is more effective than human IL-1β in stimulating PGE$_2$ synthesis in rat brain slices [15], but murine IL-1β also had no effect on cyclic AMP efflux. PGE$_2$ was the only putative mediator of fever found in this study to increase cyclic AMP release from rat brain and thereby have this second messenger implicated in its central action.

REFERENCES

1. Dascombe, M.J.: The pharmacology of fever. Prog. Neurobiol. **25**:327-373 (1985).
2. Dinarello, C.: Interleukin-1. Rev. Infect. Dis. **6**:51-95 (1984).
3. Stitt, J.T.: Prostaglandin E as the neural mediator of the febrile response. Yale J. Biol. Med. **59**:137-149 (1986).
4. Dascombe, M.J.: Cyclic nucleotides and fever. In Milton, *Pyretics and Antipyretics*, pp. 219-255 (Springer-Verlag, Berlin 1982).
5. Tovey, K.C., Oldham, K.G. & Whelan, J.A.M.: A simple direct assay for cyclic AMP in plasma and other biological samples using an improved competitive protein binding technique. Clinica chim. Acta **56**:221-234 (1974).
6. Dascombe, M.J. & Milton, A.S.: The effects of cyclic adenosine 3´,5´-monophosphate and other adenine nucleotides on body temperature. J. Physiol. (Lond.) **250**:143-160 (1975).
7. Philipp-Dormston, W.K. & Siegert, R.: Adenosine 3´,5´-cyclic monophosphate in rabbit cerebrospinal fluid during fever induced by *E. coli*-endotoxin. Med. Microbiol. Immun. **161**:11-13 (1975).
8. Dascombe, M.J. & Milton, A.S.: Cyclic adenosine 3´,5´-monophosphate in cerebrospinal fluid during thermoregulation and fever. J. Physiol. (Lond.) **263**:441-463 (1976).
9. Dascombe, M.J.: Evidence against adenosine 3´,5´-monophosphate as a mediator of fever in the brain. Neuropharmacology **25**:309-313 (1986).
10. Davoren, P.R. & Sutherland, E.W.: The effect of 1-epinephrine and other agents on the synthesis and release of adenosine 3´,5´-phosphate by whole pigeon erythrocytes. J. Biol. Chem. **238**:3009-3015 (1963).
11. Gill, D.M.: Mechanism of action of cholera toxin. Adv. Cyclic Nucleotide Res. **8**:85-118 (1977).
12. Farrar, W., Kilian, P.L., Ruff, M.R., Hill, J.M. & Pert, C.B.: Visualization and characterization of interleukin 1 receptors in brain. J. Immunol. **139**:459-463 (1987).
13. March, C.J., Mosley, B., Larsen, A., Cerretti, D.P., Braedt, G., Price, V., Gillis, S., Henney, C.S., Kronheim, S.R., Grabstein, K., Conlon, P.J., Hopp, T.P. & Cosman, D.: Cloning, sequence and expression of two distinct human interleukin-1 complementary DNAs. Nature **315**:641-647 (1985).
14. Busbridge, N.J., Dascombe, M.J., Tilders, F.J.H., van Oers, J.W.A.M., Linton, E.A. & Rothwell, N.J.: Central activation of thermogenesis and fever by interleukin-1β and interleukin-1α involves different mechanisms. Biochem. Biophys. Res. Comm. **162**:591-596 (1989).
15. Redford, E.J. & Dascombe, M.J.: Interleukin 1β and lipopolysaccharide effects on prostaglandin E$_2$ release from rat brain slices. Br. J. Pharmacol. **98**:708P (1989).

Lomax, Schönbaum (eds.) **Thermoregulation: The Pathophysiological Basis of Clinical Disorders.**
8th International Symposium Pharmacology of Thermoregulation, Kananaskis, Alberta, Canada 1991, pp. 74-78 (Karger, Basel 1992)

XIN LIANG JI, A CHINESE THERAPEUTIC DRUG, INHIBITS ENDOTOXIN-FEVER IN THE RABBIT

XIAO WEI GONG, XIAO CHEN HUANG, MASANORI NAGAI and MASAMI IRIKI

Department of Physiology, Medical University of Yamanashi, Tamaho, Nakakoma, Yamanashi 409-38 (Japan)

The onset of fever induced by lipopolysaccharide (LPS) has been studied intensively over the last decade. The first step in LPS fever is release of endogenous pyrogens (EPs) from the phagocytes. Among EPs, interleukin-1 (IL-1) and tumor necrosis factor (TNF) activate the synthesis of prostaglandins (PG) and influence thermoregulatory centres [1-3]. Antipyretics inhibit PG-synthesis. Some EPs, e.g., interferone-α (IFN-α) and macrophage inflammatory protein-1 (MIP-1), induce fever independently of PG-synthesis [4,5]. Neurophysiological evidence suggests that the action of IFN-α on temperature-sensitive neurones of the hypothalamus is mediated by endogenous opioids [6,7]. It is possible that there is a mechanism to oppose the action of EPs and induce antipyresis other than inhibition of PG-synthesis.

In Chinese medicine, a high body temperature is not considered a therapeutic objective. For example, two different types of drugs are prescribed to treat different types of complaints accompanying fever. These drugs are "Xin Liang Ji" and "Xin Wen Ji", and both possess antipyretic effect besides relieving other complaints. It is of interest to investigate how these components interact with the endogenous pyrogens in the generation of LPS fever.

METHODS: Male Japanese white rabbits, weighing 2.5-3.0 kg, were used and had been adapted to the experimental restraint chamber for at least 3 h a day. This adaptation was carried out over 2 days, so any effects of restraint stress on body temperature were eliminated. Experiments were performed at an ambient temperature of 25.0 $\pm$ 1.0°C. Core and ear temperatures were continuously measured with copper-constantan thermocouples. LPS extracted from E. coli 0111:B4 was dissolved in sterile saline and injected into the ear vein. The dose of LPS was 200 ng/kg, and the injection volume was 0.2 ml/kg.

The composition of "Xin Liang Ji" and "Xin Wen Ji" are shown in Table I and Table II. "Xin Liang Ji" was prepared as a modified "Yin Qiao San", and "Xin Wen Ji" was made up as conventional "Ma Gui Ge Ban Tang". "Yin Qiao San" and "Ma Gui Ge Ban Tang" are representative prescriptions of "Xin Liang Ji" and "Xin Wen Ji". All constituents of "Xin Liang Ji" and "Xin Wen Ji" were soaked in 600 ml water for 8 h, and then boiled for 20 min. The yield was 120 ml infusion. Drugs were administered *per os* in 50 ml, 15 min before LPS injection. In control animals, 50 ml water was administered *per os* 15 min before LPS injection.

Statistical significance of the data was evaluated with Student's t-test.

TABLE I: The composition of "Xin Liang Ji" made up as modified "Yin Qiao San"

Yin Hua	9 g	flower of Japanese honeysuckle (*Lonicerae japonica*)
Lian Qiao	9 g	weeping forsythia (*Forsythia suspensa*)
Zhi Zi	6 g	fruit of the capejasmine (*Gardenia jasminoides*)
Yuan Shen	30 g	root of Japanese figwort (*Scrophularia ningpoensis*)
Zhi Mu	9 g	rhizome of *Anemarrhena asphodeloides*
Dan Pi	9 g	root bark of the tree peony (*paeonia suffruticosa*)
Niu Zi	9 g	fruit of the great burdock (*Arctium lappa*)
Huang Qin	6 g	root of Baikal skullcap (*Scutellaria baicalensis*)
Gan Cao	6 g	root of the liquorice (*Glycyrrhiza uralensis*)

TABLE II: The composition of "Xin Wen Ji" used in the present experiments.   "Xin Wen Ji" was prescribed as "Ma Gui Ge Ban Tang"

Ma Huang	3 g	herbaceous stem of Chinese Ephedra (*Ephedra sinica*)
Gui Zhi	9 g	twig of the cassia (*Cinnamomum cassia*)
Xing Ren	6 g	seed of the apricot (*Prunus salicina*)
Bai Shao	9 g	root of the white peony (*Paeonia lactiflora*)
Da Zao	3 pics.	Chinese date (*Ziziphus jujuba*)
Gan Cao	6 g	root of the liquorice (*Glycyrrhiza uralensis*)

RESULTS: Fig. 1 shows the time course of LPS fever and the effect of "Xin Liang Ji" on LPS fever. In control animals, intravenous injection of LPS, caused a febrile response with a typical biphasic pattern. The two peaks of fever were accompanied by vasoconstriction of the ear skin vasculature as indicated by a fall in ear skin temperature. In the animals receiving "Xin Liang Ji" prepared as modified "Yin Qiao San" (Table I) 15 min before LPS injection, the generation of fever was significantly inhibited. This inhibitory effect was apparent 20 min after LPS injection, and persisted throughout the course of the LPS fever. The time course of ear skin temperature did not significantly differ between control and test animals. In 2 of 8 test animals changes of ear skin temperature were completely suppressed, but the degree of suppression varied between animals. The fever was constantly suppressed, even in animals in which vasoconstriction of the ear skin vasculature was less inhibited. Before LPS injection rectal temperature was 39.1 ± 0.2°C (mean and standard errors, n, 5) in the control animals, and 38.7 ± 0.2°C (n, 8) in animals received "Xin Liang Ji" (not statistically different). Ear skin temperature before LPS injection was 35.3 ± 1.0°C in the control animals, and 34.8 ± 1.5°C in the test animals (not statistically different). Thus, we confirm the antipyretic effect of modified "Xin Liang Ji" in the rabbit. However, "Xin Liang Ji", made up as a conventional "Yin Qiao San" (Table III) did not reveal any effect on LPS fever.

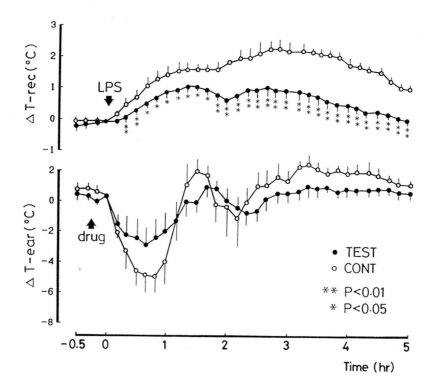

FIGURE 1: The effect of "Xin Liang Ji" prepared as modified "Yin Qiao San" on LPS fever. Changes in rectal temperature (Δ T-rec) and ear skin temperature (Δ T-ear) for drug and for control administered *per os* 15 min before LPS injection. Mean and standard errors in 5 control animals (CONT) and in 8 drug treated animals (TEST). Asterisks show data statistically different (Student's t-test: *P < 0.05; **P < 0.01).

The effect of "Xin Wen Ji" (Table II) on LPS fever was also examined in 6 animals. Prepared as convertional "Ma Gui Ge Ban Tang", it did not significantly affect LPS fever.

In the prescription of modified "Xin Liang Ji", there are nine constituents (Table I). Among these "Yuan Shen" (the root of Japanese figwort, *Scrophularia ningpoensis*) is considered to play a major role. Therefore, we subtracted "Yuan Shen" from the prescription of "Xin Liang Ji" and found that the antipyretic effect on LPS fever was lost (Fig. 2A). However, "Yuan Shen" alone did not exhibit any antipyretic effect on LPS fever (Fig. 2B).

TABLE III: The composition of "Xin Liang Ji" made up as conventional "Yin Qiao San"

Yin Hua	9 g	flower of Japanese honeysuckle
		(*Lonicerae japonica*)
Lian Qiao	9 g	weeping forsythia
		(*Forsythia suspensa*)
Jie Geng	6 g	root of the balloonflower
		(*Platycodon grandiflorum*)
Bo He	6 g	herb of the field mint
		(*Mentha haplocalyx*)
Din Zhu Ye	4 g	leef of *Lophatherum gracile*
Niu Zi	9 g	fruit of the great burdock
		(*Arctium lappa*)
Gan Cao	5 g	root of the liquorice
		(*Glycyrrhiza uralensis*)
Jing Jie	5 g	herb of *Echizonepeta tenuifolia*
Dou Chi	5 g	soybeen
		(*Glycine max*)

These results show that only "Xin Liang Ji" significantly suppressed LPS fever in the rabbit. It is also concluded that "Yuan Shen" is indispensible for the antipyretic effect of "Xin Liang Ji", but interactions among the constituents are necessary for "Yuan Shen" to act effectively.

DISCUSSION: Most of Chinese drugs are administered *per os*. This makes it very difficult to analyse their mechanism of action in animal experiments: the digestive system, absorption, constitution of the enterobacterial systems, and enzyme systems are certainly different between humans and animals. Indeed, the antipyretic effect of a Chinese drug has never been successfully observed in animal experiments. In the present experiments, we have demonstrated for the first time the antipyretic effect of "Xin Liang Ji" on LPS fever in the rabbit. This will facilitate the analysis of the mechanism(s) by which Chinese drugs act to cause an antipyretic effect.

ACKNOWLEDGEMENT: From October 1988 to April 1990, X.-W. Gong was a recipient of support of Takaku Foundation, Tokyo, Japan.

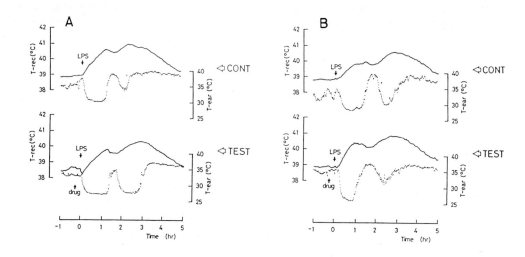

FIGURE 2: The effect of "Xin Liang Ji" without "Yuan Shen" (A) and "Yuan Shen" alone (B) on LPS fever.

REFERENCES

1. Milton, A.S.: Pyretics and antipyretics. In Milton, *Handbook of Experimental Pharmacology, Vol. 60*, pp. 257-303 (Springer Verlag, Berlin 1982).
2. Hashimoto, M., Bando, T., Iriki, M. & Hashimoto, K.: Effect of indomethacin on febrile response to recombinant human interleukin 1- in rabbits. Am. J. Physiol. **255:**R527-R533 (1988).
3. Watanabe, M., Hashimoto, M., Iriki, M. & Shimada, Y.: Arachidonate metabolites related to TNF-induced fever. Jpn. J. Physiol. **39(Suppl. 781):** (1989).
4. Dinarello, C.A., Bernheim, H.A. & Duff, G.W.: Mechanisms of fever induced by recombinant human interferon. J. Clin. Invest. **74:**906-913 (1984).
5. Davatelis, G., Wolpe, S.D., Sherry, B., Dayer, J.-M., Chicheportiche, R. & Cerami, A.: Macrophage inflammatory protein-1: a prostaglandin-independent endogenous pyrogen. Science **243:**1066-1068 (1989).
6. Nakashima, T., Hori, T., Kuriyama, K. & Matsuda, T.: Effects of interferon-alpha on the activity of preoptic thermosensitive neurons in tissue slices. Brain Res. **454:**361-367 (1988).
7. Nakashima, T., Hori, T., Kuriyama, K. & Kiyohara, T.: Naloxone blocks the interferon-alpha induced changes in hypothalamic neuronal activity. Neurosci. Lett. **82:**332-336 (1987).

Lomax, Schönbaum (eds.) **Thermoregulation: The Pathophysiological Basis of Clinical Disorders.**
8th International Symposium Pharmacology of Thermoregulation, Kananaskis, Alberta, Canada 1991, pp. 79-83 (Karger, Basel 1992)

CHARACTERISTICS OF THE TEMPERATURE AND SYMPATHETIC NERVOUS RESPONSES TO HYPOTHALAMIC MICROINJECTION OF PGE$_2$ IN THE RABBIT

XIAO CHEN HUANG, XIAO WEI GONG, MASANORI NAGAI and MASAMI IRIKI

Department of Physiology, Medical University of Yamanashi, Tamaho, Nakakoma, Yamanashi 409-38 (Japan)

Cutaneous sympathetic nervous activity is increased, and renal sympathetic nervous activity is in turn decreased, by cold stimulation and during fever [1,2]. This pattern of differentiation in sympathetic nervous responses is commonly observed in fever induced with exogenous pyrogens, e.g. lipopolysaccharide (LPS), and endogenous pyrogens, e.g. interleukin-1 (IL-1) and tumor necrosis factor (TNF) [3]. Fever has been suggested to follow the sequence: fever genesis, LPS first activates phagocytes, and activated phagocytes release endogenous pyrogens; endogenous pyrogens influence the thermoregulatory centres by activating prostaglandin (PG) synthesis. Intracerebroventricular injection of prostaglandin E$_2$ (PGE$_2$) causes fever and elicits the same response pattern in the sympathetic nervous system [4].

We have examined the effect of microinjection of PGE$_2$ into the hypothalamic regions of the rabbit on body temperature and sympathetic nervous activity. The aim of this study is to determine whether there are specific loci in the hypothalamus which are responsible for fever and the consequent pattern of sympathetic nervous responses.

METHODS: The experiments were carried out on 20 male rabbits (body weight 2.8-3.5 kg) anaesthetized with urethane (1.7 g/kg ip initially, supplemented with 0.1 g/kg/h iv).

Animals were placed in a stereotaxic instrument, and glass micropipettes, 10-15 μm in tip diameter, were located in the hypothalamic region according to the stereotaxic coordinates by Sawyer *et al.* [5]. Glass micropipettes were filled with PGE$_2$ solution (500 ng/100 nl), connected to a microinjector and the injection pressure was adjusted to attain the injection volume of 100 or 200 nl in 5 sec. After the experiments, the site of microinjection was then histologically verified.

Renal sympathetic nervous activities (RSNA) were recorded as multi-unit discharges by means of a bipolar silver wire electrodes, and was evaluated by an integrated value of discharges of 5 sec intervals.

Rectal temperature (T$_{re}$) and ear skin temperature (T$_{ear}$) were measured with thermistor probes. Heart rate and arterial blood pressure were also measured. The ambient air temperature was 24-26°C during the experiments. Rectal temperature before PGE$_2$ injection was maintained at 38.0-39.0°C by means of a heating pad.

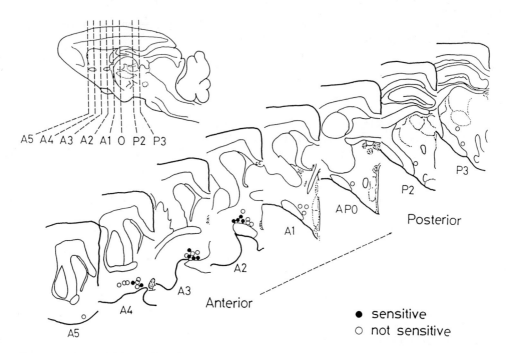

A5 A4 A3 A2 A1 0 P2 P3

P3

P2

APO

Posterior

A1

A2

A3

Anterior

A4

A5

● sensitive
○ not sensitive

FIGURE 1: Representation of the sites of PGE$_2$ microinjection on the serial cross sections of the rabbit brain. Closed circles show the loci where PGE$_2$ caused an increase in body temperature of more than 0.3°C, and open circles show the loci where PGE$_2$ was not effective.

RESULTS: Fig. 1 shows thirty-one brain loci of the hypothalamic regions in which the effect of PGE$_2$ microinjection was investigated. We determined that PGE$_2$ effectively caused fever in which the rectal temperature increased by more than 0.3°C in 1 h after PGE$_2$ microinjection. By this criterium, 10 out of 31 loci were identified as PGE$_2$ sensitive. These loci were mainly located in the rostral hypothalamus and preoptic area.

Microinjection of PGE$_2$ induced the pattern of responses associated with the sympathetic nerves at 6 loci out of 10 where PGE$_2$ effectively increased rectal temperature. At these 6 loci, microinjection of PGE$_2$ significantly increased rectal temperature by 0.5°C within 1 h, from 38.9 ± 0.2 to 39.4 ± 0.2°C (mean ± S.E.M.; $p < 0.05$ Wilcoxon matched-paired signed rarks test). Ear skin temperature decreased from 36.3 ± 0.6 to 34.5 ± 0.8°C ($p < 0.05$), and renal sympathetic neuronal activity decreased from 101.0 ± 0.4 to $89 \pm 2.2\%$ ($p < 0.05$) 3-5 min after injection of PGE$_2$. Mean arterial blood pressure and heart rate tended to increase. Respiratory rate increased from 80.0 ± 4.4 to 94.0 ± 8.7/min, 40-60 min after PGE$_2$ microinjection as rectal temperature increased. Fig. 2 shows a typical response to PGE$_2$ microinjection. Thus, the typical pattern of the differentiation of the sympathetic nervous responses during fever, i.e. an activation of the cutaneous sympathetic neurons and an inhibition of the renal sympathetic neurons, was induced by microinjection of PGE$_2$ into the hypothalamus.

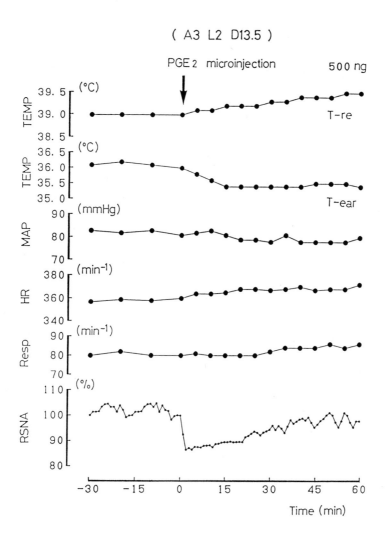

FIGURE 2: Changes in rectal and ear temperatures (T_{re}, T_{ear}), renal sympthetic nervous activity (RSNA), mean arterial blood pressure (MAP), heart rate (HR), and respiratory rate (Resp) during fever induced by PGE_2 microinjection. At a time zero (indicated by an arrow), PGE_2 (500 ng) was microinjected. The site of injection histologically identified after the experiments is indicated on the top of the figure according to the stereotaxic coordinates.

At 4 out of 10 loci the differentiation pattern of the sympathetic nervous responses was not obvious, although rectal temperature was still increased by PGE_2 microinjection. However, at these loci the increase in rectal temperature was at most 0.3°C, whereas the increase in rectal temperature was more than 0.5°C at the loci where a differentiation pattern was confirmed.

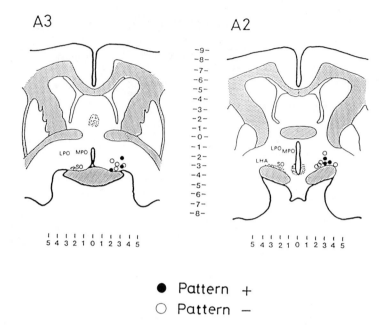

● Pattern +

○ Pattern −

FIGURE 3: Diagrammatic representation of the brain sites where PGE_2 microinjection caused the pattern responses of the sympathetic nerves (●) and the sites where PGE_2 did not induce the pattern responses (O). LHA: lateral hypothalamic area. LPO: lateral preoptic area. MPO: medial preoptic area. SO: supraoptic nucleus.

The loci where PGE_2 microinjection caused fever of over 0.5°C and a differentiation pattern of the sympathetic responses distributed within a restricted area of the rostral hypothalamus and preoptic areas, in the vicinity of the supraoptic nucleus of the hypothalamus (Fig. 3).

DISCUSSION: In the present experiments, we have confirmed that microinjection of PGE_2 caused fever and the patternized responses of the sympathetic neurons in anaesthetized rabbits. Microinjection of PGE_2 effectively caused fever at the loci in the anterior hypothalamus and preoptic areas. The distribution of these sensitive sites to PGE_2 well coincides with that in conscious animals [6]. And high incidence of PGE_2 receptors is also confirmed in these areas. Previous observations [3,4] have suggested that intracerebroventricular injection of PGE_2 causes differentiation pattern of the sympathetic responses as does the intravenous injection of LPS and IL-1 (Table I). Therefore, it is possible that PGE_2 is a mediator of patternized response of the sympathetic neurons during fever. By the present results, we have clearly shown that the sites which are sensitive to PGE_2 and initiate sympathetic differentiation are distributed in a rather restricted area of the hypothalamus, in the vicinity of the supraoptic nucleus (Fig. 3). This shows that the mechanisms to cause fever and to cause sympathetic differentiation during fever are closely related.

ACKNOWLEDGEMENT: This work was supported by a Grant-in-Aid from the Ministry of Education, Science and Culture of Japan (grant No. 02304032).

TABLE I: Summary of the sympathetic nervous responses during fever

	Tre	Skin	RSNA
PGE$_2$ (PO/AH)	↑	+	-
LPS (iv)	↑	+	-
IL-1 (iv)	↑	+	-
PGE$_2$ (icv)	↑	+	-

↑ : Fever   + : Activation   - : Inhibition   Skin : Skin sympathetic nerve activity
RSNA : Renal sympathetic nerve activity

Upper row shows the present results. The results of intravenous injection of LPS and IL-1 and intracerebroventricular injection of PGE$_2$ were taken from our previous reports [3,4].

REFERENCES

1. Iriki, M. & Simon, E.: Regional differentiation of sympathetic efferents. In Ito, *Integrative Control Function of the Brain*, pp. 221-238 (Kodansha, Tokyo 1978).
2. Riedel, W., Kozawa, E. & Iriki, M.: Renal and cutaneous vasomotor and respiratory rate adjustments to peripheral cold and warm stimuli and to bacterial endotoxin in conscious rabbits. J. Autonom. Nerv. Syst. **5:**177-194 (1982).
3. Saigusa, T. & Iriki, M.: Regional differentiation of sympathetic nerve activity during fever caused by intracerebroventricular injection of PGE$_2$. Pflügers Arch. **411:**121-125 (1988).
4. Saigusa, T.: Participation of interleukin-1 and tumor necrosis factor in the responses of the sympathetic nervous system during lipopolysaccharide-induced fever. Pflügers Arch. **416:**225-229 (1990).
5. Sawyer, C.H., Everett, J.M. & Green, J.D.: The rabbit diencephalon in stereotaxic coordinates. J. Com. Neurol. **101:**801-824 (1954).
6. Stitt, J.T.: Prostaglandin E$_1$ fever induced in rabbits. J. Physiol. **232:**163-179 (1973).

Lomax, Schönbaum (eds.) **Thermoregulation: The Pathophysiological Basis of Clinical Disorders.**
8th International Symposium Pharmacology of Thermoregulation, Kananaskis, Alberta, Canada, 1991, pp. 84-87 (Karger, Basel 1992)

CIRCADIAN VARIATION OF BODY TEMPERATURE IN MAN

B.W. JOHANSSON[1], K-A. KRISTIANSSON[2], K.I. PAPADOPOULOS[3], L.G. SALFORD[2] and B. SPORRONG[4]

[1]Section of Cardiology, General Hospital, S-214 01 Malmö (Sweden), [2]Department of Neurosurgery, Lund University Hospital, S-221 85 Lund (Sweden), [3]Department of Endocrinology, General Hospital, S-214 01 Malmö (Sweden) and [4]Department of Obstetrics and Gynecology, General Hospital, S-214 01 Malmö (Sweden)

Diurnal variations were known even to ancient mythology. The heliotrope plant, which raises its leaves by day and lowers them by night, was said to represent the immortal incarnation of the unrequited love of Clytie, daughter of the King of Babylon, for the sun god Helios, as Helios rode his chariot into the eastern sky. Clytie raised her arms in greeting; as Helios disappeared in the west, she dropped her arms forlornly, to await his return. Two hundred and fifty years ago the French astronomer Jean-Jaques d'Ortous de Mairan [1] placed a heliotrope plant in his closet, isolated from diurnal variations in illumination, and was surprised to find that the plant continued to raise and lower its leaves on schedule. Linné could determine the time of the day from a flower clock. In 1832 Augustin de Candolle [1] demonstrated that under constant conditions the period of the daily cycle of leaf movements in plants ceased to be precisely 24 h. The characteristic period, which approximates but does not equal 24 h, is the basis for the term circadian from "circa", meaning approximately, and "dies", meaning day.

Diurnal changes in the body temperature in humans were reported by Gierse in his thesis in 1842 as a result of studies on himself. Routine measurement of body temperature in clinical medicine was established in the middle of the 19th century by Bärensprung, Traute and Wunderlich. In addition to the diurnal variation with a low in the early morning hours and a high in the afternoon, several patterns in fever have been reported but in most instances rhythmical changes are apparent. The circadian body temperature pattern develops gradually after birth [2].

In the pioneering studies of human beings in environments free from external time cues, Aschoff [3] and Wever [4] studied rest-activity cycles and the rhythm of body temperature, and in some cases observed internal desynchronization between the two with a rest-activity cycle having a period of approximately 33 h, whereas the body temperature rhythm had a 24.5 h period. Subsequent research has demonstrated that when internally desynchronized circadian rhythms develop in a subject, the various physiologic and behavioral indexes cluster into two groups, tracking either with the rest-activity cycle or with the body temperature rhythm. It has been proposed that under normal conditions physiological systems receive signals from both pacemakers, which are referred to as "X" (body temperature driving) and "Y" (rest-activity cycle driving). Circadian rhythms observed in each variable are the net result of signals from both sources. However, under constant conditions, the X and Y systems can dissociate and the physiologic variables tied to each system assume the respective period.

Thus, for example slow wave sleep and growth hormone release follow the Y pacemaker, whereas the propensity for rapid-eye-movement sleep and cortisol secretion follow the X pacemaker. Although the different parameters show diurnal changes the curves can differ considerably in appearance.

Richter [5] provided the first evidence that specific neuroanatomic sites act as circadian pacemakers. Further studies pointed to the importance of the suprachiasmatic nuclei for the behavioral rhythms of activity, feeding, and drinking. But the body temperature rhythm was found to persist after the suprachiasmatic nuclei had been destroyed in squirrel monkeys, thus suggesting that the X pacemaker may be located outside the suprachiasmatic nuclei, whereas the Y pacemaker is contained within it [1].

Although body temperature measurement is used routinely in clinical practice the exact location of the pacemaker has not yet been determined and the mechanism behind the diurnal variation of body temperature is not known.

The location of the biological clock determining body temperature rhythms may vary in different species: Binkley et al. [6] reported that in sparrows the pineal organ is essential to the normal function of the biological clock controlling both activity and body temperature rhythms, whereas Richter [5] reported that removal of the pineal gland in blinded rats failed to disrupt the rats' free-running activity rhythm.

Most studies on circadian body temperature rhythms have been performed on experimental animals or healthy human volunteers. We therefore started a series of experiments in human patients in an effort to find out to what extent, if any, disorders of the endocrinological system and cerebral disease influenced the diurnal body temperature rhythm.

METHODS: Oral temperature was measured every hour from 08:00 to 12:00 h after 5 min rest and during night with 4 h interval during 24 h. In the operated patients these measurments were performed preoperatively and on the fourth day postoperatively. In the nonoperated patients temperature was measured at least during 24 h but in the majority of patients during two or more days, continuously or intermittently.

RESULTS: The body temperature rise after ovulation is produced by progesterone and a concomitant increase in heat production [7]. To find out if progesterone could be instrumental also in the diurnal variation, oral temperature was measured according to the schedule described above after oöphorectomy in 6 female patients, mean age 52, range 48-61 years, with a diagnosis of myoma (4 patients) and cancer of the uterus, respectively. The diurnal temperature rhythm with a low night value remained after both ovaries had been removed.

Body temperature was measured in 4 pregnant women during week 19, 27, 32 and 35, two of whom with premature labor. In all the typical diurnal body temperature pattern with low night values was apparent.

Three postmenopausal women aged 69, 77 and 80 years with a diagnosis of prolapse, cancer of the uterus and ovarian cancer, respectively, all showed the typical diurnal temperature pattern at an age when not only estrogen and progesterone but also gonadotrophin levels are low. Two of the patients showed a two-peaked curve with a maximum around 12:00 and 18:00 h (Fig. 1). Children of both sexes often show such a two-peaked curve but this has not been described in adult females.

These results suggest that ovarian production of sex hormones does not influence the diurnal body temperature rhythm. However, estrogen can be produced by other tissues, such as liver and adipose tissue by conversion of steroids produced by, for example, the adrenal glands.

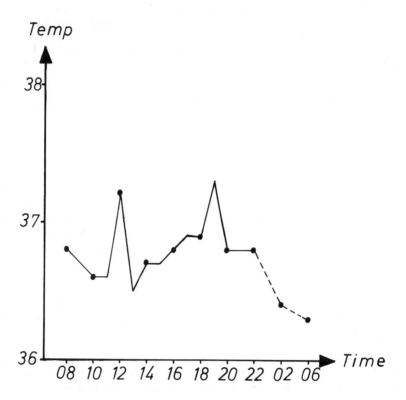

FIGURE 1: Two-peaked body temperature in postmenopausal women.

Seven female patients with acute salpingitis, mean age 23, range 17-30 years, on different days of the menstrual cycle all showed the diurnal temperature variation, although with different amplitude. The rhythm was not influenced by oral contraceptives. In two of the patients repeated determinations of the plasma estrogen to progesterone ratio were made; there was no correlation between this ratio and the body temperature.

Body temperature measurement over 24 h as described above was done in patients with different diseases of the endocrine system in an attempt to find out if other than the sexual hormones could be mediators of the circadian body temperature rhythm. Temperature curve analysis revealed the typical diurnal variation in 4 patients with thyroid disease, 3 patients with hyperparathyroidism, 1 with myasthenia gravis, 5 with hypogonadism, 8 with prolactinoma, 3 with hypopituitarism, 5 with acromegaly, 2 with adrenal malfunction, and 1 patient with hirsutism. Four patients with ophthalmopathy showed a two-peaked pattern with low values both around 10:00 h and during the night; a similar pattern was found in a patient with a suspected phaeochromocytoma and a patient with malabsorption.

Serious brain damage is necessary to eradicate the diurnal body temperature rhythm. This occurred at a consciousness level of 4 and 5 grade 1-5 in 3 patients after circulatory arrest (2 patients) and postoperatively after a hematoma in the frontal lobe. One of the patients was followed at a level of consciousness of 2 and 4: at level 2 the circadian rhythm in body temperature was apparent but disappeared when she entered level 4. These findings are in conformance with those reported by Reinberg *et al.* [8] in patients suffering from deep coma following attempted suicide by overdose of one or several drugs. These patients recovered but the circadian body temperature rhythm disappeared during the comatose state.

A 70 year old male patient with cardiac decompensation secondary to ischemic heart disease with myocardial infarctions, essential hypertension, and diabetes mellitus showed a reverse temperature pattern with lower rectal temperature values in the afternoon than in the morning in some days during the weeks before his death.

The location of the body temperature biological clock in man is not known. One approach to locating it would be temperature recordings around the clock in patients with a tumor located in specific areas of the brain. Preliminary findings indicate that pacemakers X and Y may be located close to each other. A 59 year old female patient with a tumor confined to the hypothalamic region showed most of the time a disappearance of the circadian temperature rhythm as was the case in a 69 year old man with a hematoma in the same region. Another patient, a 42 year old male, with a large pineal tumor showed a reverse rhythm with higher morning than evening temperature; but this was not the case in other patients with tumors in the pineal gland. A normal circadian temperature rhythm was observed in patients with tumors in the pituitary.

DISCUSSION: Circadian rhythmicity has been shown to be a ubiquitous phenomenon, both across phylogeny and within individual organisms. Circadian rhythms relate to clinical medicine in several ways. Its recognition has required a reassessment of many clinical diagnostic and therapeutic procedures. There is a growing recognition that disorders of circadian timekeeping may underlie a number of important diseases [1]. *Locus minoris resistentiae* has long since been established in clinical medicine. Recent knowledge on biological rhythms will be a reason for us to coin the expression *Tempus minoris resistentiae* [9]. An indication of the importance of the biological clock could be that remarkably few chemical agents influence the endogenous free-running period [1]; it is of interest that this can also be influenced by a weak electromagnetic field [4].

REFERENCES

1. Moore-Ede, M.C., Czeisler, C.A. & Richardson, G.S.: Circadian timekeeping in health and disease. New Engl. J. Med. **309:**469-476 and 530-536 (1983).
2. Menzel, W.: *Menschliche Tag-Nacht-Rhytmik und Schichtarbeit.* (Benno Schwabe & Co. Verlag, Basel 1962).
3. Aschoff, J.: Circadian rhythms in man: a self-sustained oscillator with an inherent frequency underlies human 24-hour periodicity. Science **148:**1427-1432 (1965).
4. Wever, R.A.: *The Circadian System of Man: Results of Experiments Under Temporal Isolation.* (Springer Verlag, New York 1979).
5. Richter, C.P.: *Biological Clocks in Medicine and Psychiatry.* (Charles C. Thomas, Springfield 1965).
6. Binkley, S., Kluth, E.& Menaker, M.: Pineal function in sparrows: Circadian rhythms and body temperature. Science **174:**311-314 (1971).
7. Schmidt, Th.H.: *Thermoregulatorische Grössen in Abhängigkeit von Tageszeit und Menstruationszyklus.* Thesis, München 1972.
8. Reinberg, A., Gervais, P., Pollak, E., Abulker, Ch. & Dupont, J.: Circadian rhythms during drug induced coma. Intern. J. Chronobiol. **1:**157-162 (1973).
9. Johansson, B.W.: Biologiska rytmer. Observanda Medica **4:**27-32 and 57-60 (1977).

Lomax, Schönbaum (eds.) **Thermoregulation: The Pathophysiological Basis of Clinical Disorders.**
8th International Symposium Pharmacology of Thermoregulation, Kananaskis, Alberta, Canada 1991, pp. 88-92 (Karger, Basel 1992)

THERMOREGULATORY EFFECTS OF NIMODIPINE ON COLD EXPOSED AND HYPOTHERMIC RATS

MICHAEL L. JOURDAN, TZE FUN LEE and LAWRENCE C.H. WANG

Department of Zoology, University of Alberta, Edmonton, Alberta, T6G 2E9 (Canada)

Even though the clinical features and physiological changes in different body systems during either accidental or clinically induced hypothermia have been well reviewed [1,2], little is known concerning the status of the thermoregulatory system during deep hypothermia. A significant reduction in metabolic rate has been observed in hypothermic hamsters [3] and ground squirrels [4]. In deep hypothermia, these animals appear to be poikilothermic; their core body temperatures (T_b) follow the ambient temperature (T_a) and they are incapable of rewarming without the aid of exogenous heat. It is, however, unclear whether thermoregulation would invariably fall below a critical T_b or whether thermoregulatory function persists even in hypothermia but shows gradual deterioration with the progression of hypothermia.

It has been suggested that calcium ion plays a functional role in the mechanism of thermoregulation [5]. Intracerebroventricular (icv) perfusion of excess Ca^{2+} ions causes a fall in T_b, whereas reduction of brain Ca^{2+} level by chelation with EGTA in the perfusion fluid elicits a rise in T_b in the euthermic animal [5]. In order to examine whether the thermal set point of the hypothermic rat was still operating, a selective Ca^{2+} channel antagonist, nimodipine, was used to alter endogenous Ca^{2+}-mediated thermoregulatory functions at different time points of the hypothermic bout. These responses were compared to those of the euthermic animal receiving similar nimodipine treatment under cold stress.

METHODS: Adult male Sprague-Dawley rats weighing approximately 400 g were used. Under halothane anesthesia, guide cannula (23 gauge stainless steel tubing) were implanted into the lateral ventricle of each rat utilizing the following stereotaxic coordinates: AP = 6.0 mm, L = 1.5 mm, H = 2.0 mm below the dura matter [6]. The tip of each guide tube was beveled and positioned 1.0 mm above the ventricle in order to minimize damage to the actual injection site. The precise anatomical location of the injection site was subsequently verified histologically according to standard procedures.

To test the thermoregulatory response of euthermic animals to either intraperitoneal or icv injection of nimodipine, rats were transferred to a metal metabolism chamber and exposed to -10°C under helium-oxygen (79% He; 21% O_2) for 120 min. Oxygen consumption and CO_2 production were continuously recorded and heat production (HP) was calculated from oxygen consumption and respiratory quotient. The integrated HP for each 15 min period was used as the rate of HP and the sum of HP from 7 consecutive 15 min periods (min 16-120) constituted the total HP. T_b was measured with a colonic thermocouple immediately before saline or test compound injection and immediately after cold

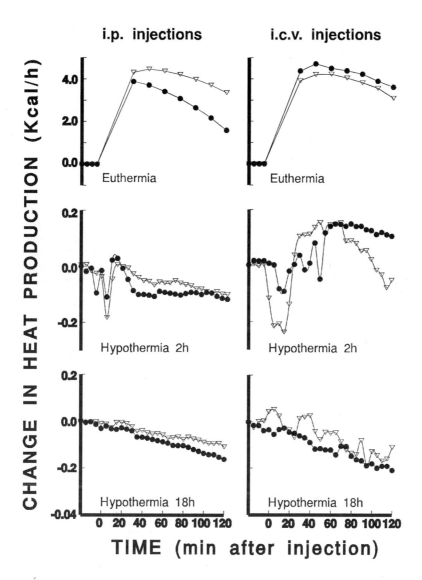

FIGURE 1: Net changes in heat production after either ip or icv injection of DMSO (∇; 1 ml/kg ip and 5 μl icv) or nimodipine ($\bullet$; 3 mg/kg ip and 1.25 μg icv) in euthermic rats exposed to He-O$_2$ at -10°C (at time 0) cold or hypothermic rats at 2 h and 18 h after hypothermic induction. Each point represents the mean from 4-7 animals. The s.e. of the mean is not shown for clarity.

exposure, the change in T$_b$ was used as an index for cold tolerance. Dimethyl sulfoxide (DMSO) or optimal dose of nimodipine, based on our preliminary studies, was administered either icv in a volume of 5 μl 10 min or ip in a volume of 1 ml/kg 15 min prior to cold exposure.

Hypothermia was induced by the method of Jourdan and Wang [7]. Briefly, rats were cooled in a water jacketed plexigas chamber at 0°C under halothane (1.5%) and He-O_2. During the initial rapid cooling halothane was decreased by approximately 0.5%/3°C drop in T_b. When T_b dropped to 28°C, halothane was discontinued and cooling continued under He-O_2 to 19°C. Hypothermia was maintained for 20 h via a feedback loop using T_b as the reference for adjustment of the circulating water bath temperature. HP was recorded continuously throughout the hypothermic bout by the method described above for the euthermic animals. Nimodipine was given either icv or ip 2 h or 18 h after hypothermic induction.

Comparisons of the thermoregulatory responses to nimodipine of rats under different physiological conditions was by either unpaired t-test or ANOVA and significance was set at $p < 0.05$ unless otherwise stated.

RESULTS: The thermoregulatory responses to either icv or ip injection of nimodipine in euthermic rats exposed to He-O_2 at -10°C and hypothermic rats at 2 h and 18 h after hypothermic induction are summarized in Fig. 1. Injection of nimodipine (3 mg/kg ip) significanty reduced both the maximal (5.34 $\pm$ 0.16 kcal/h) and total HP (30.70 $\pm$ 0.89 kcal/105 min) of euthermic rats in the cold as compared to the DMSO (1 ml/kg ip) control values (max. HP = 5.95 $\pm$ 0.06 kcal/h; total HP = 38.61 $\pm$ 0.64 kcal/105 min). Consequently, the fall in T_b was significantly greater at the end of the experiment (nimodipine: -10.33 $\pm$ 0.51°C; DMSO: -5.28 $\pm$ 0.49°C). In contrast, icv injection of nimodipine (1.25 μg) significantly enhanced both the maximal (6.21 $\pm$ 0.17 kcal/15 h) and total HP (39.88 $\pm$ 1.08 kcal/105 min) of the rat above control values (max. HP = 5.73 $\pm$ 0.09 kcal/h; total HP = 37.06 $\pm$ 0.45 kcal/105 min). However, the final decrease in T_b of the nimodipine treated rat (-5.43 $\pm$ 0.65°C) was only slightly less than that of the control (-6.43 $\pm$ 0.38°C).

Two hours after hypothermic induction, the HP of the hypothermic rat (0.62 $\pm$ 0.03 kcal/h) was significantly lower than the resting metabolic rate (1.47 $\pm$ 0.23 kcal/h) of the euthermic rat kept at room temperature. Injection of nimodipine (3 mg/kg ip) slightly reduced the HP of the hypothermic rat as compared to that observed after receiving DMSO (Fig. 1). In contrast to systemic injection, icv infusion of DMSO (5 μl) significantly increased HP which reached its peak within about 50-60 min and then declined back to its baseline value (Fig. 2). Infusion of nimodipine (1.25 μg icv) also increased HP of the hypothermic rat to the same level as that observed after DMSO injection. However, the thermogenic effect of nimodipine persisted for more than 5 h before it declined back to the pre-injection value (Fig. 2).

The metabolic rate of the hypothermic rat at 18 h after hypothermic induction (0.41 $\pm$ 0.03 kcal/h) was significantly lower than that observed at 2 h after induction. Either ip or icv injection of nimodipine failed to induce any significant changes in metabolic rate of the hypothermic rat at this stage (Fig. 1).

DISCUSSION: It is well documented that different routes of administration of Ca^{2+} channel antagonists elicits opposite thermoregulatory responses in euthermic animals kept at T_a of 20°C: systemic injection causes hypothermia whereas central administration elicits hyperthermia [8,9]. However, little is known about the thermoregulatory effect of Ca^{2+} channel antagonists in animals exposed to extreme cold. Systemic injection of nimodipine significantly attenuated HP and consequently the final T_b was lower than that of the control. At present the exact mechanism by which the Ca^{2+} channel antagonists decrease the thermogenic capacity of the animal remains unknown. In contrast to systemic injection, icv infusion of nimodipine increased HP but only increased slightly the final T_b of the rat under cold exposure. In comparison to the marked increase in T_b reported after icv injection of Ca^{2+} channel antagonists in animals kept at room temperature [8,10], the observed minimum increase in T_b may be due to the greater increase in heat loss under He-O_2 cold exposure. It is generally believed that the Ca^{2+} channel antagonists have profound effects on Ca^{2+}-mediated functions in the hypothalamus, including alteration of the ionic set-point and its consequent thermoregulatory responses [5,8].

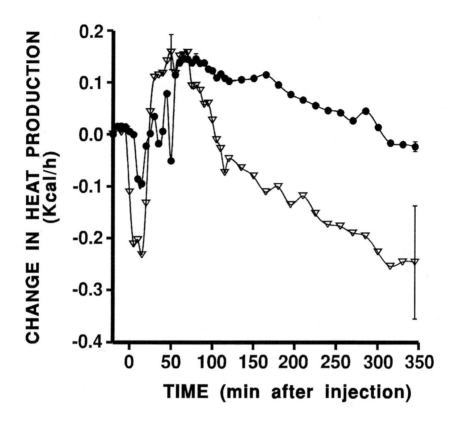

FIGURE 2: Effect of icv injection of either DMSO (5 μl, ∇) or nimodipine (1.25 μg, $\bullet$) on the metabolic rate of the hypothermic rat at 2 h after hypothermic induction. Each point represents the mean from 5 animals. The s.e. of the mean, which is indicated by vertical bars, is shown only at the max. and the last HP values for clarity.

The thermoregulatory responses of the hypothermic rat to nimodipine appears to be time dependent. At the early stage of the hypothermia bout (2 h after hypothermic induction), nimodipine elicited a similar metabolic response to that seen in the euthermic animals under cold stress. Even though the magnitude of thermogenic changes was significantly less than that of the euthermic animals, icv administration of nimodipine elicited a prolonged increase in HP whereas ip injection of the same drug elicited short and slightly reduced metabolic rate. Similar long-lasting increase in thermoregulatory response to icv injection of other Ca^{2+} channel antagonists has been previously reported in cats kept at room temperature [10]. The relatively lower thermoregulatory responses to nimodipine of the hypothermic rats as compared to the euthermic control may be due to the general decrease of cellular function [1,2] and sensitivity to exogenous stimulus [11] under the lower T_b.

In contrast to those observed in the euthermic state, either icv or ip administration of nimodipine at the later stage of the hypothermic bout (18 h after induction) failed to elicit any significant change in thermoregulatory response. One possibility for the lack of responsiveness to nimodipine may be the temperature dependent properties of the Ca^{2+} channel antagonists as it has been shown that their anti-ischemic and negative inotropic effects are reduced under hypothermic condition [12]. However, this may not be the case as the animal still responded to nimodipine at the early stage of hypothermia. On the other hand, our results may indicate that the hypothermic rat is no longer capable of regulating its T_b at this stage. This suggestion is further supported by the observation that both the thermogenic capacity and the T_b resistance (difference between T_b and T_a) at 18 h of hypothermia were significantly lower than those at the earlier stage (e.g. 2 h) of the hypothermic bout [13].

Taken together, the results indicate that the hypothermic animal is able to maintain its thermoregulatory function, even though reduced in magnitude, at low T_b. Prolonged hypothermia in the rat results in an energy deficient state [13], the lack of responsiveness of the hypothermic rat at this later stage may be a reflection of time dependent deterioration of homeostatic control functions in prolonged hypothermia.

ACKNOWLEDGEMENT: This work was supported by a NSERC operating grant A6455 to L.C.H. Wang.

REFERENCES

1. Bristow, G.K.: Clinical aspects of accidental hypothermia. In Heller, Musacchia & Wang, *Living in the Cold*, pp. 513-521 (Elsevier, New York 1986).
2. Paton, B.C.: Accidental hypothermia. Pharmac. Ther. **22:**331-377 (1983).
3. Resch, G.E. & Musacchia, X.J.: A role of glucose in hypothermic hamsters. Am. J. Physiol. **231:**1729-1734 (1976).
4. Wang, L.C.H., McArthur, M.D., Jourdan, M.L. & Lee, T.F.: Depressed metabolic rates in hibernation and hypothermia: can these be compared meaningfully? In Sutton, Coates & Remmers, *Hypoxia: The Adaptations*, pp. 78-83 (B.C. Decker, Toronto 1990).
5. Myers, R.D.: The role of ions in thermoregulation and fever. In Milton, *Handbook of Experimental Pharmacology, Vol. 60. Pyretics and Antipyretics*, pp. 151-186 (Springer, Berlin 1982).
6. Pellegrino, L.J., Pellegrino, A.S. & Cushman, A.J.: *A Stereotaxic Atlas of the Rat Brain* (Plenum Press, New York 1979).
7. Jourdan, M.L. & Wang, L.C.H.: An improved technique for the study of hypothermia physiology. J. Thermal Biol. **12:**175-178 (1987).
8. Palmi, M. & Sgaragli, G.: Hyperthermia induced in rabbits by organic calcium antagonists. Pharmac. Biochem. Behav. **34:**325-330 (1989).
9. Benedek, G. & Szikszay, M.: Potentiation of thermoregulatory and analgesic effects of morphine by calcium antagonists. Pharmac. Res. Comm. **16:**1009-1018 (1984).
10. Beleslin, D.B., Jovanovic-Micic, D. & Samardzic, R.: Nature of hypo- and hyperthermia induced by the calcium antagonist nicardipine. Arch. Int. Physiol. Biochim. **95:**347-353 (1987).
11. Hoo-Paris, R., Jourdan, M.L., Moreau-Hamsany, C. & Wang, L.C.H.: Plasma glucagon, glucose and fatty acids concentrations and secretion during prolonged hypothermia in the rat. Am. J. Physiol. (in press).
12. Hearse, D.J., Yamamoto, F. & Shattock, M.J.: Calcium antagonists and hypothermia: the temperature dependency of the negative inotropic and anti-ischemic properties of verapamil in the isolated rat heart. Circulation **70:**154-164 (1984).
13. Jourdan, M.L., Hoo-Paris, R. & Wang, L.C.H.: Characterization of hypothermia in a non-hibernator: the rat. In Malan & Canguilhem, *Living in the Cold II*, pp. 289-296 (John Libbey Eurotext, Montrouge 1989).

Lomax, Schönbaum (eds.) **Thermoregulation: The Pathophysiological Basis of Clinical Disorders.**
8th International Symposium Pharmacology of Thermoregulation, Kananaskis, Alberta, Canada 1991, pp. 93-99 (Karger, Basel 1992)

ROLE OF CALCIUM IN AN ANIMAL MODEL FOR THE HOT FLUSH

MICHAEL J. KATOVICH, ORIT SHECHTMAN and KIMBERLY HANLEY

Department of Pharmacodynamics, Box J-487, JHMHC, College of Pharmacy, University of Florida, Gainesville, Florida 32610 (USA)

One of the most frequent manifestations of the menopause is the hot flush. This episodic thermoregulatory disturbance is characterized by the sensation of heat and is followed by vasomotor and neuroendocrine manifestations. A transient tachycardia precedes an elevation of skin temperature, while a surge in luteinizing hormone (LH) and a fall in core temperature accompany the flush. We have observed [1-5] that administration of an opioid antagonist to morphine-dependent rats results in a prompt rise in tail skin temperature (TST) and a subsequent fall in colonic temperature (Tc). Additionally, an elevated heart rate and hypersecretion of LH also are manifested in this animal model [2]. These physiological changes are similar in magnitude, duration and temporal association with those exhibited in women undergoing a flushing episode. These flushing episodes are more pronounced in ovariectomized rats [4], and are attenuated with administration of estrogen [4,5] or alpha adrenergic agents [1,3]. These same therapeutic agents have been used effectively to alleviate the flushes observed in women [6-9]. Recently we have demonstrated that similar flushing episodes can be produced in naive rats following administration of an LHRH agonist [10] or 2-deoxyglucose (2DG,11). Likewise these two flush responses can be significantly attenuated by pre-administration of alpha adrenergic agents (12, and unpublished observations). Thus, it appears that some adrenergic activation may be a common pathway by which we can induce flushing episodes in animals. Therefore, it is conceivable that by utilizing these animal models other possible therapeutic drugs could be evaluated in their ability to reduce this "flushing episode".

Calcium has an unique role in muscle and nerve cells in that it is a carrier of positive charge that contributes to both excitability and an intracellular second messenger which is responsible for a variety of cellular responses. In particular, calcium is a cellular messenger critical to stimulus response events which include excitation-contraction and stimulus secretion coupling [13]. Calcium, thus, is involved in regulation of the cell and in turn is regulated by the cell. Cellular calcium movements are regulated by a variety of mechanisms which include both chemically and electrically gaited calcium channels. Of particular interest are the voltage dependent calcium selective ion channels, which are activated and inactivated by changes in membrane potential. These channels are the sites of action of a major therapeutic group of drugs, the calcium channel antagonists. The purpose of these studies was to evaluate the effects of a calcium channel blocker in each of these three models utilized to exhibit 'flushing' episodes in animals.

METHODS: Female Charles Rivers CD rats, initially weighing 175-225 g were housed in groups of 2 in hanging stainless steel cages in a room maintained at 25 $\pm$ 1°C and illuminated from 05:00 to 19:00 h. Food and water were provided *ad libitum*. All animals were ovariectomized 2-3 weeks prior to the temperature studies.

TABLE I: Effect of verapamil on tail skin temperature (TST) and colonic temperature (Tc) in morphine dependent female rats

Experimental Group	Baseline TST (°C)	Mean Maximal Δ TST (°C)	Area under the 60 min TST Curve (°C-min)	Baseline Tc (°C)	Mean Maximal Δ Tc (°C)	Area under the 60 min Tc Curve (°C-min)
Experiment 1						
Control (n=6)	27.7±0.3[†]	5.9±0.3	243.5±17.1	39.2±0.2	-3.5±0.4	-111.5± 5.9
Verapamil-treated (10 mg/Kg,sc,n=6)	27.4±0.3	4.5±0.9	152.3±30.6*	39.3±0.4	-3.9±0.5	-120.2±20.8
Experiment 2						
Control (n=6)	26.9±0.3	6.5±0.5	237.3±17.9	39.6±0.3	-4.5±0.3	-145.2±13.7
Verapamil-treated (20 mg/Kg,sc,n=6)	26.2±0.2	3.9±0.7*	157.4±30.4*	39.0±0.5	-2.7±0.3*	-83.9±10.9*
Experiment 3						
Control (n=6)	26.8±0.2	4.5±0.7	175.1±24.9	39.8±0.2	-4.0±0.2	-140.7± 9.0
Verapamil-treated (40 mg/Kg,sc,n=6)	26.0±0.2	0.9±0.4*	26.3±14.8*	39.1±0.3	-2.7±0.4*	-77.5±12.6*

[†]mean±standard error of mean; * significantly different from respective control $p<0.05$.

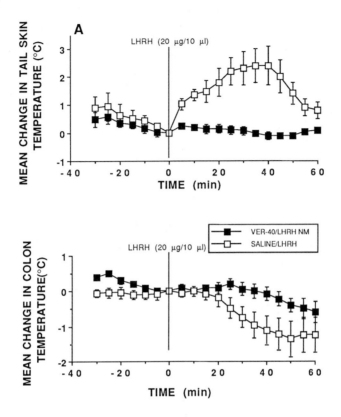

FIGURE 1: Effect of systemic administration of LHRH (20 αg/10 μl icv) at time zero on changes in mean tail skin temperature (A) and changes in mean colonic temperature (B) in non-morphine (NM), naive rats. Animals were pretreated with verapamil (40 mg/kg sc, filled squares), or saline (1 ml/kg sc, open squares) 30 min prior to LHRH. Each point represents the mean of 6 animals and the vertical bar represents one standard error of the mean.

Morphine dependency was produced as described previously [1-5] in some rats by subcutaneous implantation of a pellet containing 75 mg of morphine on day 1 and 2 additional 75 mg pellets on day 3. All temperature experiments were conducted 2 days afer the last morphine pellets were implanted. For central drug administration of the LHRH ([Des-Gly[10], im-Bz-D-His[6],Pro[6]]-LHRH ethylamide, Bachem, Inc.), standard stereotaxic techniques were used to implant cannula guides into the lateral cerebral ventricles (icv) one week prior to the temperature experiments.

On the day of the experiment, animals were lightly restrained in wire mesh cages. Colonic temperature (Tc) was measured with a copper-constantan thermocouple inserted 6 cm beyond the anus and taped to the base of the tail. Tail skin temperature (TST) was measured with a second copper constantan thermocouple taped to the dorsal region of the tail. Temperatures for all 12 animals (6 control and 6 experimental for each study) were measured simultaneously with a data acquisition and control system (CYBORG) interfaced to an Apple IIe computer. Temperatures were recorded at 5 min intervals. All rats were allowed a one hour adjustment period after they were placed in the restraining cages to obtain baseline temperatures. In all studies the animals were administered verapamil (at 10, 20, or 40 mg/kg sc, Knoll Pharmaceutical Co.) or the vehicle (saline) thirty min prior to administration of the agent used to induce the flush. In the morphine-dependent rats this agent was naloxone (0.5 mg/kg sc, Sigma) and in the naive animals either 2-deoxyglucose (2-DG, 750 mg/kg sc, Sigma) or LHRH (20 μg/10 μl icv) was utilized. Temperatures were monitored at 5 min intervals until TST values were restored to baseline conditions (1 or 2 hours). All temperature studies were performed between 9 and 12 AM in a room maintained at 26 $\pm$ 1°C.

Data were summarized by calculating the maximal changes in temperature and the area under the temperature curves manifested by each rat for each of the groups and analyzed by students 'T-test' with significance set at 95% confidence limits.

RESULTS: Table I summarizes the results from the effects of 3 doses of verapamil on the thermal response to naloxone in morphine-dependent rats. In all three of the studies basal TST and Tc were similar between the 2 groups. There also was no effect of verapamil alone on the basal temperatures. The maximal rise in TST in the control groups ranged from 4 to 6°C and the maximal fall in Tc ranged between 3.5 and 4.1°C. Pretreatment with systemically administered verapamil at a dose of 10 mg/kg did not effect the rise in TST or the fall in Tc. Administration of the intermediate dose of verapamil (20 mg/kg sc) significantly reduced both the rise in TST and the fall in Tc by about 50%. Whereas, administration of the highest dose of verapamil virtually abolished the rise in TST (the 'flush' response) in the morphine-dependent rat with no further alterations in Tc. These results are similarly manifested when the area under the temperature curves are evaluated, except that there was a significant reduction in the TST curve with the lowest dose of verapamil.

Central administration of LHRH to naive rats results in a more moderate flush response as manifested by a 3.0 $\pm$ 0.5°C rise in TST and a fall in Tc of 1.5 $\pm$ 0.5°C. Systemic administration of verapamil (40 mg/kg sc) significantly attenuated both of these responses (Fig. 1). Basal skin temperatures (26.4 $\pm$ 0.1 and 26.6 $\pm$ 0.2°C) and colonic temperatures (38.0 $\pm$ 0.2 and 38.6 $\pm$ 0.4°C) were similar in the verapamil and control treated rats, respectively. Area under the TST curve also revealed a significant attenuated response in the verapamil treated group (4.8 $\pm$ 4.0°C min) compared to the control group (124.7 $\pm$ 29.7°C min) administered LHRH alone. Fig. 2 summarizes the results of administration of 2DG to naive rats. Control animals responded to 2DG administration with an elevation of TST (3.3 $\pm$ 0.7°C) and a corresponding fall in Tc (-1.5 $\pm$ 0.4°C). Pretreatment with verapamil (40 mg/kg sc) abolished the rise in TST without having an appreciable effect on the fall in Tc. Basal TST and Tc were similar in both the control and verapamil treated groups. Area under the TST curve also revealed a significant effect of verapamil (30.9 $\pm$ 21.7°C min) when compared to the control animals administered only 2DG (142.4 $\pm$ 33.0°C min).

DISCUSSION: We previously reported that the morphine-dependent rat may be a useful model to study the mechanisms involved in the menopausal hot flush since administration of naloxone to these dependent animals [2] produce thermal, cardiac and endocrine manifestations similar in magnitude, duration and temporal association to those manifested in women undergoing a hot flush. We have also demonstrated that the thermal response is more sensitive to the absence of estrogens [4] and can be abolished by central [3] or peripheral [1] administration of clonidine and other alpha$_2$-adrenergic agonists and that adrenalectomized rats [1] also produce an attenuated flush response.

Lomax et al. [14] previously reported that central administration of LHRH resulted in a marked rise in skin temperature in the rat. Recently we also have demonstrated that central administration of LHRH resulted in an elevated tail skin temperature which is more sensitive in morphine-dependent animals [10]. This thermal response is centrally mediated and not associated with secretion of LH. From our studies we suggested that LHRH may act as a neuromodulator to some thermosensitive neurons and activation of these pathways could result in a flush-like response. A recent report [12] has demonstrated that this LHRH flush response is also abolished by treatment with phentolamine or clonidine indicating an adrenergic component to the flush response.

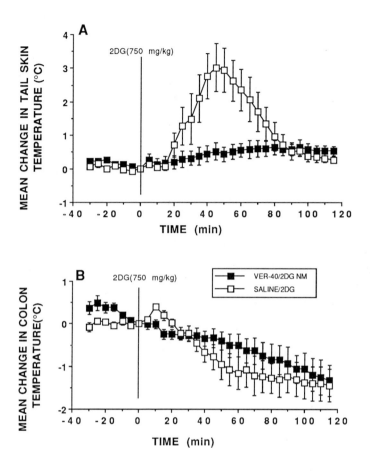

FIGURE 2: Effect of systemic administration of 2 deoxyglucose (2DG, 200 mg/kg sc) at time zero on changes in mean tail skin temperature (A) and changes in mean colonic temperature (B) in non-morphine (NM), naive rats. Animals were pretreated with verapamil (40 mg/kg sc, filled squares) or saline (1 ml/kg sc, open squares) 30 min prior to 2DG. Each point represents the mean of 6 animals and the vertical bar represents one standard error of the mean.

The thermosensitive neurons of the hypothalamus are known to be gluco-, osmo-, and steroid-sensitive which suggests that temperature-sensitive neurons have multiple interactions with various regulatory systems. We have demonstrated that cellular hypoglycemia, induced by 2DG [11] or administration of insulin [15], does result in a flush response. Similar reports have been observed in man [16]. Additionally, we have reported that hyperglycemia can reduce the flush response in morphine-dependent animals administered naloxone [15]. We feel that this hypoglycemic condition results in an activation of the adrenergic system in a similar manner as in the other two animal models and suggests that the adrenergic system is a common pathway for any flush-like response.

The results reported here suggest that another common therapeutic agent for cardiovascular disorders may also be an effective agent in alleviating the symptoms of the menopausal hot flush.

Calcium channel blockers have been shown to inhibit the expression of naloxone-precipitated morphine abstinence syndrome *in vivo* after either peripheral or central administration in rats [18-20]. Both behavioral and neurochemical signs of morphine withdrawal were observed in a dose dependent manner with administration of verapamil [18]. These studies concluded that the effects of verapamil were mediated by inhibiting neurotransmitter release; however, the possibility that peripheral sites of action can contribute to the differential effects of calcium channel inhibitors cannot be overlooked. Receptor studies have demonstrated that the effects of calcium antagonists do not seem to be mediated through alpha-adrenoreceptor [17], nor to opiate receptor stimulation [18]. Thus, the mechanism of the response differs from those of opioids or alpha-adrenoreceptor agonists. Interestingly, there has been no reports demonstrating *in vivo* effects of verapamil on neurotransmitter release in naive animals. In the current study the tail skin temperature surge to administration of LHRH and 2DG in naive rats were both attenuated by verapamil in the same manner as the thermal effects were observed during morphine withdrawal. Thus, there appears to be a similar calcium dependent mechanism involved in the three methods utilized to produce a rise in skin temperature (flush). From the results presented the precise mechanism of verapamil in alleviating the flush-like response in rats cannot be stated with certainty. The most logical targets for the calcium antagonist in this thermal response is via a central or peripheral release of some neurotransmitter or possibly due to some peripheral vascular event. However, it should also be noted that this drug may have effects at sites other than calcium channels. Further studies are required to elucidate the precise mechanism. Currently, calcium channel blockers are used as therapeutic agents for numerous nonrelated disease states. Data from the current studies may indicate another possible therapeutic treatment in women exhibiting hot flush episodes.

ACKNOWLEDGEMENTS: The authors wish to thank Ms. Billie Jean Goins for preparation of the manuscript and Phylis Raynor for technical assistance. This work was supported by NIH grant HD-18133.

REFERENCES

1. Katovich, M.J., Pitman, D.L. & Barney, C.C.: Mechanisms mediating the thermal response to morphine withdrawal in rats. Proc. Soc. Exp. Biol. Med. **193**:129-135 (1990).
2. Simpkins, J.W., Katovich, M.J. & Song, I-C.: Similarities between morphine withdrawal in the rat and the menopausal hot flush. Life Sci. **32**:1957-1966 (1983).
3. Katovich, M.J., Simpkins, J.W. & Barney, C.C.: Alpha-adrenergic mediation of the tail skin temperature response to naloxone in morphine-dependent rats. Brain Res. **426**:55-61 (1987).
4. Katovich, M.J. & Simpkins, J.W.: Further evidence for an animal model for the hot flush. In Lomax & Schönbaum, *Thermoregulation: Research and Clinical Applications*, pp. 101-106 (Karger, Basel 1989).
5. Katovich, M.J. & O'Meara, J.: Effect of chronic estrogen on the skin temperature response to naloxone in morphine-dependent rats. Can. J. Physiol. Pharmacol. **65**:563-567 (1987).
6. Tulandi, T., Samarthji, L. & Kinch, R.A.: Effect of intravenous clonidine on menopausal flushing and luteinizing hormone secretion. Brit. J. Obstet. Gynec. **990**:854-857 (1983).
7. Freedman, R.R., Woodward, S. & Sabharwal, S.C.: α-adrenergic mechanism in menopausal hot flushes. Obstet. Gynecol. **76**:573-578 (1990).
8. Sherwin, B.B. & Gelfand, M.M.: Effects of parenteral administration of estrogen and androgen on plasma hormone levels and hot flushes in the surgical menopause. Am. J. Obstet. Gynecol. **148**:552-557 (1984).
9. Ravnikar, V.: Physiology and treatment of hot flushes. Obstet. Gynecol. **75**:3s-8s (1990).
10. Katovich, M.J., Simpkins, J.W. & O'Meara, J.: Effects of acute central LHRH administration on the skin temperature response in morphine dependent rats. Brain Res. **494**:85-94 (1989).

11. Simpkins, J.W., Andreadis, D.K., Millard, W.J. & Katovich, M.J.: The effects of celular glucoprivation on skin temperature regulation in the rat. Life Sci. **47:**107-115 (1990).

12. Katovich, M.J. & Simpkins, J.W.: Adrenergic modulation of the LHRH flush response in rats. Physiologist **33:**A105 (1990).

13. Janis, R.A., Silver, P. & Triggle, D.J.: Drug action and cellular regulation. Adv. Drug Res. **16:**309-591 (1987).

14. Lomax, P., Bajorek, J.G., Chesarek, W. & Tataryn, I.V.: Thermoregulatory effects of luteinizing hormone releasing hormone in the rat. In Cox, Lomax, Milton & Schönbaum, *Thermoregulatory Mechanisms and Their Therapeutic Implications*, pp. 208-211 (Karger, Basel 1980).

15. Simpkins, J.W., Katovich, M.J. & Millard, W.J.: Glucose modulation of skin temperature responses during morphine withdrawal in the rat. Psychopharmacol. **102:**213-220 (1990).

16. Santiago, J.V., White, N.H., Skor, D.A., Levandoski, L.A., Bier, D.M. & Cryer, P.E.: Defective glucose counterregulation, limits intensive therapy of diabetes mellitus. Am. J. Physiol. **247:**E215-E220 (1984).

17. Van Meel, J.A.C., Qian, J., Timmermans, P.B.M.W.M. & Van Zwieten, P.A.: Differential inhibition of α_2-adrenoceptor mediated pressor response by (+) and (-) verapamil in pithed rats. J. Pharm. Pharmacol. **35:**500-504 (1983).

18. Bongianni, F., Carla, V., Moroni, F. & Pellegrini-Giampietro, D.E.: Calcium channel inhibitors suppress the morphine-withdrawal syndrome in rats. Br. J. Pharmac. **88:**561-567 (1986).

19. Pellegrini-Giampietro, D.E., Bacciottini, L., Carla, V. & Moroni, F.: Morphine withdrawal in cortical slices: suppression by Ca^{2+}-channel inhibitors of abstinence-induced [^{3}H] noradrenaline release. Br. J. Pharmac. **93:**535-540 (1988).

20. Baeyens, J.M., Esposito, E., Ossowska, G. & Samanin, R.: Effects of peripheral and central administration of calcium channel blockers in the naloxone-precipitated abstinence in morphine-dependent rats. Eur. J. Pharmacol. **137:**9-13 (1987).

Lomax, Schönbaum (eds.) **Thermoregulation: The Pathophysiological Basis of Clinical Disorders.**
8th International Symposium Pharmacology of Thermoregulation, Kananaskis, Alberta, Canada 1991, pp. 100-104 (Karger, Basel 1992)

CAN COLD TOLERANCE BE IMPROVED BY REDUCING SEPTAL ADENOSINE ACTIVITY IN RATS?

TZE FUN LEE and LAWRENCE C.H. WANG

Department of Zoology, University of Alberta, Edmonton, Alberta, T6G 2E9 (Canada)

Previous studies have shown that acute systemic pretreatment with aminophylline (AMPY) significantly elevated maximum thermogenesis and improved cold tolerance in rats [1,2] and man [3] in severe cold. The thermogenic effect of AMPY is via antagonism of endogenously produced adenosine since 1) pretreatment with a specific adenosine receptor antagonist, but not a phosphodiesterase inhibitor, significantly improved cold tolerance as observed with AMPY [4]; 2) treatment with adenosine deaminase (AD), which inactivates endogenous adenosine activity by converting adenosine to inosine, resulted in significant increases in thermogenesis and cold tolerance [5]. Further, using selective antagonists, the improvement of cold tolerance can be elicited by pretreatment with selective A_1, but not A_2, adenosine receptor antagonists [6].

Central administration of adenosine has been shown to cause a dose-related hypothermia in mice [7] whereas increases in both heat production and body temperature (T_b) were observed after icv injection of adenosine antagonists [8]. This raises the possibility that an increase in thermogenesis observed in our previous studies after systemic pretreatment with adenosine antagonist could result from blockade of the negative thermal effect of the central adenosine activity. To test this possibility we microinjected adenosine antagonists into the preoptic/hypothalamic area but observed no beneficial effect in improving cold tolerance [9]. Since specific receptor sites for adenosine exist in numerous areas of the CNS [10], it is possible that extrahypothalamic sites could be involved in its thermoregulatory response. To investigate this AMPY and AD were microinjected directly into the lateral septum, within which thermosensitive neurons have been shown to exist [11], and the effects of these treatments on thermogenesis and cold tolerance were assessed.

METHODS: Adult male Sprague-Dawley rats weighing approximately 400 g were housed individually at 21°C in a walk in environmental chamber under 12L:12D photoperiod. Food was rationed daily to maintain body weight around 400 g throughout the whole experimental period. Water was available at all times. Under halothane anesthesia, guide cannulae (23-gauge stainless steel tubing) were implanted bilaterally into the lateral septum of each rat utilizing the following stereotaxic coordinates: AP=7.6 mm, L=1.0 mm, H=4.0 mm below the dura matter [12]. The tip of each guide tube was beveled and positioned 1.0 mm above the septum in order to minimize damage to the actual injection site. After completion of the experiments, the precise anatomical location of the injection site was subsequently verified histologically.

On the day of experiment, each rat was transferred to a metal metabolism chamber and exposed to -10°C under helium-oxygen (79% He; 21% O_2) for 120 min. The He-O_2 (1.5 1/min STP) was used to facilitate heat loss. Oxygen consumption and CO_2 production were continuously recorded and integrated by an on-line computerized data acquisition system. Heat production (HP) was calculated from oxygen consumption and respiratory quotient using Kleiber's equation [13]. The integrated HP for each 15 min period was used as the rate of HP. The colonic temperature (T_b; 6 cm from anus) was measured immediately before saline or test compound injection and immediately after cold exposure and the change in T_b was used as an index for cold tolerance. Vehicle or test compound was administered either intraseptally in a volume of 1 μl/site 10 min prior, or intraperitoneally in a volume of 1 ml/kg 15 min prior to cold exposure. To avoid habituation and possible acclimation, at least 7 days was allowed between successive cold exposures, and vehicle or test compound treatment was randomized in each animal in a self-control design.

Aminophylline and adenosine deaminase (Type VI) were used and each drug was prepared immediately before an experiment in a pyrogen-free artificial CSF. Each test solution was always passed through a 0.22 μM Millipore filter for sterility. For statistical comparisons on the effects of treatments in individuals of the same group, Wilcoxon's Signed Ranks test was used. Significance was set at $p < 0.05$ unless otherwise stated.

RESULTS: The mean absolute increases in total and maximal HP and the changes of T_b in rats receiving either intraperitoneal or bilateral intraseptal injection of vehicle or various doses of AMPY are shown in Table I. Similar to earlier reports [1,2], acute systemic injection of optimal dose of AMPY (10 mg/kg ip) significantly increased both the maximal and total HP by 12.8% and 16.7%, respectively. Consequently, the final fall in T_b was significantly lower than that of the control. After intraseptal injection with CSF, the thermogenic pattern was similar to those observed with ip injection of saline and the final T_b dropped about 6°C after a 2 h exposure to the cold. In contrast, both the total and maximal thermogenesis were significantly enhanced after intraseptal injection of AMPY (25 μg/site) 8.0% and 7.2% respectively above control values. Further increases in dosage of AMPY, up to 50 μg/site, did not cause any further increase in HP. As compared with the same group of animals receiving ip AMPY (10 mg/kg), intraseptal injection of AMPY (25 μg/site) resulted in lower total and maximal HP by 6.4% and 2.4%, respectively, and significantly lower final T_b (Table I). Further, a noticeable increase in behavioral activity was observed only in rats which received AMPY intraseptally (25-50 μg/site), but not in those with intraperitoneal injection of AMPY, before placing into the metabolism chamber.

To investigate further whether the thermogenic capacity of the rat can be enhanced by reducing the endogenous adenosine activity, adenosine deaminase (AD) was used and the results are summarized in Table I. The pattern of thermogenic response in rats after receiving AD was similar to that observed with AMPY. Intraseptal injection of AD caused dose-related increases in both heat production adn cold tolerance. The highest thermogenic response was observed after receiving AD 200 μunit/site. However, systemic injection of AD (200 unit/kg ip) into the same group of rats elicited significantly higher total and maximal HP, by 8.8% and 6.8%, respectively, and significantly higher final T_b (Table I). Similar to that observed after intraseptal injection of AMPY rats were more active after receiving AD intraseptally.

DISCUSSION: Even though the thermogenic effect of adenosine receptor antagonists is not mediated through blocking the hypothalamic adenosine receptor, it cannot be entirely ruled out that the adenosine antagonist may act on other CNS thermoregulatory sites. To resolve this issue, AMPY was injected directly into the septum and its thermogenic action assessed. Intraseptal injections of various doses of AMPY caused a dose-related enhancement in HP and increased the cold tolerance of the rat. However, both the total and maximal HP elicited by intraseptal injection of AMPY were significantly lower than those observed in the same group of rats receiving systemic injection of AMPY. The failure of intraseptal AMPY to elicit a similar thermogenic capacity cannot be due to an insufficient dosage, as further increasing the dose to 50 μg/site failed to enhance the thermogenic response beyond that seen at 25 μg/site. This finding suggests that a comparable beneficial thermal effect of systemically administered AMPY is not achievable by blocking the septal adenosine receptors. Further, a general behavioral excitation was noted in rats after intraseptal, but not systemic, injection; it is probable that the increase in metabolic rate and T_b after intraseptal administration of AMPY is a secondary effect due to behavioral excitation following CNS adenosine receptor antagonism. The similar increases in HP and T_b associated with behavioral excitation have been reported earlier in rats after icv injection of theophylline (200 μg) [8].

TABLE I: Effects of intraseptal or intraperitoneal injection of aminophylline (AMPY) or adenosine deaminase (AD) on maximal HP, total HP and change in final T_b on rats exposed to cold

Dosage	N	Maximal HP (Kcal/15 min)*	Total HP (Kcal/105 min)*	T_b Changes (°C)
Intraseptal (dose/site)				
CSF 1.0 μl	7	1.53±0.04	9.84±0.37	-6.26±0.71
AMPY 12.5 μg	7	1.56±0.07[1]	10.13±0.52[1]	-5.62±0.68[1]
AMPY 25.0 μg	7	1.64±0.04[2]	10.64±0.35[1,2]	-4.82±0.56[1,2]
AMPY 50.0 μg	7	1.62±0.03[2]	10.55±0.46[1,2]	-4.73±0.62[1,2]
CSF 1.0 μl	8	1.52±0.03	9.79±0.35	-5.93±0.54
AD 100 μunit	8	1.49±0.04[1]	9.81±0.32[1]	-5.50±0.60[1]
AD 200 μunit	8	1.62±0.04[1,2]	10.57±0.44[1,2]	-4.12±0.51[1,2]
AD 400 μunit	8	1.58±0.04[1,2]	10.45±0.41[1,2]	-4.37±0.55[1,2]
Intraperitoneal				
Saline 1.0 ml/kg	7	1.49±0.06	9.69±0.62	-5.81±0.66
AMPY 10.0 mg/kg	7	1.68±0.04[2]	11.31±0.35[2]	-3.50±0.57[2]
Saline 1.0 ml/kg	8	1.56±0.05	10.19±0.41	-5.64±0.68
AD 200 unit/kg	8	1.73±0.06[2]	11.50±0.44[2]	-2.95±0.45[2]

*1 Kcal = 4.18 KJ
[1]Significantly different from group receiving same drug intraperitoneally, p < 0.05
[2]Significantly different from corresponding vehicle control group, p < 0.05

Another approach to demonstrate the physiological involvement of an endogenous substance is to alter the concentration of the endogenous substance. The enzyme AD, which attenuates the effects of endogenously produced adenosine by converting it to inosine, was chosen to alter septal adenosine activity. Intraseptal injection of AD significantly elevated thermogenesis and final T_b of the rat, indicating that reducing endogenous adenosine activity within the septum enhances thermogenic capacity of the animal. Similar to that observed with AMPY, ip injection with AD was more effective than intraseptal injection in eliciting thermogenic response of the rat under cold exposure.

Based on our results, it is apparent that reducing septal adenosine activity leads to enhanced HP in the rat. Since a noticeable increase in behavioral activity was observed immediately after intraseptal injection of either AMPY or AD before placing the rat in the metabolism chamber, it is possible that the thermogenic response is secondary to the increase in activity. Further, since the total HP elicited after intraseptal administration of either drug is significantly lower than that after ip injection of the same drug, it seems that reducing the septal adenosine activity may have only limited contribution towards the overall beneficial effect of using adenosine antagonist in improving cold tolerance.

Considering the present results and those obtained after intrahypothalamic injection where adenosine antagonist failed to elicit any thermogenic response [9], it is quite possible that the adenosine antagonists' effects in improving cold tolerance is peripheral in origin. This proposition is supported by the finding that adenosine has been shown to be a potent inhibitor not only on lipolysis [14] and gluconeogenesis [15], but also on reducing glucose utilization in skeletal muscle [16]. Blocking the adenosine receptor activity will, therefore, result in increased substrate utilization in the shivering muscle under cold stimulation. Further, numerous studies have shown that adenosine can inhibit neurotransmitter release presynaptically [17]; this could lead to reduced neural stimulation in the shivering muscle and result in lower capacity in heat production under cold stress. Peripheral injection of adenosine antagonist in enhancement of thermogenesis may thus also involve attenuating the inhibitory effect of adenosine in neurotransmission. In spite of these possibilities, it is apparent that further studies using adenosine antagonists which cannot cross the blood-brain barrier would be required to firmly establish that the beneficial effect of adenosine antagonists on cold tolerance is indeed peripheral in action.

ACKNOWLEDGEMENTS: This research was supported by a Medical Research Council of Canada Operating Grant to L. Wang.

REFERENCES

1. Wang, L.C.H.: Effects of feeding on aminophylline induced supra-maximal thermogenesis. Life Sci. **29:**2459-2466 (1981).
2. Wang, L.C.H. & Anholt, E.C.: Elicitation of supramaximal thermogenesis by aminophylline in the rat. J. Appl. Physiol. **53:**16-20 (1982).
3. Wang, L.C.H., Man, S.F.P. & Belcastro, A.N.: Metabolic and hormonal responses in theophylline-increased cold resistance in males. J. Appl. Physiol. **63:**589-596 (1987).
4. Wang, L.C.H., Jourdan, M.L. & Lee, T.F.: Mechanisms underlying the supramaximal thermogenesis elicited by aminophylline in rats. Life Sci. **44:**927-934 (1989).
5. Wang, L.C.H. & Lee, T.F.: Enhancement of maximal thermogenesis by reducing endogenous adenosine activity in the rat. J. Appl. Physiol. **68:**580-585 (1990).
6. Lee, T.F., Li, D.J., Jacobson, K.A. & Wang, L.C.H.: Improvement of cold tolerance by selective A_1 adenosine receptor antagonists in rats. Pharmac. Biochem. Behav. **37:**107-112 (1990).
7. Yarbrough, G.G. & McGuffin-Clineschimidt, J.C.: In vivo behavioral assessment of central nervous system purinergic receptors. Eur. J. Pharmacol. **76:**137-144 (1981).
8. Lin, M.T., Chandra, A. & Liu, G.G.: The effects of theophylline and caffeine on thermoregulatory functions of rats at different ambient temperatures. J. Pharm. Pharmac. **32:**204-208 (1980).
9. Wang, X.L., Lee, T.F. & Wang, L.C.H.: Do adenosine antagonists improve cold tolerance by reducing hypothalamic adenosine activity in rats? Brain Res. Bull. **24:**389-393 (1990).
10. Lee, K.S. & Reddington, M.: Autoradiographic evidence for multiple CNS binding sites for adenosine derivatives. Neuroscience **19:**535-549 (1986).

11. Nakashima, T., Hori, T. & Kiyohara, T.: Intracellular recording analysis of septal thermosensitive neurons in the rat. In Mercer, *Thermal Physiology*, pp. 69-72 (Elsevier, New York 1989).

12. Pellegrino, L.J., Pellegrino, A.S. & Cushman, A.J.: *A Stereotaxic Atlas of the Rat Brain*, (Plenum Press, New York 1979).

13. Wang, L.C.H.: Factors limiting maximum cold-induced heat production. Life Sci. **23:**2089-2098 (1978).

14. Ohisalo, J.J.: Regulatory function of adenosine. Med. Biol. **65:**181-191 (1987).

15. Lavoinne, A., Buc, H.A., Claeyssens, S., Pinosa, M. & Matray, F.: The mechanism by which adenosine decreases gluconeogenesis from lactate in isolated rat hepatocytes. Biochem. J. **246:**449-454 (1987).

16. Challis, R.A.J., Leighton, B., Lozeman, F.J. & Newsholme, E.A.: The hormone-modulatory effects of adenosine in skeletal muscle. In Gerlach & Becker, *Topics and Perspectives in Adenosine Research*, pp. 275-285 (Springer-Verlag, Berlin 1987).

17. Fredholm, B.B. & Dunwiddle, T.V.: How does adenosine inhibit transmitter release? Trends Pharmac. Sci. **9:**130-134 (1988).

Lomax, Schönbaum (eds.) **Thermoregulation: The Pathophysiological Basis of Clinical Disorders.**
8th International Symposium Pharmacology of Thermoregulation, Kananaskis, Alberta, Canada, 1991, pp. 105-108 (Karger, Basel 1992)

HYPOTHERMIA AND MYOCARDIAL PRESERVATION DURING CARDIOVASCULAR SURGERY

M. LEVY[1] and M. BANSINATH

Department of Anesthesiology, School of Medicine, New York, University Medical Center, 550 First Avenue, New York, New York 10016 (USA)

Body temperature is an important factor which affects the pharmacology of many drugs including inhalational and intravenous anesthetics [1]. Hypothermia is deliberately induced during cardiovascular surgery to decrease general metabolic activity [2]. For some surgical procedures, cardioplegia is used as an adjuvant to hypothermia. During cardiovascular surgery, myocardial preservation is dependent both on the temperature [3] and the cardioplegic method used [4]. The formulation of clinically used cardioplegic solutions differs markedly [5-7]. These differences are in the concentration of ions like potassium, magnesium, sodium and calcium as well as in the osmotic agent, buffering capacity of the solution and calcium antagonists used. To date, the ideal cardioplegic solution and the temperature to be used during cardiovascular surgery have not been clearly defined. In this retrospective study, variations in the cardioplegic method and temperature as possible factors affecting the surgical outcome were evaluated.

METHODS: From the Medline data base, using cardioplegia and hypothermia as the key words for the search strategy, studies published during 1980-1990 were selected. From this list, reports using data from experimental animals were excluded. The list was then edited to include clinical reports in which results on coronary artery bypass grafting were discussed. From this edited list, ten studies which included data on postoperative complications, such as the mortality incidence, infarction and arrhythmias, were selected. With the help of this final list of clinical studies, data on adverse reactions were compiled to evaluate if the temperature and cardioplegic method used could be the basis for the incidence of the adverse reactions reported.

RESULTS: The results of the present retrospective analysis are presented in Tables I and II, the range of temperature used varied from 25-28°C. The percentage of mortality ranged between 0-5.3% when hypothermia was the only method used for myocardial preservation. The percentage of mortality was 0-4% in studies which used hypothermia (25-28°C) as an adjuvant to the cardioplegic solution (Table II). The incidence of infarction in hypothermia alone groups ranged from 1.2-20% while in studies which used hypothermia and cardioplegia the incidence ranged from 0-20.8%. The formulation of the cardioplegic solutions used by different investigators was not the same.

---

[1]Visiting Assistant Professor, Department of Anesthesiology, Hospices Civils, 1 Place de l'Hôpital, 67000, Strasbourg, France

TABLE I: Percentage of adverse reactions in aorta-coronary artery bypass grafting

Reference	No. of Cases	Temperature (°C)	Mortality	Infarction	Arrhythmias
No cardioplegic solution					
Akins [9]	500	28	2.4	1.8	1.4
Olinger [10]	1088	--	1.7	1.2	---
Bonchek [11]	500	28	1.0	3.6	---

TABLE II: Percentage of adverse reactions in aorta-coronary artery bypass grafting

Reference	No. of Cases	Temperature (°C)	Mortality H/H+Cplg	Infarction H/H+Cplg	Arrhythmias H/H+Cplg
Potassium crystalloid					
Berger [12]	950	25	5.3/1.9	8.9/3.8	---/---
Roberts [13]	40	25	---/---	5.0/5.0	---/---
Jacocks [14]	50	--	---/---	15.4/20.8	---/---
St. Thomas					
Flameng [15]	72	25	4.7/4.0	4.5/4.0	6.0/12.0
Pepper [16]	50	28	---/---	4.0/4.0	---/---
Bretschneider					
Beyersdorf[17]	37	28	---/---	15/8.0	25/17.0
Hjelms [18]	20	28	0.0/0.0	20/0.0	---/---

Note: The authors generally mentioned only the name but not the formulation of the cardioplegic solution. When the formulation was mentioned, it was not always the uniform, e.g. Studies which used, St. Thomas solution, formulation I or II was not mentioned. H = Hypothermia, Cplg = Cardioplegia, --- = Not mentioned.

DISCUSSION: The results indicate that the incidence of adverse reactions were essentially similar when hypothermia alone was used as well as when cardioplegic solutions were used in addition to hypothermia. However, using retrospective analysis, it is difficult to correlate the incidence of adverse reactions with the method used for cardioplegia. The primary reason appears to be the many variables used in different investigations. A similar conclusion was drawn in the past, when articles published prior to 1985 were analyzed [8]. The basic limitation of this previous analysis was the arbitrary assignment of positive and negative effect on the outcome of surgery. Therefore, we used objective end points such as, death, arrhythmia and infarction to evaluate the positive effect of a cardioplegic method. Due to the inherent complexities involved in the *in vivo* studies, a discussion of an *in vitro* study wherein variables are controlled could be of value. One such study has evaluated cytotoxicity of 11 cardioplegic solutions using tissue culture [5]. The results of this study indicated that the percentages of dead cells were dependent on the duration and temperature of the incubation but not on the composition of the cardioplegic solution. Therefore, with the *in vitro* test paradigm used, ranking of the cardioplegic solutions based on their toxicity was not possible.

Another important factor observed in our retrospective assessment was that little significance appears to have been attached to the chronic pathophysiological risk factors. Factors such as diabetes, hypertension, the type and duration of medication the patients might have had before surgery could affect the results of myocardial preservation. It is concluded that a controlled prospective study using a standard protocol is warranted to identify the ideal temperature and composition required for effective myocardial preservation.

REFERENCES

1. Bansinath, M., Turndorf, H. & Puig, M.M.: Influence of hypo- and hyperthermia on disposition of morphine. J. Clin. Pharmacol. **28**:860-864 (1988).
2. Sealy, W.C.: Hypothermia: its possible role in cardiac surgery. Ann. Thorac. Surg. **47**:788-791 (1989).
3. Balderman, S.C.: The most appropriate temperature for myocardial preservation. In Roberts, *Myocardial Protection in Cardiac Surgery*, Cardiothoracic Surgery, Series Z, pp. 303-359 (Marcel Dekker, NY 1987).
4. Gebhard, M.M.: Myocardial protection and ischemia tolerance of the globally ischemic heart. Thorac Cardiovasc. Surg. **38**:55-59 (1990).
5. Carpentier, S., Murawsky, M. & Carpentier, A.: Cytotoxicity of cardioplegic solutions: evaluation by tissue culture. Circulation **64(Suppl. II)**:90-95 (1981).
6. de Jong, J.W.: Cardioplegia and calcium antagonists: a review. Ann. Thorac. Surg. **42**:593-598 (1986).
7. Fromme, G.A., White, R.D. & Housmans, P.R.: Myocardial preservation. In Roberts, *Myocardial Protection in Cardiac Surgery*, pp. 395-408 (Marcel Dekker, NY 1987).
8. McGoon, D.C.: The ongoing quest for ideal myocardial protection. A catalog of the recent English literature. J. Thorac Cardiovasc. Surg. **89**:639-653 (1985).
9. Akins, C.W.: Noncardioplegic myocardial preservation for coronary revascularization. J. Thorac Cardiovas. Surg. **88**:174-181 (1984).
10. Olinger, G.N.: Intermittent ischemic arrest. In Roberts, *Myocardial Protection in Cardiac Surgery*, pp. 207-219 (Marcel Dekker, NY 1987).
11. Bonchek, L.I. & Burlingame, M.W.: Coronary artery bypass without cardioplegia. J. Thorac Cardiovasc. Surg. **93**:261-267 (1987).
12. Berger, R.L., Davis, K.B., Kaiser, G.C., Foster, E.D., Hammond, G.L., Tong, T.G.L., Kennedy, J.W., Sheffield, T., Ringqvist, I., Wiens, R.D., Chaitman, B.R. & Mock, M.: Preservation of the myocardium during coronary artery bypass grafting. Circulation **64(Suppl. II)**:61-66 (1981).

13.   Roberts, A.J., Sanders Jr., J.H., Moran, J.M., Kaplan, K.J., Lichtenthal, P.R., Spies, S.M. & Michaelis, L.L.: Nonrandomized matched pair analysis of intermittent ischemic arrest versus potassium crystalloid cardioplegia during myocardial revascularization. Ann. Thorac Surg. **31:**502-511 (1981).

14.   Jacocks, M.A., Fowler, B.N., Chaffin, J.S., Lowenstein, E., Lappas, D.G., Pohost, G.M., Boucher, C.A., Okada, R.D., Hanna, N., Daggett, W.M., Butler, J., Balkas, C.: Hypothermic ischemic arrest versus hypothermic potassium cardioplegia in human beings. Ann. Thorac Surg. **34:**157-165 (1982).

15.   Flameng, W., Van-der-Vusse, J.G., DeMeyere, R., Borgers, M., Sergeant, P., Meersch, E.V., Geboers, J. & Suy, R.: Intermittent aortic cross-clamping versus St. Thomas' hospital cardioplegia in extensive aorta-coronary bypass grafting. J. Thorac Cardiovasc. Surg. **88:**164-173 (1984).

16.   Pepper, J.R., Lockey, E., Cankovic-Darracott, S. & Braimbridge, M.V.: Cardioplegia versus intermittent ischaemic arrest in coronary bypass surgery. Thorax **37:**887-892 (1982).

17.   Beyersdorf, F., Krause, E., Sarai, K., Sieber, B., Deutschlander, N., Zimmer, G., Mainka, L., Probst, S., Zegelman, M., Schneider, W. & Satter, P.: Clinical evaluation of hypothermic ventricular fibrillation, multi-dose blood cardioplegia and single-dose Bretschneider cardioplegia in coronary surgery. Thorac Cardiovasc. Surg. **38:**20-29 (1990).

18.   Hjelms, E. & Steiness, E.:Myocardial protection in coronary artery bypass surgery. A study comparing cold cardioplegia and intermittent aortic cross clamping. J. Cardiovasc. Surg. **23:**403-406 (1982).

Lomax, Schönbaum (eds.) **Thermoregulation: The Pathophysiological Basis of Clinical Disorders.**
8th International Symposium Pharmacology of Thermoregulation, Kananaskis, Alberta, Canada 1991, pp. 109-113 (Karger, Basel 1992)

CARDIAC FUNCTION AND MYOCARDIAL CALCIUM REGULATION AT VARYING BODY TEMPERATURES

BIN LIU, DARRELL D. BELKE, MICHAEL L. JOURDAN and LAWRENCE C.H. WANG

Department of Zoology, University of Alberta, Edmonton, Alberta, T6G 2E9 (Canada)

Survival in hypothermia, and recovery during rewarming, requires adequate cardiac output to provide sufficient blood flow to organs and tissues. Many studies have dealt with isolated hearts under Langendorff perfusion in order to investigate the effect of low temperature on cardiac function [1,2]. Since the isolated heart does little external work under the Langendorff perfusion these studies may not be functionally relevant to the *in vivo* situation as a continuous increase in systemic vascular resistance occurs during hypothermia [3,4]. Development of the isolated working heart model has provided a useful method for examining cardiac function under the increased work load characteristic of deep hypothermia.

Previous studies in our laboratory have demonstrated that rats can recover fully after experiencing prolonged hypothermia at a body temperature (T_b) of 19°C for 20-24 h [5-7]. Beyond this time period, more than 50% of the rats die in hypothermia or cannot fully recover on rewarming. Whether this is due to a gradual failure of cardiac function, pumping against high peripheral resistance in hypothermia, is unknown. The aim of the present study was to examine the capability of the working heart after it has endured the insult of prolonged hypothermia. The effect of hypothermia on cardiac activator Ca^{2+} was also investigated since cellular Ca^{2+} plays an important role in the contraction of cardiac muscle, thus directly affecting cardiac performance in hypothermia.

METHODS: Male Sprague Dawley rats (400 g) were divided into two groups: 1) euthermic; maintained at 22°C ambient temperature and T_b near 37°C, and without food for 24 h. 2) hypothermic; induced and maintained at a T_b of 19°C for 20 h by the method of Jourdan and Wang [5] prior to sacrifice. All experimental manipulations of the rats were approved by the University of Alberta Animal Use Committee.

Both euthermic and hypothermic rats were sacrificed by cervical dislocation. The heart was rapidly excised and put into cold (4°C) Krebs-Henseleit solution containing (mM): NaCl (118), KCl (4.7), $MgSO_4$ (1.6), KH_2PO_4 (1.2), $NaHCO_3$ (25.0), Na_2-EDTA (0.5), $CaCl_2$ (2.5), glucose (11.0) and Na-pyruvate (2.0), gassed with 95% O_2 and 5% CO_2 (pH 7.4). The aorta and pulmonary vein were cannulated as described by Lopaschuk *et al.* [8]. The heart was initially perfused at 19°C for 30 min as a Langendorff preparation at an aortic pressure of 60 mm Hg, and then switched to working mode with 15 cm H_2O preload on left atrium and various aortic afterloads. An 18 gauge needle was inserted into left ventricle through the apex of the heart. Left ventricular systolic pressure (LVSP) was measured with a pressure transducer and recorded on a polygraph. After obtaining measurements of LVSP at different afterloads in the working mode, the heart was switched back to the Langendorff perfusion. The perfusion temperature was then increased to 25 or 37°C and the same pressure measurements were made after a 20-30 min equilibrium at each temperature. The heart was electrically paced with a stimulator through a pair of bipolar platinum electrodes placed on the right atrium. The pace frequency was 1.5 Hz at 19°C, 2.0 Hz at 25°C and 4.0 Hz at 37°C.

The left ventricular papillary muscle was excised at 19°C in aerated Krebs-Henseleit solution without Na_2-EDTA and Na-pyruvate, and mounted vertically in a 5 ml thermostated bath chamber. The ventricular base of the muscle was tied with 5-0 thread to the holder of an electrode while the tendinous end of the muscle was tied to the hook of a force transducer. The muscle was first equilibrated and stimulated (30 beats/min) at 19°C for 60 min. A special stimulation protocol, as described previously [9], was then used to construct a mechanical restitution curve (i.e., the amplitude of first contraction after a pause as the function of the duration of the pause) in order to evaluate the level of activator Ca^{2+} available in the myocytes.

RESULTS: Fig. 1 shows the changes of LVSP at different afterloads for both hypothermic and euthermic hearts. At all temperatures, and in both groups, LVSP increased as the afterload was raised from 40 to 100 mm Hg. At 19°C, there was no difference in LVSP of hypothermic hearts (n, 8) from the euthermic ones (n, 7) when the afterload was increased from 40 to 60 mm Hg; however, LVSP was lower in hypothermic hearts when the afterload was increased to 70 and 80 mm Hg. A further increase in the afterload to 90 and 100 mm Hg at 19°C resulted in a significantly ($p < 0.05$) reduced LVSP in the hypothermic hearts. Raising the temperature to 25 or 37°C had similar effects on both hypothermic and euthermic hearts; however, LVSP was always lower in hypothermic rat hearts than that in euthermic hearts, although no statistical difference was observed between the two groups.

The mechanical restitution of the papillary muscles was investigated at 19°C (Fig. 2). After the steady state contraction was reached with a constant stimulation, the stimulus was stopped for a measured period and started again. The first contraction (F_1) varies with the duration of the pause. It can be seen in Fig. 2 that the amplitude of F_1 after a pause from 15 sec up to 5 min was significantly ($p < 0.05$) lower in the papillary muscles (n, 19) from hypothermic hearts than that in the papillary muscles (n, 15) from euthermic hearts.

DISCUSSION: In recent studies from our laboratory the haematocrit was observed to increase significantly in rats after 24 h of hypothermia at a T_b of 19°C [6,7]. This, and other observations, indicate a marked increase in systemic vascular resistance during hypothermia [3,4]. It is expected that the heart must overcome this high peripheral resistance during hypothermia to supply adequate blood flow to organs and tissues. As shown in Fig. 1, LVSP at 19°C was significantly lower in hypothermic hearts than that in euthermic hearts when the afterload was in the range of 90 and 100 mm Hg. This implies that with the progression of hypothermia over 20 h at a T_b of 19°C, the decrease in LVSP of the hypothermic heart may not be able to provide sufficient output, under the high peripheral resistance characteristic of hypothermia, in order to maintain adequate organ perfusion.

Since cellular Ca^{2+} plays an important role in cardiac excitation-contraction coupling, the availability of activator Ca^{2+} in myocytes was also evaluated in the present study by assessing the post-rest contraction of the papillary muscle from euthermic and hypothermic hearts. Changes in amplitude of the first contraction (F_1) after a specific rest interval reflects the amount of activator Ca^{2+} released during excitation of the cardiac myocyte [10]. A lower amplitude of F_1 at 19°C in the mechanical restitution of papillary muscles from hypothermic hearts (Fig. 2) indicates that a decreased level of activator Ca^{2+} is available in the hypothermic heart. As the sarcoplasmic reticulum (SR) is the primary source of activator Ca^{2+} for contraction in the rat cardiac myocyte [11], the decrease in activator Ca^{2+} and LVSP (especially under high afterloads) at 19°C could reflect a deterioration in the ability of the SR to accumulate, store, and release Ca^{2+} after prolonged hypothermia [12]. Further studies on these aspects should reveal the limiting mechanisms for sustained cardiac function under prolonged hypothermia.

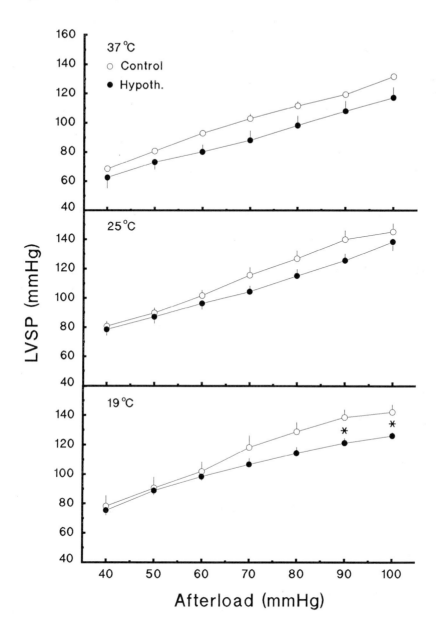

FIGURE 1: Left ventricular systolic pressure (LVSP) as a function of afterload at 37, 25 and 19°C in hypothermic and euthermic (control) rat hearts. Symbols represent mean, bars represent standard error (hypothermic n, 8, control n, 7). (*, Significant difference, p < 0.05).

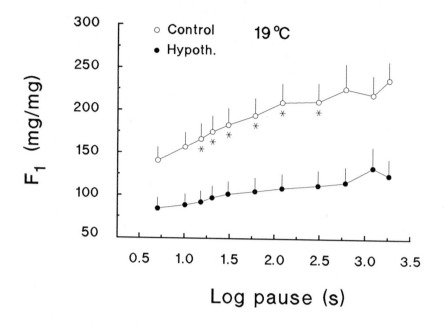

FIGURE 2: The first post-rest contraction (F_1) in papillary muscles from hypothermic and euthermic (control) rat hearts at 19°C. Symbols represent mean, bars represent standard error (hypothermic n, 19; control n, 15). (*, Significant difference, $p < 0.05$).

ACKNOWLEDGEMENTS: We thank Mrs. Li-ying Zhang for her assistance. This study was supported by grants from the Alberta Heart and Stroke Foundation and the National Science and Engineering Research Council of Canada to Dr. L.C.H. Wang. B. Liu is the recipient of a studentship from the Alberta Heritage Foundation for Medical Research.

REFERENCES

1. Zataman, M.L.: Renal and cardiovascular effects of hibernation and hypothermia. Cryobiology **21:**593-614 (1984).
2. Jones, S.B. & Romano, F.D.: Functional characteristics and responses to adrenergic stimulation of isolated heart preparations from hypothermic and hibernating subjects. Cryobiology **21:**615-626 (1984).
3. Popovic, V.P. & Kent, K.M.: Cardiovascular responses in prolonged hypothermia. Am. J. Physiol. **209:**1069-1074 (1965).
4. Morray, J.P. & Pavlin, E.G.: Oxygen delivery and consumption during hypothermia and rewarming in the dog. Anesthesiology **72:**510-516 (1990).
5. Jourdan, M.L. & Wang, L.C.H.: An improved technique for the study of hypothermia physiology. J. Therm. Biol. **12:**175-178 (1987).

6. McArthur, M.D., Jourdan, M.L. & Wang, L.C.H.: Effects of hypothermia and rewarming on plasma metabolites in rats. In Lomax & Schönbaum, *Thermoregulation: The Pathophysiological Basis of Clinical Disorders*, 8th International Symposium Pharmacology of Thermoregulation, Kananaskis, Canada 1991, pp. 119-123 (Karger, Basel 1992).

7. Jourdan, M.L., Hoo-Paris, R. & Wang, L.C.H.: Characterization of hypothermia in non-hibernator: the rat. In Malan & Canguilhem, *Living in the Cold II*, pp. 289-296 (John Libbey Eurotext, Ltd., Montrouge, France 1989).

8. Lopaschuk, G.D., Hansen, C.A. & Neely, J.R.: Fatty acid metabolism in hearts containing elevated levels of CoA. Am. J. Physiol. **250:**H351-H359 (1986).

9. Liu, B., Wohlfart, B.& Johansson, B.W.: Mechanical restitution at different temperatures in papillary msucles from rabbit, rat and hedgehog. Cryobiology **27:**596-604 (1990).

10. Wohlfart, B. & Noble, M.I.M.: The cardiac excitation-contraction cycle. Pharmacol. Ther. **16:**1-43 (1982).

11. Bers, D.M.: Ca influx and sarcoplasmic reticulum Ca release in cardiac muscle activation during postrest recovery. Am. J. Physiol. **248:**H336-H381 (1985).

12. Hess, M.L., Krause, S.M., Robbins, A.D. & Greenfield, L.J.: Excitation-contraction coupling in hypothermic ischemic myocardium. Am. J. Physiol. **240:**H336-H341 (1981).

Lomax, Schönbaum (eds.) **Thermoregulation: The Pathophysiological Basis of Clinical Disorders.**
8th International Symposium Pharmacology of Thermoregulation, Kananaskis, Alberta, Canada 1991, pp. 114-118 (Karger, Basel 1992)

DOPAMINE ANTAGONISTS AND COCAINE INDUCED TEMPERATURE CHANGES

PETER LOMAX and KERI A. DANIEL

Department of Pharmacology, School of Medicine, and the Brain Research Institute, University of California at Los Angeles, Los Angeles, California 90024-1735 (USA)

The neuropharmacology of cocaine is complex with its actions being expressed at multiple sites in the CNS. A predominant effect of the drug is its ability to block reuptake of dopamine, leading to increased availability of the amine at the postsynaptic receptors. Thus, many of the responses to cocaine are dopaminergic in nature [see 1] and may be mediated by different receptor types, e.g., pretreatment with a dopamine D_1 antagonist (SCH 23390) protects rats from the lethal effect of cocaine but has no effect on the incidence of seizures [2].

The change in body temperature (T_b) following administration of cocaine to the rat varies with the experimental conditions. When the animal is at rest at its normal ambient temperature (T_a) (20°C) acute administration of cocaine (10-40 mg/kg) leads to a dose dependent fall in T_b [3]. Raising T_a to 35°C causes the response to revert to a dose dependent hyperthermia over the same dose range [4]. When the animals were exercising on a treadmill at T_a 22°C cocaine (30 mg/kg) did not modify the running behavior but caused a significant rise in T_b compared to the vehicle injected controls [5]. It is likely that the fall in T_b involves central dopaminergic pathways since injection of dopamine into the CNS, or systemic administration of dopaminergic agonists, such as apomorphine, cause a fall in T_b in most species [see 6].

The effect of the dopamine D_1 antagonist SCH 23390 on the thermoregulatory responses to cocaine has been investigated.

METHODS: Female Sprague-Dawley rats were housed at $22 \pm 1°C$ and ambient humidity on a standard 12 h light/dark cycle. Food and water were freely available up to the start of each experimental session. At the time of delivery from the breeders the rats had a body weight of 130-175 g and were between 6 and 8 weeks old. The animals were observed for at least 7 days prior to the experiments and during this period they were handled and allowed to adapt and stabilize to the laboratory environment. A temperature controlled cabinet was used when experiments were conducted at T_a above the normal T_a of the laboratory. All experimental sessions were started at 08:00 h to control for circadian variations. Deep body temperature was measured with a small animal thermistor probe, inserted through the rectum for at least 6 cm, and connected to a telethermometer. The readings were taken at 15 min intervals with at least a 30 min stabilization period prior to injection of drugs. Cocaine hydrochloride was dissolved in pyrogen free NaCl (0.9%) solution to the appropriate concentration to allow an injection volume of 0.1 ml/100 g body weight. Doses are given as the weight of the salt. For control injections NaCl (0.9%) was injected in the same volume (0.1 ml/100 g). All injections were made intraperitoneally. Data were analyzed using a microcomputer statistical program which calculates exact probability levels.

RESULTS: A group of 12 animals, caged at T_a $22 \pm 1\,°C$, was injected with SCH 23390 (1 mg/kg) and with the saline vehicle, in random order on separate days. During the first 60 min after injection there was no significant difference in T_b between the two groups (Fig. 1). From then on, however, the normal circadian fall in T_b was more pronounced in the SCH 23390 treated animals and the mean T_b was significantly lower than that of the control group at 120 min ($p = 0.0133$; two sample t test). The temperatures of both treatment groups were the same at 08:00 h the following day.

Under identical experimental conditions groups of 12 rats were injected with vehicle, cocaine (20 mg/kg), or cocaine (20 mg/kg) 15 min after SCH 23390 (1 mg/kg) (Fig. 1). Each treatment caused a fall in T_b within 60 min which was of similar magnitude at 30 min ($p = 0.1829$) although in both groups T_b was significantly lower than that of the control group ($p < 0.0025$; Student t test) at this time. The T_b had returned to the initial level by 60 min in the animals treated with cocaine alone but it remained at the low point for more than 120 min in those pretreated with SCH 23390. In a further group of 6 rats core temperature was recorded at intervals over 120 h after injection of SCH 23390 (1 mg/kg) followed by cocaine (20 mg/kg) 15 min later. At 24 h T_b had fallen to $36.35 \pm 0.41\,°C$ (control T_b, $38.22 \pm 0.10\,°C$; mean fall $1.98 \pm 0.14\,°C$). Thereafter the temperature recovered slowly, although at 120 h it was still significantly lower than the initial temperature ($p < 0.05$). From 24 to 120 h T_b in animals treated with SCH 23390 alone did not differ from that of the vehicle injected controls.

In groups of 6-8 rats housed at T_a $30 \pm 1\,°C$ for the duration of the recordings neither 0.9% NaCl nor SCH 23390 (1 mg/kg) changed T_b significantly ($p > 0.9$; Wilcoxon Rank-sum with Mann-Whitney U test) comparing time 0 and 30 min (Fig. 2). At this T_a cocaine (20 mg/kg) caused a significant rise in T_b within 30 min after injection ($p = 0.0088$) (Fig. 2). When SCH 23390 (1 mg/kg) was injected 15 min prior to cocaine (20 mg/kg) however, T_b declined and at 30 min was significantly different from that in animals treated only with cocaine ($-0.75 \pm 0.26\,°C$ and $+0.61 \pm 0.19\,°C$, respectively; $p = 0.0082$) (Fig. 2).

DISCUSSION: In previous studies in rats and mice, carried out at a thermoneutral T_a, SCH 23390 had no effect on T_b [7], or caused variable changes which were not dose related [8]. In these, and other reports, the responses were followed over the first 60 min after drug administration; there do no appear to be any data concerning longer term effects of this dopamine D_1 antagonist on T_b. There was no significant change in T_b up to 90 min following injection of SCH 23390 in our rats (Fig. 1). Thereafter, however, T_b slowly declined and remained lower than in the controls for several hours.

Hypothermia induced by cocaine at T_a $22\,°C$ is of short duration [3] and T_b returns to the initial level within 60 min (Fig. 1). In animals pretreated with the D_1 antagonist, although the initial fall was similar to that occurring after cocaine alone, T_b did not recover immediately (Fig. 1) and was below normal for more than 120 h. Comparing T_b after SCH 23390 with that following SCH 23390 + cocaine (Fig. 1), there was no significant difference at 120 min ($37.63 \pm 0.08\,°C$ and $37.50 \pm 0.11\,°C$; $p = 0.3139$). At 24 to 120 h T_b continued to be low after the combined treatment but had returned to normal levels in rats receiving only SCH 23390. These findings proffer two possible interpretations: blockade of the D_1 receptors delays recovery from cocaine induced hypothermia, or cocaine prolongs the long term fall in T_b caused by SCH 23390.

In contrast, at a T_a above the thermoneutral zone for the rat cocaine caused hyperthermia with a time course of 30-60 min (Fig. 2)[3]. Although, by itself, SCH 23390 did not alter T_b at T_a $30\,°C$, it not only prevented the rise but it converted the response to cocaine to a fall in T_b which persisted for more than 90 min (Fig. 2).

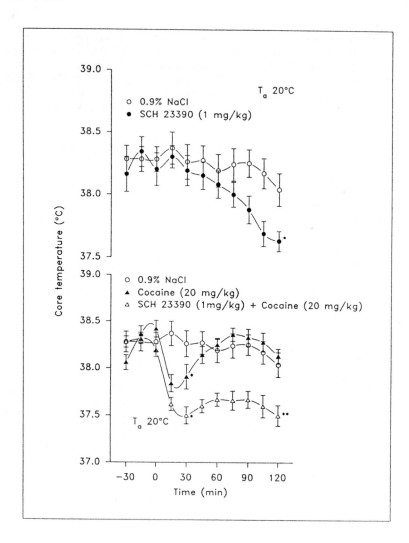

FIGURE 1: Time course of the changes in T_b in rats at T_a 20°C following drug injection at time -15 min (pretreatment with SCH 23390). Upper graph: *p = 0.0133 compared to control. Lower graph: *p < 0.0025 compared to vehicle control; **p < 0.0001 compared to cocaine alone and to vehicle control.

If the thermoregulatory effects of cocaine are indeed mediated by central dopaminergic systems these findings are consistent with earlier conclusions, using selective agonists and antagonists [7-9], that D_1 receptor activation leads to a rise in T_b and D_2 activation causes a fall. The direction of the temperature change when both receptor subtypes are triggered would seem to be a function of the ambient conditions and the consequent ongoing state of the thermoregulatory system. At a higher T_a the hyperthermic response is dominant but when the D_1 receptors are blocked hypothermia, mediated by the D_2 receptors, occurs.

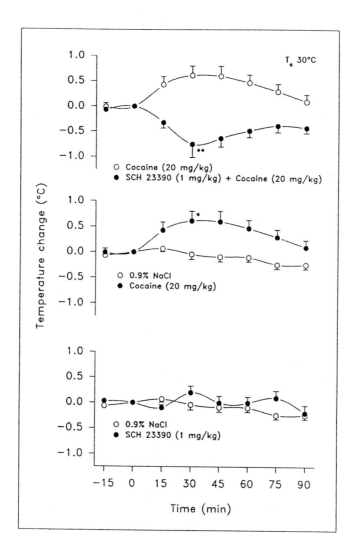

FIGURE 2: Time course of the changes in T_b in rats at T_a 30°C following drug injection at time 0 or at time -15 min (pretreatment with SCH 23390). *p = 0.0088 compared to vehicle control; **p = 0.0082 compared to cocaine alone.

The CNS has a relatively high density of dopamine D_1, compared to D_2, receptors (of the order of 3-5:1), in addition to a probable distinct D_3 receptor in the limbic system [10]. The majority of identified drug effects are manifest at the D_2 receptor with the D_1 receptor being something of a mystery protein. One suggestion for the role of the D_1 receptor is as a modulator of the D_2 receptor, possibly by expression of a signal protein. This regulation could occur over an extended time frame which would account for the delayed and prolonged effect on T_b seen after D_1 blockade by SCH 23390.

There is increasing evidence, in a large number of cases of severe toxicity among cocaine abusers, that stress related heat stroke may be the terminal event [for references see 4]. The mortality rate from all forms of stress induced heat stroke is very high, exceeding 80% unless expeditious and skilled emergency treatment is available. In patients presenting with hyperthermia secondary to cocaine poisoning, dopamine D_1 antagonists may prove to be useful adjuvants to body cooling in order to reduce T_b.

ACKNOWLEDGEMENTS: This research is supported by NIDA Grant DA 04904.

REFERENCES

1. Fisher, S., Raskin A. & Uhlenhuth, E.H. (eds): *Cocaine: Clinical and Biobehavioral Aspects*. (Oxford University Press, New York, 1987).
2. Witkin, J.M., Goldberg, S.R. & Katz, J.L.: Lethal effects of cocaine are reduced by the dopamine-1 receptor antagonist SCH 23390 but not by haloperidol. Life Sci. **44**:1285-1291 (1989).
3. Lomax, P. & Daniel, K.A.: Body temperature changes induced by cocaine in the rat. In Mercer, *Thermal Physiology 1989*, pp. 265-271 (Excerpta Medica, Amsterdam 1989).
4. Lomax, P. & Daniel, K.A.: Cocaine and body temperature in the rat: effects of ambient temperature. Pharmacol. **40**:103-109 (1990).
5. Lomax, P. & Daniel, K.A.: Cocaine and body temperature in the rat: effect of exercise. Pharmacol. Biochem. Behav. **36**:889-892 (1990).
6. Cox, B.: Dopamine. In Lomax & Schönbaum, *Body Temperature*, pp. 231-255 (Dekker, New York 1979).
7. Sánchez, C: The effects of dopamine D-1 and D-2 receptor agonists on body temperature in male mice. Eur. J. Pharmacol. **171**:201-206 (1989).
8. Chipkin, R.E.: Effects of D1 and D2 antagonists on basal and apomorphine decreased body temperature in mice and rats. Pharmacol. Biochem. Behav. **30**:683-686 (1988).
9. Vasse, M., Chagraoui, A., Henry, J.-P. & Protais, P: The rise of body temperature induced by stimulation of dopamine D_1 receptors is increased in acutely reserpinized mice. Eur. J. Pharmacol. **181**:23-33 (1990).
10. Sokoloff, P., Giros, B., Martres, M.-P., Bouthenet, M.-L. & Schwartz, J.-C.: Molecular cloning and characterization of a novel dopamine receptor (D_3) as a target for neuroleptics. Nature (Lond.) **347**:146-151 (1990).

Lomax, Schönbaum (eds.) **Thermoregulation: The Pathophysiological Basis of Clinical Disorders.**
8th International Symposium Pharmacology of Thermoregulation, Kananaskis, Alberta, Canada 1991, pp. 119-123 (Karger, Basel 1992)

EFFECTS OF HYPOTHERMIA AND REWARMING ON PLASMA METABOLITES IN RATS

M. DAWN McARTHUR, MICHAEL L. JOURDAN and LAWRENCE C.H. WANG

Department of Zoology, University of Alberta, Edmonton, Alberta, T6G 2E9 (Canada)

Hypothermia is a state of low body temperature (T_b) which occurs when heat loss exceeds heat production and from which animals cannot rewarm without exogenous heat. The hypothermic animal survives by virtue of its innate cellular cold tolerance but eventually will die if not rewarmed. The limitations to survival in hypothermia are still unclear but appear to include perturbations of cardiovascular and respiratory function, tissue perfusion and O_2 delivery, and substrate mobilization and utilization [1,2]. During rewarming, rising T_b may cause further imbalances that jeopardize maintenance of homeostasis [1]. In particular, the availability of glucose has often been cited as a primary factor in hypothermic survival [1-3].

Recently, Jourdan and Wang [4] have developed a method that provides rapid induction and prolonged maintenance of stable hypothermia, which enables rats to survive at $T_b = 19°C$ for 24 h and ground squirrels to survive at $T_b = 7°C$ for 72 h. With this model, the hypothermic animal is given free reign over physiological function, allowing the study of the factors that control and may limit survival during prolonged hypothermia and/or subsequent rewarming [5-7]. We have observed that animals that do not survive rewarming from prolonged hypothermia generally succumb when T_b reaches 22-25°C. This suggests that critical failures occur in this T_b range, although the primary disturbance may have occurred earlier in the bout. In order to assess some of the differences between survivors and non-survivors, we have compared the metabolite profiles of these two groups of rats during induction, maintenance and rewarming from prolonged hypothermia.

METHODS: Male Sprague-Dawley rats, housed individually at an ambient temperature (T_a) of $22 \pm 1°C$ under 12L:12D or natural photoperiod, were fed lab chow rationed to maintain mass near 400 g and given water *ad libitum*. The animals were not fasted prior to induction of hypothermia.

Cannulation (right jugular vein and left common carotid artery) and induction of hypothermia were as previously described [4-7]. Briefly, following surgery the halothane anaesthetized rat was transferred to a water-jacketed Plexiglas chamber at T_a 0°C under He-O_2 (79% He; 21% O_2) in an open flow system. The halothane concentration was decreased by $\approx 0.1\%$ per 1°C drop in T_b; the anaesthetic was removed when T_b reached 28°C. When T_b reached 23°C, the He-O_2 was replaced by normal air. In hypothermia, T_b was maintained at 19°C by a computerized feedback loop using rectal temperature as the reference for the adjustment of T_a. Rewarming was initiated by raising T_a to 30°C after approximately 18 h at $T_b = 19°C$. The animals were grouped as either Group A (surviving to $T_b > 26°C$) or Group B (surviving to $T_b = 22-26°C$ (Table I).

TABLE I: Body temperatures (T_b) and time-course data for Group A and B rats

Sample	Group	N	T_b (°C)	Time (h)
Post-surgery	A	4	34.4 ± 0.3	-3.3 ± 1.0
	B	5	34.3 ± 0.9	-4.3 ± 1.2
Initial hypothermia	A	4	19.7 ± 0.4	0
	B	5	19.4 ± 0.2	0
Final hypothermia	A	5	19.3 ± 0.3	17.6 ± 0.5
	B	5	19.2 ± 0.2	16.3 ± 0.4
Rewarm T_b = 22°C	A	4	22.7 ± 0.5	18.4 ± 2.2 (0.8)
	B	5	22.5 ± 0.4	17.6 ± 0.2 (1.3)
Rewarm T_b = 26°C	A	5	25.8 ± 0.6	19.6 ± 2.2 (2.0)
	B	3	26.1 ± 0.3	18.7 ± 0.1 (2.4)
Rewarm T_b = 30°C	A	5	30.6 ± 1.0	22.2 ± 3.1 (4.6)
	B	0	---	---

Group A = animals surviving to T_b > 26°C during rewarming;
Group B = animals surviving to T_b 22-26°C during rewarming.
Times in parentheses indicate mean time from onset of rewarming.
Values are mean ± sem; no significant differences were found between groups A and B.

Blood samples for metabolites were taken from the arterial cannula before and after cooling and at several times during hypothermia and rewarming (Table I). 250 μl blood samples were centrifuged immediately and the plasma frozen at -70°C until assayed for glucose and FFA concentrations. Plasma glucose was measured using the glucose-oxidase method (Sigma kit 510) and plasma FFA by a colorimetric method [8]. A 150 μl aliquot of whole blood was deproteinized in 300 μl perchloric acid (0.4%), centrifuged, and lactate measured spectrophotometrically using LDH-linked reduction of NAD^+.

RESULTS: All rats survived induction and maintenance of hypothermia. During rewarming, all animals survived until T_b reached 22°C, but only half survived to T_b > 26°C. On average, Group B rats rewarmed somewhat more quickly than did Group A rats (Table I).

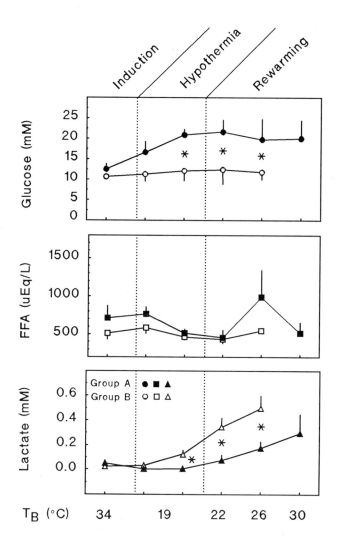

FIGURE 1: Plasma concentrations of glucose, FFA, and lactate during induction, hypothermia, and rewarming in rats. Group A: animals surviving rewarming to $T_b > 26°C$; Group B: animals surviving rewarming to $T_b = 22-26°C$. Times, actual T_b, and N are given in Table I. Values are mean $\pm$ sem; * significantly different ($P < 0.05$, ANOVA) between groups A and B.

As can be seen in Fig. 1, the most striking differences in the metabolite profiles of Groups A and B rats were indicated by the changes in plasma glucose and lactate. Plasma glucose did not differ between the survivors and non-survivors before cooling (12.3 $\pm$ 1.9 mM vs. 10.7 $\pm$ 0.9 mM). During hypothermia and rewarming Group A rats maintained a consistently high plasma glucose that was approximately twice that of Group B rats ($\approx$ 20 mM vs. $\approx$ 12 mM) (Fig. 1). Plasma lactate was very low in both groups initially, and increased over 18 h at $T_b = 19°C$ only in Group B rats. During rewarming lactate rose more rapidly in non-survivors, so that the final lactate concentration of Group

B rats was greater than that of Group A rats (Fig. 1). Plasma FFA was slightly higher in Group A during induction and early hypothermia but decreased by 18% over 18 h to the level of Group B. Plasma FFA was similar in the two groups at the first rewarming sample but rose substantially higher in Group A at $T_b \approx 26°C$, before falling at $T_b \approx 30°C$ to the final level of Group B (516 ± 144 μEq/l vs. 545 ± 38 μEq/l) (Fig. 1).

TABLE II: Plasma glucose, FFA and lactate values for euthermic rats maintained at T_a 23°C

Sample (time following surgery)	Glucose (mM)	FFA (μEq/l)	Lactate (mM)
Immediately	12.1 $\pm$ 1.6 (6)	588 $\pm$ 67 (6)	1.0 $\pm$ 0.3[1] (5)
60 min	9.5 $\pm$ 0.4 (6)	677 $\pm$ 82 (6)	0.3 $\pm$ 0.1 (5)
24 h	9.5 $\pm$ 1.2 (6)	429 $\pm$ 18 (5)	0.1 $\pm$ 0.03 (5)

Values are mean $\pm$ sem (N);
[1]Significantly greater than 60 min and 24 h ($P < 0.05$, ANOVA).

DISCUSSION: Compared to survivors, rats that do not survive rewarming have lower plasma glucose and FFA concentrations during hypothermia as well as lower glucose and higher lactate concentrations during rewarming (Fig. 1). The potential capability of the hypothermic animal to rewarm successfully may be related to its responsiveness to cooling during induction of hypothermia. Increases in glucose and FFA are attributed to both stress and cold exposure responses, which include decreased insulin and increased catecholamine, glucagon, and corticosterone levels [1,6,9]. This leads to mobilization of glucose via glycogenolysis in heart, liver and muscle, and of fat via lipolysis in adipose tissue. Rats in Group B showed a less vigorous response to lowered T_b than did rats in Group A, and thus began the hypothermic bout with lower glucose and FFA levels (Fig. 1). It should be noted, however, that the glucose and FFA levels of even non-survivors are similar to those of euthermic animals and theoretically should be adequate to sustain the low metabolic rate of the hypothermic animal.

The differences in FFA profiles of survivors and non-survivors are less obvious than those of glucose or lactate profiles. The decreases in FFA observed in both group A and B rats (Fig. 1) suggests that FFA are an important substrate during hypothermia, as is true of cold-exposed animals and hypothermic humans and rabbits [9]. The initial rise in FFA in Group A rats between $T_b \approx 22°C$ and $\approx 26°C$ suggests that survivors retain a better capacity to respond to the increased demand for metabolic fuel during rewarming.

In hamsters hypothermic survival at $T_b = 5°C$ is positively correlated with glucose concentration and survival in both hypothermia and rewarming are augmented by glucose administration or pretreatment with glucocorticoids [1,2]. This does not appear true of rats, since glucose administration has no beneficial effect (unpublished). Hypothermic survival in rats appears instead to be more dependent on the balance of hormones (e.g. insulin and glucagon) and the ability of tissues to use substrates [1,3,5,6]. The striking difference between Group A and B rats suggests a correlation between survival and glucose concentration, and seems at odds with these observations. Unlike hypothermic hamsters, however, Group B rats were not hypoglycemic compared to euthermic animals (Table II). In contrast, Group A rats became hyperglycemic during hypothermia (Fig. 1). Hyperglycemia is suggested to protect the hypothermic heart from ventricular fibrillation by reducing plasma K^+ and may play a role in balancing osmotic stress [1] so as to be beneficial during both hypothermia and rewarming.

Despite availability of substrate, glucose and FFA oxidation rates may be decreased by an overall depression of aerobic metabolism. Plasma lactate increased during rewarming in both survivors and non-survivors, but the rise occurred earlier and to a greater extent in non-survivors than in survivors (Fig. 1). In Group B rats this increase in anaerobic metabolism is concomitant with decreased cardiovascular/respiratory function, as these animals had higher hematocrit ratios (55-60% vs. 45-50% in group A rats), lower arterial P_{O2}, higher arterial P_{CO2}, and lower arterial pH than did the survivors [7]. This pattern suggests that low tissue blood flow, and hence decreased oxygen and substrate delivery, rather than substrate availability *per se*, may be the primary causative factors in the suppression of oxidative metabolism in hypothermia and rewarming. Remedial measures directed towards maintenance of cardiovascular function and peripheral blood flow may therefore be more effective than augmentation of substrate in improving the survival of hypothermic animals.

ACKNOWLEDGEMENTS: We thank J. Westly and X. Yin for their technical assistance. This work was supported by a grant from the NSERC of Canada to L.C.H. Wang and by a Studentship from the Alberta Heritage Foundation for Medical Research to M.D. McArthur.

REFERENCES

1. Jourdan, M.L., Lee, T.F. & Wang, L.C.H.: Survival and resuscitation from hypothermia: what natural hibernation can tell us about mammalian response to hypothermia. In Groat & Fuller, *Clinical Applications of Cryobiology* (CRC Press 1991) (in press).

2. Musacchia, X.J.: Comparative physiological and biochemical aspects of hypothermia as a model for hibernation. Cryobiology 21:583-592 (1984).

3. Steffen, J.M.: Glucose, glycogen, and insulin responses in the hypothermic rat. Cryobiology 25:94-101 (1988).

4. Jourdan, M.L. & Wang, L.C.H.: An improved technique for the study of hypothermia physiology. J. Therm. Biol. 12(2):175-178 (1987).

5. Hoo-Paris, R., Jourdan, M.L., Wang, L.C.H. & Rajotte, R.V.: Insulin secretion and substrate homeostasis in prolonged hypothermia in rats. Am. J. Physiol. 255:R1035-R1040 (1988).

6. Hoo-Paris, R., Jourdan, M.L., Moreau-Hamsany, C. & Wang, L.C.H.: Plasma glucagon, glucose, and free fatty acid concentrations and secretion during prolonged hypothermia in the rat. Am. J. Physiol. 260:R480-R485 (1991).

7. McArthur, M.D., Jourdan, M.L. & Wang, L.C.H.: Prolonged stable hypothermia: effects on blood gases and pH in rats and ground squirrels. Am. J. Physiol. (submitted 1990).

8. Duncombe, W.G.: The colorimetric micro-determination of long-chain fatty acids. Biochem. J. 88:7-10 (1963).

9. Nesbakken, R.: Aspects of free fatty acid metabolism during induced hypothermia. Scand. J. Clin. Lab. Invest. 31(131):5-72 (1973).

Lomax, Schönbaum (eds.) **Thermoregulation: The Pathophysiological Basis of Clinical Disorders.**
8th International Symposium Pharmacology of Thermoregulation, Kananaskis, Alberta, Canada 1991, pp. 124-127 (Karger, Basel 1992)

CONTROVERSIAL INFLUENCES OF PEPTIDES ON AVA AND CAPILLARY BLOOD FLOW IN THE SHEEP LIMB

K.C. MOGG[1], J.R.S. HALES[2], A.A. FAWCETT[3] and C.C. POLLITT[4]

[1]NSW Department of Agriculture & Fisheries, P.O. Box K220, Haymarket, NSW 2000 (Australia), [2]School of Physiology & Pharmacology, University of New South Wales, Kensington, NSW 2033 (Australia), [3]C.S.I.R.O., Ian Clunies Ross Animal Research Laboratory, Prospect, NSW 2149 (Australia) and [4]C.A.M.S., University of Queensland, St. Lucia, Queensland 4067 (Australia)

For body temperature regulation it is essential that skin blood flow (BF) be varied markedly, sometimes including changes in the partition of total BF between capillaries and arteriovenous anastomoses (AVAs) [1]. Adrenergically mediated variations in skin vasoconstrictor tone, particularly of AVAs, are known [2,3] and non-adrenergic, non-cholinergic mechanisms have been demonstrated [see 4]. However, although electron microscope and immunocytochemical techniques have identified vasoactive peptides in the walls of AVAs [see 4], the recent focus of attention on these transmitters or cotransmitters [5] does not appear to have included their possible influences on BF through skin AVAs. Also, few if any studies, besides those on humans, have involved conscious animals.

The present study represents pilot observations in conscious sheep, employing one dose level for each of three well known vasodilator peptides, viz., substance P (SP), calcitonin gene related peptide (CGRP) and vasoactive intestinal polypeptide (VIP); the α-adrenergic receptor antagonist, phentolamine, was also tested.

METHODS: Probes for continually monitoring total BF by an ultrasonic transit time method were implanted chronically on each femoral artery. Catheters were implanted in an external jugular vein and in the pulmonary and each femoral artery for drug administration and radioactive microsphere measurements. By simultaneously injecting a dose of microspheres into a femoral artery and another dose bearing a different nuclide label into a jugular vein, while sampling from the pulmonary artery and monitoring total femoral BF, measurements were obtained of total limb BF passing through AVAs and skin capillary BF in the areas under the TPM probes [6]. The sheep stood in a climatic room with dry bulb temperature adjusted to 13-18°C so that metatarsal skin surface temperature indicated slight skin vasoconstriction. Two TPM probes were mounted on the lateral limb surface at about the midpoint of the metatarsus to provide an index of changes in local skin BF called the "Tissue Perfusion Index" (TPI). Although this instrument has not been fully evaluated, it is designed to measure only the pulsatile portion and to discard the non-pulsatile portion of the BF; it exhibits an excellent correlation with microsphere measurements of skin capillary BF [6] and unpublished data indicate that it is also sensitive to BF through AVAs and therefore provides an index of total local skin BF.

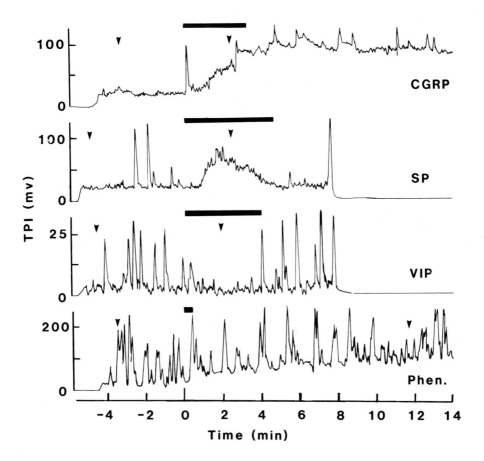

FIGURE 1: Example effects of the four drugs tested on the Tissue Perfusion Index (TPI) of BF in metatarsal skin of conscious sheep. Black bar indicates period of drug administration. First arrow indicates "control" and second, the "drug" injection of microspheres. Outstanding spikes are movement artefacts. Near the start and/or end of observations, the TPM was switched to check zero.

When the total femoral BF and local TPI were stable, control microsphere measurements were made; the drug was then administered i.a. and when femoral BF or TPI showed a distinct change or at a time based on published responses (if there was no clear change in our parameters), the "drug" microsphere measurements were made.

Drugs were: CGRP, rat sequence, 300 pmol/min for approx. 5 min; SP, 2 pmol/min for approx. 5 min; VIP, porcine sequence, 300 pmol/min for approx. 5 min; phentolamine mesylate, 10 mg bolus; we tried to use the maximum doses with minimal effect on blood pressure.

RESULTS & DISCUSSION: Example records of TPI are given in Fig. 1 and data representing relative changes in the measured parameters are summarized in Table I. The peptides were tested in one leg of each of 5, and phentolamine of 4 sheep.

TABLE I: **Relative effects of the four drugs tested**

	MAP	Total Femoral BF	Total Limb AVA BF	Skin Capillary BF	TPI
CGRP	↓?	↑↑	↑↑↑	↑?	↑↑↑
SP	0	0	↓?	↓?	↑↑↑
VIP	0	↑?	*	↓	0
Phen.	↓?	↑	↑↑↑	↓	↑↑

↑, increase; ↓, decrease; 0, no change; ? these limited data indicate a small, insignificant change; *see text re. VIP.

The three peptides tested are regarded as potent dilators of the vasculature of many animal and human tissues [5,7]. Thus, the CGRP-induced increases in total femoral BF and in local skin TPI were expected, however, our microsphere data further demonstrate a marked preferential partition of the increased BF through AVAs with little or no increase in capillary perfusion.

SP is a very widely studied vasodilator peptide and was expected to increase skin BF according to venous occlusion plethysmography and venous oxyhaemoglobin saturation measurements in the human forearm [8] and venous outflow measurements in the anaesthetized dog's paw [9]. Therefore, our data are contradictory in finding no change in total femoral, total limb AVA and skin capillary BF. The sole effect of SP is noteworthy, viz., a marked although transient increase in TPI; had we not been using the recently developed TPM, a complete lack of any detectable effect of SP would have been concluded. The half-life of SP effects appears to be only about 15 sec [10] and therefore it might be suggested that our microsphere measurements missed such effects. However, the "drug" microsphere injection illustrated in Fig. 1 was clearly during the local TPI increase even though the peak had passed. Two possible explanations for the SP-induced increase in TPI with no change in any of the other BF parameters are: (a) there was an increase in local AVA BF, detected by the TPM but not by local microspheres, which was completely negated in the microsphere measurement of total limb AVA BF by decreased AVA BF elsewhere in the limb; (b) there was an increase in the pulsatile component of local skin capillary BF (the component detected by the TPM), which was offset by an equal decrease in the non-pulsatile component, resulting in unchanged local skin capillary BF as measured by the microspheres.

The absence of any clear vasodilator effects of VIP is unexpected in view of the marked vasodilatory action found for tissues previously studied [see 5]. We are unaware of any reports for skin, for which the present study demonstrated a small but consistent (to 23-78%) decrease in capillary BF. The effect of VIP on total limb AVA BF was highly variable, i.e., two decreased, two increased and one remained unchanged. This was our only test substance which had no effect on TPI.

Phentolamine is well known to be an extremely potent dilator of limb AVAs [2,3] and was included in the present study principally to confirm the validity of methods in view of the number of unexpected results yielded by the peptides. Further, the marked increase in TPI while capillary BF decreased slightly, demonstrates that the TPM is sensitive to BF through AVAs.

In conclusion, the present data indicate the possibility of major effects of CGRP and SP (but not VIP) on skin BF. However, discrepancies with previous work point to the need for cautious interpretation of results in view of the variation in data obtained by different methods to measure different aspects of BF, and also species and tissue differences in responses. The vasodilator effects observed in other *in vivo* studies were associated with decreased arterial pressure and therefore the general absence of this in the present study may indicate that our dose levels chosen to be the maximum which would not evoke general systemic or central effects were too low to elicit responses comparable with those other studies.

ACKNOWLEDGEMENTS: This work was partly supported by the Queensland Equine Research Foundation.

REFERENCES

1. Johnson, J.M., Brengelmann, G.L., Hales, J.R.S., Vanhoutte, P.M. & Wenger, C.B.: Regulation of the cutaneous circulation. Fed. Proc. **45**:2841-2850 (1986).
2. Spence, R.J., Rhodes, B.A. & Wagner, H.N., Jr.: Regulation of arteriovenous anastomotic and capillary blood flow in the dog leg. Am. J. Physiol. **222**:326-332 (1972).
3. Hales, J.R.S., Foldes, A., Fawcett, A.A. & King, R.B.: The role of adrenergic mechanisms in thermoregulatory control of blood flow through capillaries and arteriovenous anastomoses in the sheep hind limb. Pflügers Arch. **395**:93-98 (1982).
4. Hales, J.R.S. & Molyneux, G.S.: Control of cutaneous arteriovenous anastomoses. In Vanhoutte, *Vasodilatation: Vascular Smooth Muscle, Peptides, Autonomic Nerves and Endothelium*, pp. 321-332 (Raven Press, New York 1988).
5. Owman, C., Hanko, J., Hardebo, J.E. & Kåhrström, J.: Neuropeptides and classical autonomic transmitters in the cardiovascular system: Existence, coexistence, action, interaction. In Christensen, Henriksen & Lassen, *The Sympatho-adrenal System*, Alfred Benzon Symposium 23, pp. 340-383 (Munksgaard, Copenhagen 1986).
6. Hales, J.R.S., Stephens, F.R.N., Fawcett, A.A., Daniel, K., Sheahan, J., Westerman, R.A. & James, S.B.: Observations on a new non-invasive monitor of skin blood flow. Clin. Exp. Pharm. Physiol. **16**:403-415 (1989).
7. Euler, U.S. von and Pernow, B. (Eds.): *Substance P* (Raven Press, New York 1977).
8. Löfström, E., Pernow, B. & Wahren, J.: Vasodilating action of substance P in the human forearm. Acta Physiol. Scand. **63**:311-324 (1965).
9. Burcher, E., Atterhög, J-H., Pernow, B. & Rosell, S.: Cardiovascular effects of substance P: Effects on the heart and regional blood flow in the dog. In Euler and Pernow, *Substance P*, pp. 261-268 (Raven Press, New York 1977).
10. McEwan, J.R., Benjamin, N., Larkin, S., Fuller, R.W., Dollery, C.T., MacIntyre, I. & Path, F.R.C.: Vasodilation by calcitonin gene-related peptide and by substance P: A comparison of their effects on resistance and capacitance vessels of human forearms. Circulation **77**:1072-1080 (1988).

Lomax, Schönbaum (eds.) **Thermoregulation: The Pathophysiological Basis of Clinical Disorders.**
8th International Symposium Pharmacology of Thermoregulation, Kananaskis, Alberta, Canada 1991, pp. 128-132 (Karger, Basel 1992)

INVOLVEMENT OF BROWN ADIPOSE TISSUE IN THERMOGENIC RESPONSE TO TRH IN MONOSODIUM GLUTAMATE TREATED MICE

TERUKO NOMOTO, YOKO UCHIDA and YOSHIE SHIBATA

Department of Pharmacology, Tokyo Women's Medical College, Tokyo 162 (Japan)

Thyrotropin releasing hormone (TRH), the first hypothalamic hormone identified, affects thermoregulation in many species [1-3]. Previous studies have shown that TRH induced hyperthermia in mice is abolished by hypophysectomy [4]. In a subsequent study, wet weights of brown adipose tissue (BAT) were decreased by 50-60% in hypophysectomized mice as compared with control mice.

BAT has a role in both heat production of non-shivering thermogenesis [5] and the regulation of energy balance in states of diet-induced thermogenesis [6]. BAT thermogenesis is regulated primarily by the sympathetic nervous system in response to cold or diet [5]. It has been shown that defective control of BAT thermogenesis results in obesity [7,8]. However, the thermogenic response of BAT to a cafeteria diet is known to be normal in mice with monosodium glutamate (MSG) induced obesity [6]. The present study was designed to examine whether BAT thermogenesis, as well as the sympathetic nervous system, in mice with MSG induced obesity, are influenced by TRH administration.

METHODS: ICR strain male mice were used for these experiments. The 180 mice were divided into three groups: group 1 received saline injections (control); groups 2 and 3 were injected with MSG (2 or 4 mg/g sc) on alternate days for the first 10 days after birth (MSG 2 and MSG 4). They were maintained in an air-conditioned animal room at 23°C and were weaned at 28 days of age. Drugs used were: TRH (pGlu-His-ProNH$_2$) and MSG (monosodium-L-glutamate). The drugs were dissolved in physiological saline and injected ip except MSG. At 9 weeks of age, each of the three groups was divided into three groups which were injected with either saline (0.1 ml/10 g ip) or TRH (10 or 30 mg/kg ip).

The core temperature (T_r) was measured with a thermocouple probe inserted 2 cm into the rectum. T_r were measured just before TRH of saline administration and every 15 min for 1 h thereafter. Blood samples were collected from the jugular vein 5 min after TRH or saline administration under light ether anesthesia and centrifuged at 3,000 x g. The plasma was stored at -20°C until catecholamine measurement, using HPLC with an electrochemical detector according to the method of Mefford [9].

To analyze the results statistically, Student's t-test was used.

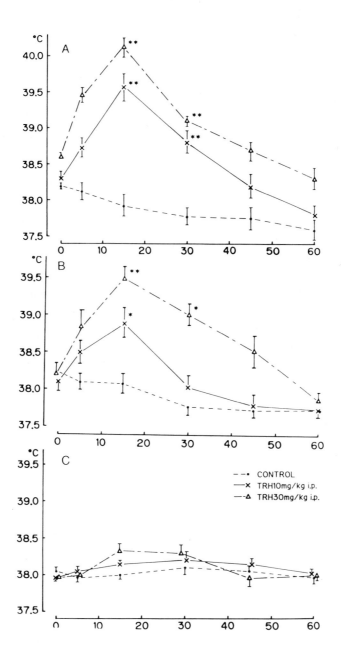

FIGURE 1: Time course (min) of the rectal temperature change (°C) produced by injection of (0) saline, (X) TRH (10 mg/kg) and (Δ) TRH (30 mg/kg) in mice neonatally pretreated by saline (A), MSG 2 mg/g (B) and MSG 4 mg/kg (C). Each point represents the mean of 9 to 12 mice, the vertical line indicating the S.E.M. *P < 0.05; **P < 0.01 vs. saline treated mice (Student's t-test)

RESULTS: The effects of the two doses of TRH (10 or 30 mg/5 ml/kg ip) and saline on T_r were investigated in the three groups. Fig. 1-A shows the effects of saline and TRH (10 or 30 mg/kg ip) on T_r in control mice. A significant, dose-dependent rise in T_r was observed 15 min after TRH administration: 1.5°C with TRH (30 mg/kg) and 1.2°C with TRH (10 mg/kg). Fig. 1-B shows the effects of TRH induced hyperthermia in MSG 2 mice. The greatest change was observed 15 min after administration, as in controls. Thus, peak responses to TRH (10 or 30 mg/kg) were lower than in controls, but not significantly so. However, as Fig. 1-C shows, there was no change nor any appreciable thermogenic effect observed in MSG 4 mice. In addition, these results demonstrated no difference between the hyperthermic effects of the two doses of TRH.

As for plasma catecholamines, there was no significant difference in the basal level of either norepinephrine (NE) or epinephrine (E) among the three groups examined. Neither was there any significant difference between controls and MSG 4 after TRH administration. However, all MSG 2 mice has higher plasma concentrations of E than NE.

DISCUSSION: It was well known that BAT is a site of thermogenesis. The key element in BAT heat production is the capacity of the abundant mitochondria of this tissue to increase respiration. A unique uncoupling protein (UCP) or thermogenin is present in the inner membrane of BAT mitochondria. The UCP increase rapidly following NE or cold exposure in intact animals, which is accounted for by a proportional increment in UCP mRNA [10,11].

In this study, TRH injection (30 mg/kg ip) induced hyperthermia in control mice (40.1 ± 0.12°C), the MSG 2 mice (39.5 ± 0.15°C) and the MSG 4 mice (38.3 ± 0.10°C), in decreasing order. However, as shown in Fig. 2, plasma catecholamine levels were not significantly different, after TRH administration, among the three groups examined. These results indicate that TRH induced hyperthermia depends on BAT induced thermogenic activity.

The administration of MSG to mice in the neonatal period induces destructive lesions in the arcuate and ventromedial nuclei of the hypothalamus, resulting in an obesity syndrome and diminished oxygen consumption with less locomotor activity [12]. On the other hand, the sympathetic nervous system activity in interscapular BAT of MSG mice was significantly lower than in control mice [13]. Since the protein content in BAT mitochondria in MSG treated mice was lower than in the control mice, the heavier BAT weight in MSG treated mice increased plasma NE and E after injection of TRH.

The present study indicates enhanced BAT thermogenesis in control and MSG 2 mice after TRH administration. However, MSG 4 mice showed no change in thermoregulation, other than an increase in plasma catecholamines, after TRH administration. This indicates an impaired TRH induced response, although the exact mechanisms are not presently clear.

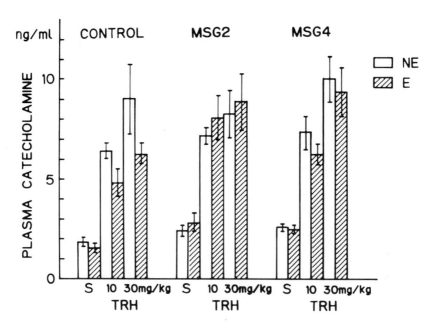

FIGURE 2: Effects of TRH (10 or 30 mg/kg ip) on plasma catecholamine (ng/ml). Each column represents the mean of 6 to 10 samples; vertical lines show the S.E.M.

REFERENCES

1. Boschi, G. & Rips, R.: Tyrotropin releasing hormone (TRH) induced hyperthermia and its potentiation in the mouse: peripheral or central origin. IRCS Med. Sci. **9**:200-201 (1981).
2. Horita, A., Carino, M.A. & Lai, H.: Pharmacology of thyrotropin-releasing hormone. Ann. Rev. Pharmacol. Toxicol. **26**:311-332 (1986).
3. Clark, W.G. & Lipton, J.M.: Brain and pituitary peptides in thermoregulation. Pharmac. Ther. **22**:249-297 (1983).
4. Nomoto, T., Uchida, Y. Boschi, G. & Rips, R.: Thyroid hormone involvement in TRH induced hyperthermia in mice with various thyroid states. In Lomax & Schönbaum, *Thermoregulation: Research adn Clinical Applications*, pp. 152-155 (Karger, Basel 1986).
5. Foster, D.O. & Frydman, M.L.: Nonshivering thermogenesis in the rat. I. Measurements of blood flow with microspheres point to brown adipose tissue as the dominant site of calorigenesis induced by noradrenaline. Can. J. Physiol. Pharmacol. **56**:110-122 (1978).
6. Rothwell, N.J. & Stock, M.J.: A role for brown adipose tissue in diet-induced thermogenesis. Nature **281**:31-35 (1979).
7. Moss, D., Ma, A. & Cameron, D.P.: Defective thermoregulatory thermogenesis in monosodium glutamate-induced obesity in mice. Metabolism **34**:626-630 (1985).
8. Duloo, A.G. & Miller, D.S.: Unimpaired thermogenic response to noradrenaline in genetic (ob/ob) and hypothalamic (MSG) obese mice. Bioscience Reports **4**:343-349 (1984).

9. Mefford, I.N., Ward, M.M., Miles, L., Taylor, B., Chesney, M.A., Keegan, D.L. & Barchas, J.D.: Determination fo plasma catecholamines and free 3,4-dihydroxyphenylacetic acid in continuously collected human plasma by high performance liquid chromatography with electrochemical detection. Life Sci. **20:**477-483 (1981).

10. Silva, J.E.: Full expression of uncoupling protein gene requires the concurrence of norepinephrine and triiodothyronine. Mol. Endocrinol. **2:**706-713 (1988).

11. Bianco, A.C., Sheng, X. & Silva, J.E.: Triiodothyronine amplifies norepinephrine stimulation of uncoupling protein gene transcription by a mechanism not requiring protein synthesis. J. Biol. Chem. **263:**18168-18175 (1988).

12. Dawson, R. Jr. & Lordon, J.F.: Behavioral and neurochemical effects of neonatal administration of monosodium L-glutamate in mice. J. Comp. Physiol. Psychol. **95:**71-84 (1981).

13. Yoshida, T., Nishioka, H., Nakamura, Y. & Kondo, M.: Reduced norepinephrine turnover in mice with monosodium glutamate-induced obesity. Metabolism **33:**1060-1063 (1984).

Lomax, Schönbaum (eds.) **Thermoregulation: The Pathophysiological Basis of Clinical Disorders.**
8th International Symposium Pharmacology of Thermoregulation, Kananaskis, Alberta, Canada 1991, pp. 133-137 (Karger, Basel 1992)

LOWER ENVIRONMENTAL TEMPERATURE INDUCED REGULATION OF BODY TEMPERATURE: INVOLVEMENT OF GABAERGIC DOPAMINERGIC INTERACTION

SUCHANDRA BISWAS and MRINAL K. PODDAR

Department of Biochemistry, University of Calcutta, 35 Ballygunge Circular Road, Calcutta 700 019 (India)

Homeotherms can maintain body temperature (BT) at a fairly constant value despite variations in the environmental temperature by *in situ* thermoregulatory centre, located in the hypothalamic nuclei of the brain, through the regulation of heat production and heat loss [1-4]. Constant control of BT is regulated by central cholinergic, dopaminergic or serotonergic systems [5-8]. Many drugs are also known to interfere with the temperature regulation [9-11]. The hypothalamus contains high amounts of γ-aminobutyric acid (GABA) and its synthesizing enzyme glutamate decarboxylase [12].

It is not unlikely that GABA may play a role in thermoregulation. Intraventricular, intracisternal or intraperitoneal injection of GABA to conscious rat alters BT [11,13,14]. The reduced oxygen consumption and rectal temperature caused by injection of GABA into the preoptic-anterior hypothalamus of cats [15] are consistent with an inhibitory role for GABA. GABA induced hypothermia is antagonized by pretreatment with atropine [11] suggesting that GABA induced hypothermia may be mediated partly by ACh release. Thus, interaction of GABA with other neurons may play an important role in thermoregulation. Recently, we have shown that GABA acts through the cholinergic system during thermoregulation at high ambient temperatures [16]. Further, it has been observed [17,18] that exposure to low environmental temperatures (LET) produces a region specific changes in GABAergic activity in mammalian brain. This information led to a study of the interaction between GABA and cholinergic or dopaminergic neurons in the regulation of BT at low ambient temperature.

METHODS: Adult male albino rats (body weight 120-130 g) of Charles Foster strain were kept in 12 h light - 12 h dark cycle at room temperature ($28 \pm 1°C$) with constant relative humidity ($80 \pm 5\%$) and were maintained on standard laboratory diet and water *ad libitum*. Experiments were carried out between 10:30 h and 12:30 h.

Physostigmine, muscimol, haloperidol and atropine sulfate were solubilized in distilled water. Bicuculline was dissolved in HCl (0.01 N). L-DOPA and carbidopa were suspended in distilled water and were given orally. All other drugs were administered intraperitoneally.

Animals were divided into different groups of 6 animals each. Rats of group 1-16 were kept at room temperature ($28 \pm 1°C$) and were administered saline or drugs viz, bicuculline (1 mg/kg ip); muscimol (1 mg/kg ip); L-DOPA (100 mg/kg po) + carbidopa (10 mg/kg po); haloperidol (1 mg/kg ip); physostigmine (0.2 mg/kg ip); atropine (5 mg/kg ip); L-DOPA + carbidopa + bicuculline or muscimol or physostigmine; muscimol + haloperidol or atropine; bicuculline + haloperidol or physostigmine or atropine; haloperidol + physostigmine. The animals of group 17-32 were exposed to LET (12 $\pm$ 0.5°C) in a cold chamber with controlled ventilation at a fixed relative humidity (80 $\pm$ 5%) for 2 h and received saline or drugs(s) at their respective dose(s) through the same route. Bicuculline, muscimol, atropine, haloperidol were injected 30 min, L-DOPA + carbidopa 1 h, physostigmine 15 min, before measurement of rectal temperature of rats exposed to either 38°C or 12°C.

Rectal temperature was recorded with a thermister probe inserted 2 cm into the rectum of normal and LET-exposed rats. The rectal temperature of LET exposed rats was measured at the end of the 2nd hour of exposure.

The statistical significance between two mean values was assessd by two-tailed student 't' test.

RESULTS: Table I shows that exposure of rats to LET (12°C) did not significantly alter the BT as compared to that of normal rats kept at room temperature (28°C). Treatment with bicuculline (1 mg/kg ip) enhanced, while muscimol (1 mg/kg ip) reduced BT of both control and LET exposed rats. The muscimol induced decrease or bicuculline induced increase in BT of cold exposed rat was comparatively smaller than that observed in control rats kept at 28°C treated under similar conditions. L-DOPA (100 mg/kg po) + carbidopa (10 mg/kg po) produced slight hypothermia in control rats kept at 28°C, but enhanced BT of cold exposed rat. Haloperidol (1 mg/kg ip), on the other hand, reduced BT of cold exposed rats. Treatment with physostigmine (0.2 mg/kg ip) enhanced, while atropine (5 mg/kg ip) reduced BT of control rats kept at 28°C. These drugs did not significantly alter BT of rats exposed to 12°C. Table I also shows that muscimol or haloperidol induced decrease in BT of LET exposed rats was further reduced when both of these drugs were coadministered to LET exposed rats. Muscimol induced hypothermia in normal rats kept at room temperature was absent following treatment with haloperidol. The bicuculline or L-DOPA + carbidopa induced rise in BT of rats exposed to 12°C was increased when bicuculline and L-DOPA + carbidopa were coadministered under similar condition. Bicuculline induced hypothermia in normal rat kept at 28°C was attenuated by treatment with L-DOPA + carbidopa. Table I shows that the muscimol induced reduction and the L-DOPA + carbidopa induced enhancement of BT of cold exposed rat was prevented when both these durgs were coadministered in rat exposed to 12°C. Moreover, the bicuculline induced enhancement or the haloperidol induced reduction in BT of cold exposed rats was prevented when bicuculline and haloperidol were administered under similar conditions. At 28°C bicuculline induced hyperthermia was potentiated following cotreatment with haloperidol. It is noted that the L-DOPA + carbidopa or bicuculline or haloperidol induced change in BT of cold exposed rats was not significantly altered following treatment with physostigmine. Similarly atropine did not significantly change the muscimol or bicuculline induced change in BT of rat exposed to 12°C.

DISCUSSION: The studies show that exposure to 12°C does not alter significantly BT of normal rats maintained at 28°C. Bicuculline increases while muscimol reduces BT of normal and cold exposed rats indicating that inactivation of GABA receptor enhances, whereas activation reduces BT of normal and cold exposed rat. Muscimol induced reduction of rectal temperature suggests an inhibitory role of GABA in thermoregulation. This is in accord to the findings of Bligh [12] who suggested that GABA agonists reduce heat production and lowers rectal temperature at low ambient temperatures. Further, it is noted that the muscimol induced decrease or bicuculline-induced increase in BT of cold exposed rats is comparatively small compared to control rats kept at 28°C, indicating that inactivation of GABA receptors may prevent lowering of BT during cold exposure. Recently, we have reported that exposure of rats to 12°C for 2 h inhibits hypothalamic GABAergic activity [17]. Thus, it could be assumed that inhibition of GABA at 12°C may abolish the inhibitory role of GABA and prevent the decrease in heat production.

TABLE I: Effect of lower environmental temperature on rectal temperature of rats treated with agonists and antagonists of GABAergic, dopaminergic and cholinergic systems

Treatment(s)	Rectal Temperaure (°C) at	
	28°C	12°C
Control (Saline)*	36.2 ± 0.14	36.0 ± 0.10
Bicuculline	37.3 ± 0.20^{2}	36.9 ± 0.15^{4}
Muscimol	35.1 ± 0.10^{2}	$35.5 \pm 0.13^{4,6}$
L-DOPA + Carbidopa	35.7 ± 0.17^{3}	$36.6 \pm 0.15^{4,7}$
Haloperidol	36.6 ± 0.19	$35.6 \pm 0.15^{4,6}$
Physostigmine	37.1 ± 0.20^{2}	36.0 ± 0.18^{4}
Atropine	35.5 ± 0.15^{2}	35.8 ± 0.15
L-DOPA + Carbidopa + Bicuculline	$36.7 \pm 0.15^{3,8}$	$37.3 \pm 0.19^{5,13}$
Muscimol + Haloperidol	36.0 ± 0.15	$35.2 \pm 0.10^{4,5,11,12}$
L-DOPA + Carbidopa + Muscimiol	35.7 ± 0.15^{3}	$35.9 \pm 0.12^{4,11,13}$
Bicuculline + Haloperidol	37.6 ± 0.18^{1}	$36.2 \pm 0.13^{4,12}$
Muscimol + Atropine	35.1 ± 0.18^{1}	35.3 ± 0.12^{5}
L-DOPA + Carbidopa + Physostigmine	$36.4 \pm 0.20^{1,9}$	36.5 ± 0.14^{6}
Haloperidol + Physostigmine	$37.5 \pm 0.13^{1,13}$	$35.6 \pm 0.13^{3,4}$
Bicuculline + Physostigmine	$37.9 \pm 0.20^{1,9}$	$36.8 \pm 0.13^{4,5,9}$
Bicuculline + Atropine	$36.5 \pm 0.25^{8,10}$	$36.5 \pm 0.12^{6,10}$

Results are expressed as mean $\pm$ SEM, n = 6.
*No significant change was observed in rectal temperature when control rats were treated with saline (0.89% NaCl) either ip or po.
Significantly different from control at 28°C: [1]$p < 0.001$; [2]$p < 0.01$; [3]$p < 0.05$.
Corresponding drug treatment at 28°C: [4]$p < 0.02$.
Control at 12°C: [5]$p < 0.001$; [6]$p < 0.01$; [7]$p < 0.05$; bicuculline [8]p K 0.01; physostigmine [9]$p < 0.05$; atropine [10]$p < 0.02$; muscimol [11]$p < 0.01$; haloperidol [12]$p < 0.05$; L-DOPA + carbidopa [13]$p < 0.05$.

The increase in BT with L-DOPA + carbidopa and the lowering of BT after haloperidol in cold exposed rats suggest that a dopaminergic system is involved in thermoregulation during cold exposure. Bicuculline or L-DOPA + carbidopa induced increases in BT of cold exposed rats is potentiated when bicuculline and L-DOPA + carbidopa are coadministered. Moreover, the muscimol or haloperidol induced fall in BT of cold exposed rats is reduced when both of these drugs are administered. These results suggest that inhibition of GABA activates the dopaminergic system and regulates BT of cold exposed rats. Further, L-DOPA + carbidopa induced increases in BT in cold exposed rats is absent in muscimol treated animals indicating that although activation of dopaminergic systems raises BT in cold exposed rats, simultaneous treatment with muscimol inhibits the dopaminergic activation and prevents L-DOPA + carbidopa induced hyperthermia in cold exposed rats. Prevention of the haloperidol induced fall in BT of cold exposed rats by coadministration of bicuculline (Table I) suggests that inhibition of GABAergic systems prevents the haloperidol induced hypothermia in cold exposed rat. Activation of dopaminergic systems may be mediated through inhibition of GABA [19] in the cold exposed rats. No significant changes in BT of muscimol (or bicuculline or haloperidol or L-DOPA + carbidopa) treated rats exposed to 12°C followed cotreatment with physostigmine or atropine suggesting that cholinergic system is not involved.

It has been reported that exposure to cold activates the thyroid gland and stimulates thyrotrophin secretion [20]. Thyrotrophin is known to increase basal metabolic rate and energy production [21]. The inhibition of hypothalamic GABAergic activity [17] during exposure to 12°C may be correlated with inactivation of hypothalamic GABA receptors and stimulation of thyrotrophin secretion [22]. This may be one of the mechanisms of protection against hypothermia due to cold exposure. Thyrotrophin induced potentiation of the calorigenic action of catecholamines [22] may also be considered as another possible reason to maintain normal BT during cold exposure.

In conclusion, exposure of rats to 12° for 2 h does not significantly alter BT. Short term LET exposure activates central DA through inhibition of central GABAergic systems and prevents the lowering of BT by facilitating heat production or by reducing heat loss.

ACKNOWLEDGEMENTS: Present work was supported by Indian Council of Medical Research, New Delhi, India.

REFERENCES

1. Blatteis, C.M.: Hypothalamic substances in the control of body temperature: general characteristics. Fed. Proc. **40:**2731-2740 (1981).
2. Crawshaw, L.I.: Temperature regulation in vertebrates. Ann. Rev. Physiol. **42:**473-491 (1980).
3. Siesjo, B.K.: Hypothermia and hyperthermia. In Siesjo, *Brain Energy Metabolism*, pp. 324-344 (Wiley and Sons, New York 1978).
4. Stolwijk, J.J. & Hardy, J.D.: Control of body temperature. In Lee, *Handbook of Physiology, Section 9. Reactions to Environmental Agents* (Am. Physiol. Soc., Bethesda, Maryland 1977).
5. Lipton, J.M. & Clark, W.G.: Neurotransmitters in temperature control. Ann. Rev. Physiol. **48:**a613-623 (1986).
6. Young, A. & Dawson, N.J.: Effect of environmental temperature on the development of a noradrenergic thermoregulatory mechanism in the rat. Pflu. Arch. Eur. J. **412:**141-146 (1988).
7. Beckman, A.L. & Carlisle, H.J.: Effect of intrahypothalamic infusion of acetylcholine on behavioral and physiological thermoregulation in the rat. Nature **221:**561-562 (1969).
8. Minano, F.J., Sancibrian, M. & Serrano, J.S.: Hypothermic effect of GABA in conscious stressed rats: Its modification by cholinergic agonists and antagonists. J. Pharm. Pharmacol. **39:**721-726 (1987).
9. Lomax, P.: Drugs and body temperaure. Int. Rev. Neurobiol. **12:**1-43 (1970).
10. Weihe, W.H.: The effect of temperature on the action of drugs. Ann. Rev. Pharmacol. **13:**409-425 (1973).
11. Cox, B. & Lomax, P.: Pharmacologic control of temperature regulation. Ann. Rev. Pharmacol. Toxicol. **17:**341-353 (1977).
12. Cox, B., Ary, M. & Lomax, P.: Dopaminergic involvement in withdrawal hypothermia and thermoregulatory behavior in morphine dependents rat. Pharmacol. Biochem. Behav. **4:**259-262 (1976).
13. Bligh, J.: Aminoacids as central synaptic transmitters or modulators in mammalian thermoregulation. Fed. Proc. **40:**2746-2749 (1981).

14. Dhumal, V.R., Gulati, O.D. & Nandkumar, S.S.: Effects on rectal temperature in rats of γ-aminobutyric acid: Possible mediation through putative transmitters. Eur. J. Pharmacol. **35**:341-347 (1976).

15. Squires, R.D.: Thermoregulatory effects of injections of γ-aminobutyric acid (GABA) and picrotoxin into medial preoptic region of cats. Fed. Proc. **26**:555 (abstr.) (1967).

16. Biswas, S. & Poddar, M.K.: Does GABA act through dopaminergic/cholinergic interaction in the regulation of higher environmental tempreature-induced change in body temperature? Meth. Find. Exp. Clin. Pharmacol. **12**:303-307 (1990).

17. Biswas, S. & Poddar, M.K.: Effect of short- and long-term exposures to low environmental temperature on brain regional GABA metabolism. Neurochem. Res. **15**:821-826 (1990).

18. Otero Losada, M.E.: Changes in central GABAergic function following acute and repeated stress. Brit. J. Pharmacol. **93**:483-490 (1988).

19. Ladinsky, H., Consolo, S., Bianchi, S. & Jori, A.: Increase in striatal acetylcholine by picrotoxin in the rat: Evidence for a GABAergic-dopaminergic-cholinergic link. Brain Res. **108**:351-361 (1976).

20. Lin, M.T., Wang, P.S., Chuang, J., Fan, L.J. & Won, S.J.: Cold stress or a pyrogenic substance elevates thyrotropin releasing hormone levels in the rat hypothalamus and induces thermogenic reactions. Neuroendocrinology **50**:177-181 (1989).

21. West J.B.: Visceral control mechanism. In Best & Taylor, *Physiological Basis of Medical Practice*, pp. 1211-1234 (Williams and Wilkins, London 1985).

22. Norizzano, O.C., Karora, A., Rettori, V., Ponzio, R. & McCann, S.M.: GABAergic control of TSH secretion: Effect of bicuculline injected in the median preoptic area and the arcuate nucleus on the release of TSH in the rat. Commun. Biol. **6**:383-392 (1988).

Lomax, Schönbaum (eds.) **Thermoregulation: The Pathophysiological Basis of Clinical Disorders.**
8th International Symposium Pharmacology of Thermoregulation, Kananaskis, Alberta, Canada 1991, pp. 138-142 (Karger, Basel 1992)

THE Cl-CHANNEL OF THE INNER MITOCHONDRIAL MEMBRANE OF BROWN ADIPOCYTES CAN BE BLOCKED BY PURINE DI- AND TRINUCLEOTIDES

DETLEF SIEMEN[1] and THOMAS KLITSCH[2]

[1]Institut für Zoologie, Universität Regensburg, Postfach 397, D-8400, Regensburg (Germany) and [2]Physiologisches Instutut, Justus-Liebig-Universität, Aulweg 129, D-6300 Giessen (Germany)

In many small mammals, especially in hibernators, brown adipose tissue is the main site of nonshivering thermogenesis. It is located in the scapular and cervical region, along the aorta and around the kidneys and is innervated by noradrenergic sympathetic nerve endings. Noradrenaline (NA) stimulation of β-receptors leads to lipolysis via cAMP as a 2nd messenger. Free fatty acids activate a 32 kDal-protein (uncoupling protein, UCP) in the inner mitochondrial membrane. It can be blocked by purine di- or trinucleotides (ATP, ADP, GTP, GDP) in the absence of free fatty acids. UCP works as a proton shunt, short circuiting ATP synthesis. Thus, the respiratory chain works with zero efficiency, continuously producing heat [see 1]. Our aim was to test whether the UCP mediated currents are big enough to show up as single channel events in current recordings of the inner mitochondrial membrane.

METHODS: Interscapular and cervical brown adipose tissue were dissected from 6-8 week old male Sprague-Dawley rats, kept at room temperature and fed *ad libitum*. Preparation of brown adipocyte mitochondria was as described by Cannon and Nedergaard [3]. Stored on ice the mitochondria could be used for up to 36 h.

In order to remove the outer membrane mitochondria were transferred to 2 ml of a hypotonic solution, and after 5-10 min 0.5 ml of a solution concentrated 5 fold was added, thus restoring isotonic conditions. During swelling the outer mitochondrial membrane breaks up and the inner membrane unfolds to give delicate vesicles, 3-5 μm in diameter, called mitoplasts. Remnants of the outer membrane still adhered to the inner membrane at one point. This spot was visible by electron microscopy and as a dark cap in phase contrast microscopy [4]. We carefully avoided approaching the mitoplasts with the patch pipette from the cap side. If it did nevertheless occur there was a high probability of recording the large voltage dependent anion channel (VDAC) which is thought to be present only in the outer membrane. Due to practical considerations it was impossible to form patches with the mitoplasts at the bottom of the experimental chamber. Therefore we caught them by gentle suction close to the bottom of the chamber when they were still slowly sinking. Techniques of patch clamp were used as described by Hamill *et al.* [5]. Pipettes had a resistance of 15-35 MΩ. Further details are given elsewhere [2,6].

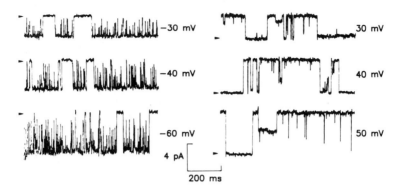

FIGURE 1: Current traces from the mitochondrial inner membrane of rat brown adipocytes. Mitoplast attached recording with KCl solution in bath and pipette. Levels at which the channel was closed are indicated by arrowheads. Potential was kept at +40 mV before the records at negative potentials were made in order to remove voltage-dependent deactivation of the channels. Occasional events with smaller amplitude presumably indicate substates of the Cl⁻ channel as they are frequently reached from the open state, 21°C.

SOLUTIONS CONTAINED (in mM): Isolation procedure: sucrose (250), K-HEPES (5), EGTA (1)g bovine serum albumine (0.1%) (BSA). Storage solution: KCl (150), K-HEPES (20), BSA (0.1%). Hypotonic solution: K-HEPES (5). Hypertonic solution: KCl (750), K-HEPES (100). Bath solution: 2 ml hypotonic solution + 0.5 ml hypertonic solution. Pipette solution: KCl (150), K-HEPES (20). pH always was 7.2.

RESULTS: Approaching the mitoplasts with the patch pipette 5-15 GΩ-seals were formed. In about one out of three patches single channel events with a conductance of 107.8 ± 8.7 pS (n, 16; 21°C) could be observed (Fig. 1). From the whole mitoplast experiments we calculated a channel density of 18.8 ± 8.1 (n, 28) channels per mitochondrion at a holding potential of +35 mV. Current-voltage relations in the mitoplast attached mode showed a straight line in isotonic KCl solution in pipette and bath. After changing the pipette solution to K gluconate, the inward currents carried by negative charge were missing thus indicating an anion channel being responsible for the current (cations were unchanged). Cl⁻ ions passed the channel better than SO_4^{2-} ions (56.3 ± 4.6 pS; n, 3). Closing of the channel was clearly voltage dependent increasing steeply at potentials more negative than 0 mV. Control measurements on mitoplasts prepared from rat liver cells showed the same type of channel.

In the mitoplast attached mode it was difficult to change the solution in the pipette as well as inside the mitoplast. Therefore the whole mitoplast mode was chosen in order to test the Cl⁻ channel for different blocking substances. We took advantage of occasional breaking of the membrane inside the rim of the pipette, leaving the GΩ seal intact. Thus it was possible to measure all channels of the "whole mitoplast" together.

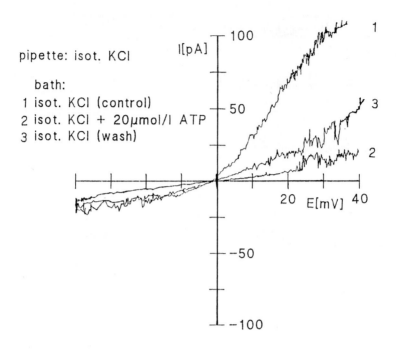

pipette: isot. KCl

bath:
1 isot. KCl (control)
2 isot. KCl + 20µmol/l ATP
3 isot. KCl (wash)

FIGURE 2: Voltage dependence of current across the mitochondrial inner membrane in the whole mitoplast mode. Almost linear part at negative voltages gives "leakage current". Assymmetrical part at positive potentials due to Cl⁻ channel. Inward flowing negative charges deflect upward. E: holding potential, I: current response, 21°C.

As a stimulus a continuous change in membrane potential was used, starting at 0 mV, increasing to +40 mV, decreasing to -40 mV, and increasing back to 0 mV within at least 2 min. These ramps had to be very slow to avoid loops of hysteresis due to time dependence of the Cl⁻ channels. Fig. 2 shows this type of experiment illustrating only the current response at changes of potential from +40 mV to -40 mV. The upper curve was measured using the normal KCl pipette solution. During the lower curve the bath contained additional 20 µM ATP and the curve in the middle represents an incomplete wash-out after 10 min. ATP (as well as ADP, GDP, and GTP) obviously blocks the assymmetrical part of the current-voltage relation, representing the Cl⁻ channel that normally turns on at positive potentials. Mean values of reduction of the assymmetrical part of the current by a 20 µM-concentration were 52.6 ± 9.1 (ATP, n, 3), 83.6 ± 7.5 (ADP, n, 3), 68.3 ± 7.2 (GTP, n, 4), and 52.9 ± 24.1 (GDP, n, 6), respectively. To our surprise GMP, considered a control, was able to block the Cl⁻ channel (81.2 ± 14.8, n, 3). cGMP or plain phosphate, however, did not.

DISCUSSION: This paper demonstrates the existence of a voltage dependent, Cl⁻ conducting anion channel in the inner mitochondrial membrane of rat brown fat and liver cells. The fact that such a channel exists in liver cells was shown by Sorgato *et al.* [4]. They discussed whether this channel could have something to do with the uncoupling protein of brown adipocyte mitochondria. They used giant mitoplasts of rats treated with the copper chelator cuprizone. As brown fat mitochondria are bigger than others, it seemed promising to test them without cuprizone. However, as a control we succeeded to show the anion channel also on untreated liver cells.

In a second attempt Sorgato *et al.* [7] tried to find a blocking substance of the channel testing 12 common blockers - without success. But the authors showed that it is insensitive to N,N'-dicyclohexylcarbodiimide (DCCD). Thus, it must not be confused with the anion uniporter found by Beavis [8]. Here we demonstrate that ATP, ADP, GTP, GDP, and GMP are able to block the anion channel in brown adipocytes. Nevertheless we do not think that this channel is identical with the UCP since (i) It is generally believed that UCP is unique to brown adipocytes [9]; the anion channel was found in liver and heart cell mitochondria [2,4,7,10]. (ii) From biochemical data of Nicholls *et al.* [9] a single channel conductance of less than 0.1 fS for one UCP was estimated, much smaller than the conductance of the channel described here. (iii) The voltage dependence of this channel shows it is active in the positive potential range, whereas nonshivering thermogenesis takes place at the negative potential range where the Cl⁻ channel normally is closed. (iv) Malan and Mioskowski [11] report a strong dependence of UCP on the pH. We did not see a pH-dependence in our experiments. (v) GMP is about 44 times less potent as a blocker of UCP than is GDP [12]. In our experiments both nucleotides had about the same potency.

It should be mentioned that there exists a model of the UCP in which proton conductance and a Cl⁻ conductance are described as two entities of the same protein [13]. However, the Cl⁻ conductance of this model was calculated to be of the same order of size as the proton conductance, i.e., in the range of fS. We thus still believe that we found a Cl⁻ channel that was previously unknown in brown adipocytes which can be blocked by purine nucleotides. It exists only in low densities and it may not be involved directly in nonshivering thermogenesis. But there is a so-called unmasking effect in brown adipocytes that appears several minutes after NA treatment or about 1 h after exposing the adipocyte to cold stress [14]. During this time an increase in GDP binding occurs without an increase in the amount of protein. At the same time the matrix volume of the mitochondria increases considerably. As one possibility the Cl⁻ channel could be involved in volume regulation during these changes of the unmasking effect.

REFERENCES

1. Nicholls, D.G. & Locke, R.M.: Thermogenic mechanisms in brown fat. Physiol. Rev. **64:**1-65 (1984).
2. Klitsch, T. & Siemen, D.: The inner mitochondrial membrane anion channel is present in brown adipocytes but is not identical with the uncoupling protein. J Membrane Biol. **122:**69-75 (1991).
3. Cannon, B. & Nedergaard, J.: Adipocytes, preadipocytes, and mitochondria from brown adipose tissue. In Hausman & Martin *Biology of the Adipocyte: Research Approaches*, pp. 21-51 (Van Nostrand Reinhold, New York 1987).
4. Sorgato, M.C., Keller, B.U. & Stühmer, W.: Patch-clamping of the inner mitochondrial membrane reveals a voltage-dependent ion channel. Nature **330:**498-500 (1987).
5. Hamill, O.P., Marty, A., Neher, E., Sakmann, B. & Sigworth, F.J.: Improved patch-clamp techniques for high resolution current recording from cells and cell-free membrane patches. Pflügers Arch. **391:**85-100 (1981).
6. Weber, A. & Siemen, D.: Permeability of the nonselective channel in brown adipocytes to small cations. Pflügers Arch. **414:**564-570 (1989).

7. Sorgato, M.C., Moran, O., de Pinto, V., Keller, B.U. & Stühmer, W.: Further investigation on the high conductive ion channel of the inner membrane of mitochondria. J. Bioenergetics Biomembranes **21:**485-496 (1989).

8. Beavis, A.D.: The mitochondrial inner-membrane anion channel possesses two mercurial-reactive regulatory sites. Eur. J. Biochem. **185:**511-519 (1989).

9. Nicholls, D.G., Cunningham, S.A. & Rial, E.: The bioenergetic mechanism of brown adipose tissue thermogenesis. In Trayhurn & Nicholls *Brown Adipose Tissue*, pp. 52-85 (Edward Arnolds, London 1986).

10. Kinnally , K.W., Campo, M.L. & Tedeschi, H.: Mitochondrial channel activity studied by patch-clamping mitoplasts. J. Bioenergetics Biomembranes **21:**497-506 (1989).

11. Malan, A. & Mioskowski, E.: pH-temperature interactions on protein function and hibernation: GDP binding to brown adipose tissue mitochondria. J. Comp. Physiol. B **158:**487-493 (1988).

12. Lin, C.S. & Klingenberg, M.: Characteristics of the isolated purine nucleotide binding protein from brown fat mitochondria. Biochem. (Wash.) **21:**2950-2956 (1982).

13. Nicholls, D.G., Snelling, R. & Rial, E.: Proton and calcium circuits across the mitochondrial inner membrane. Biochem. Soc. Trans. **12:**388-390 (1984).

14. Nedergaard, J. & Cannon, B.: Apparent unmasking of [^{3}H]GDP binding in rat brown-fat mitochondria is due to mitochondrial swelling. Eur. J. Biochem. **164:**681-686 (1986).

Lomax, Schönbaum (eds.) **Thermoregulation: The Pathophysiological Basis of Clinical Disorders.**
8th International Symposium Pharmacology of Thermoregulation, Kananaskis, Alberta, Canada 1991, pp. 143-146 (Karger, Basel 1992)

POSSIBLE INVOLVEMENT OF PROSTAGLANDIN I_2 IN MODULATING BLOOD FLOW IN RESPONSE TO NORADRENALINE IN BROWN ADIPOSE TISSUE OF RATS

YOKO UCHIDA and TERUKO NOMOTO

Department of Pharmacology, Tokyo Women's Medical College, Tokyo 162 (Japan)

The control of blood flow in brown adipose tissue (BAT) is important in the thermogenic function of the tissue [1] and its main regulator is noradrenaline (NA) [2], which induces marked increases in BAT blood flow when infused intravenously [3,4].

Prostacyclin (PGI_2) has potent antithrombotic property, dilates blood vessels and is the main metabolite of arachidonic acid in vascular tissue [5-7]. Therefore, it has been suggested that PGI_2 plays an essential role in the homeostasis of the cardiovascular system and may also play a role in the regulation of the local circulation. In addition to direct action on the vascular smooth muscle, PGI_2 alters responses to adrenergic nerve stimulation and to exogenous catecholamines by acting on prejunctional and postjunctional sites, i.e., PGI_2 is one of the potential modulators of adrenergic neuroeffector events [8-12].

However, blood flow and the thermogenic response to PGI_2 are not defined in BAT. There have been no reports indicating that PGI_2 plays a role in the regulation of regional blood flow in BAT. Therefore, the role of PGI_2 in modulating adrenergic neuroeffector events was examined by investigating the effect of PGI_2 on the increase in BAT blood flow elicited by infusion of NA in urethane anesthetized rats.

METHODS: Male Wistar-Imamichi rats weighing about 300 g were maintained on a standard diet and water *ad libitum* in an air-conditioned room (23 $\pm$ 2°C, 55 $\pm$ 5% humidity) lighted 14 h a day (06:00 to 20:00). The rats were anesthetized with urethane (1 g/kg body weight ip) 1 h before the blood flow measurement. Cannulae were inserted into the left jugular and left femoral veins to permit continuous infusion of NA and PGI_2, respectively. Various doses of NA (0.087, 0.26, 0.87, 2.6, 8.7, 26 nmol/kg/min) and PGI_2 (0.03, 0.1, 0.3 nmol/rat/min) were infused continuously at rates of 30 μl/min and 10.67 μl/min, respectively. NA was dissolved in 0.9% saline and the PGI_2 was dissolved in a glycine buffer (pH 10.5) immediately before use because of its instability in aqueous solution (pH 7.4) and then diluted with saline. The interscapular brown adipose tissue (IBAT) was carefully exposed under urethane anesthesia and the IBAT blood flow was measured using a laser-Doppler flowmeter.

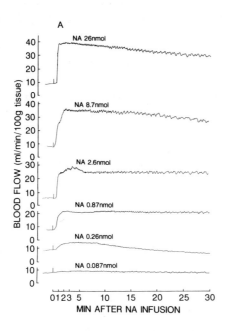
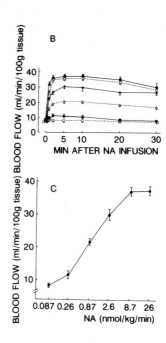

FIGURE 1: A: Actual records of IBAT blood flow in response to various doses of NA in urethane anesthetized rats. NA (0.087, 0.26, 0.87, 2.6, 8.7, 26 nmol/kg/min) were infused via a jugular vein for 30 min. B: Response to NA infused intravenously on the mean blood flow obtained from 6-8 rats. Values represent means ± SEM. When the SEM bars are not shown, they are smaller than the size of the symbols. C: Dose-related changes in the IBAT blood flow response to NA. Each symbol gives maximum response to various doses of NA. Values are represented as means ± SEM (n, 6-8).

RESULTS: Intravenous infusion of NA produced a dose-dependent increase in IBAT blood flow at infusion rates ranging from 0.26 to 8.7 nmol/kg/min (Fig. 1). The maximum increase in IBAT blood flow occurred 2-5 min after infusion. Near steady state levels were then maintained during the 30 min of NA infusion, but there was a slight gradual decline in blood flow at all doses of NA. The lowest dose of NA (0.087 nmol/kg/min) produced no significant increase in IBAT blood flow. The dose-response curve for NA shown in Fig. 1C demonstrates that the dose producing an approximate half-maximum response (ED_{50}) was 0.87 nmol/kg/min.

In an attempt to determine whether PGI_2 has a role in the regulation of regional blood flow to BAT in rats, the effect of PGI_2 and the modification of IBAT blood flow in response to NA by PGI_2 at a dose producing an approximate half-maximum response (0.87 nmol/kg/min) was determined. As shown in Fig. 2A, infusion of PGI_2 (0.03, 0.1, 0.3 nmol/rat/min, data of doses 0.03 and 0.1 are not shown) and its vehicle (glycine buffer) did not produce any significant changes in IBAT blood flow during the 30 min infusion. However, simultaneous infusion of NA with PGI_2 (0.03, 0.1 and 0.3 nmol/rat/min) attenuated the increase in IBAT blood flow induced by NA at the dose producing an approximate half-maximum response (0.87 nmol/kg/min). The patterns recorded during simultaneous infusion of PGI_2 were somewhat different from those of NA alone, especially at the low dose of PGI_2 (0.03 nmol/rat/min) (Fig. 2A), suggesting two phasic changes. At this low dose, an initial increase in

IBAT blood flow during first few minutes was not completely inhibited and furthermore, IBAT blood flow gradually returned to basal levels during the later part of the infusion. In contrast, the higher two doses (0.1, 0.3 nmol/rat/min) completely inhibited the later phase, but the first increase was greatly reduced. An infusion of PGI$_2$, 10 min later also attenuated the increased IBAT blood flow induced by NA (0.87 nmol/kg/min) (Fig. 2B).

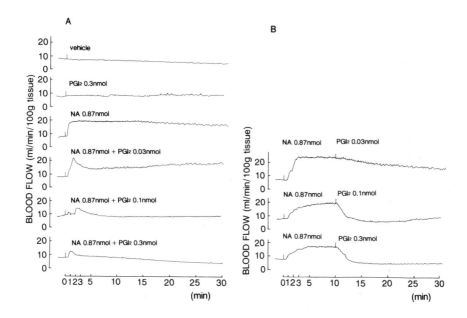

FIGURE 2: A: Effect of PGI$_2$ infusion on NA induced increase in IBAT blood flow. PGI$_2$ (0.03, 0.1, 0.3 nmol/rat/min) or vehicle (glycine buffer) were infused via a femoral vein. NA (0.87 nmol/kg/min: half-maximum response dose) was infused intravenously via a jugular vein. The three lower recordings are simultaneous infusions of NA and PGI$_2$. Bars on actual records indicate start of infusion. B: Effect of PGI$_2$ infusion on NA induced increase in IBAT blood flow. NA was infused intravenously via jugular vein during 30 min. PGI$_2$ infusion began 10 min later. The bars on actual records indicate start of infusion.

DISCUSSION: Many reports have indicated that NA infused exogenously induces a marked increase in blood flow to BAT in rats [3,4]. Furthermore, in these reports, most of the data have been recorded by microsphere techniques. However, in the present experiment, the rate of blood flow was determined by use of a laser-Doppler flowmeter. One benefit of using this method is the ability continuously to monitor changes in blood flow. Data shown in Fig. 1A are actual recordings obtained and confirm the marked increase in IBAT blood flow following infusion of NA. Little is known, however, of the detailed mechanism involved in this increase. It is well documented that the NA induced thermogenic activity in BAT, accompanied by a large increase in blood flow, is mainly mediated via β-adrenoceptors located on the adipocyte membrane [1]. β vasodilating receptors (possibly β_2 recepors) have not yet been found in the vascular bed of BAT. The effect of NA might thus be indirect and secondary to the metabolic activity of the tissue. Additionally, based on dynamic matching of supply and utilization of oxygen and the substrate, a joint regulation of adipocyte activity and tissue blood flow is necessary.

It was firstly reported by Moncada and Vane [5,6] that PGI_2 is a potent vasodilator and an inhibitor of platelet aggregation. In doses which do not affect basal blood flow to BAT, both simultaneously and 10 min after infusion, PGI_2 attenuated the increase in IBAT blood flow induced by NA. In the present study no evidence was obtained showing a role for PGI_2 on the control of resting blood flow in BAT, however our findings indicate that PGI_2 modulates the blood flow response to NA related adrenergic neuroeffector events. Therefore, it can be speculated that the contribution of PGI_2 in the regulation of regional blood flow to BAT is not essential when the tissue is not stimulated, whereas it might counteract an increase in IBAT blood flow, indicating that PGI_2 is important in feedback control for homeostasis when the tissue is fully activated by infusion of NA.

REFERENCES

1. Foster, D.O.: Quantitative role of brown adipose tissue in thermogenesis. In Trayhurn & Nicholls, *Brown Adipose Tissue*, pp. 31-51 (Edward Arnold, London 1986).
2. Girardier, L. & Seydoux, J.: Neural control of brown adipose tissue. In Trayhurn & Nicholls, *Brown Adipose Tissue*, pp. 122-151 (Edward Arnold, London 1986).
3. Foster, D.O. & Frydman, M.L.: Nonshivering thermogenesis in the rat. II. Measurements of blood flow with microspheres point to brown adipose tissue as the dominant site of the calorigenesis induced by noradrenaline. Can. J. Physiol. Pharmacol. **56:**110-122 (1978).
4. Rothwell, N.J. & Stock, M.J.: Influence of noradrenaline on blood flow to brown adipose tissue in rats exhibiting diet-induced thermogenesis. Pflügers Arch. **389:**237-242 (1981).
5. Moncada, S., Gryglewski, R., Bunting, S. & Vane, J.R.: An enzyme isolated from arteries transforms prostaglandin endoperoxides to an unstable substance that inhibits platelet aggregation. Nature **263:**663-665 (1976).
6. Bunting, S., Gryglewski, R., Moncada, S. & Vane, J.R.: Arterial walls generate from prostaglandin endoperoxides a substance (Prostaglandin X) which relaxes strips of mesenteric and coeliac arteries and inhibits platelet aggregation. Prostaglandins **12:**897-913 (1976).
7. Raz, A., Isakson, P.C., Minkes, M.S. & Needleman, P.: Characterization of a novel metabolic pathway of arachidonate in coronary arteries which generates a potent endogenous coronary vasodilator. J. Biol. Chem. **252;**1123-1126 (1977).
8. Hedqvist, P.: Actions of prostacyclin (PGI_2) on adrenergic neuroeffector transmission in the rabbit kidney. Prostaglandins **17:**249-258.
9. Susic, H. & Malik, K.U.: Prostacyclin and prostaglandin E_2 effects on adrenergic transmission in the kidney of anesthetized dog. J. Pharmacol. Exp. Ther. **218:**588-592 (1981).
10. Inokuchi, K. & Malik, K.U.: Attenuation by prostaglandins of adrenergically induced renal vasoconstriction in anesthetized rats. Am. J. Physiol. **246:**R228-R235 (1984).
11. Nakajima, M. & Toda, N.: Prejunctional and postjunctional actions of prostaglandins $F_{2\alpha}$ and I_2 and carbocyclic thromboxane A_2 in isolated dog mesenteric arteries. Europ. J. Pharmacol. **120:**309-318 (1986).
12. Neri Serneri, G.G., Castellani, S., Scart, L., Trotta, F., Chen, J.L., Carnovali M., Poggesi, L. & Masotti, G: Repeated sympathetic stimuli elicit the decline and disappearance of prostaglandin modulation and an increase of vascular resistance in humans. Circulation Res. **67:**580-588 (1990).

Lomax, Schönbaum (eds.) **Thermoregulation: The Pathophysiological Basis of Clinical Disorders.**
8th International Symposium Pharmacology of Thermoregulation, Kananaskis, Alberta, Canada 1991, pp. 147-151 (Karger, Basel 1992)

THE EFFECTS OF CENTRALLY ADMINISTERED PROSTAGLANDIN E₂ DURING PYROGENIC TOLERANCE TO *E. COLI* ENDOTOXIN

MARSHALL F. WILKINSON[1], MARCELLINO MONDA[1,2], NORMAN W. KASTING[3] and QUENTIN J. PITTMAN[1]

[1]Neuroscience Research Group, Department of Medical Physiology, University of Calgary, Health Sciences Research Centre, 3330 Hospital Drive, N.W., Calgary, Alberta T2N 4N1 (Canada); [2]Department of Human Physiology, 1st Faculty of Medicine, University of Naples, Naples 80138 (Italy) and [3]Department of Physiology, University of British Columbia, Vancouver, British Columbia V6T 1W5 (Canada)

Repeated peripheral administration of bacterial endotoxin results in a state of refractoriness known as pyrogenic or endotoxin tolerance. This tolerant condition is generally believed to be due to both the increased ability of reticuloendothelial cells to clear endotoxin from the circulation [1,2] and the reduction, by these cells, in the secretion of pyrogenic cytokines upon repeated exposure to endotoxins [3]. An additional component contributing to the mechanism of pyrogenic tolerance has been proposed. Cooper *et al.* [4] demonstrated that increases within the septum of arginine vasopressin (AVP) immunoreactivity occur in the pyrogen tolerant guinea pig and they proposed that AVP may play a role in pyrogenic tolerance in a manner similar to that seen in the near term and pregnant guinea pig [5]. When an antagonist to the AVP V_1 receptor was administered into the ventral septal area (VSA) of the endotoxin tolerant rat the pyrogenic response to intravenous endotoxin returned [6]. If endogenous AVP is released in the brain during the development of tolerance, we hypothesized that the response to centrally administered pyrogen should be similarly attenuated. Furthermore, it should be possible to measure retrieved quantities of immunoreactive AVP in the rat VSA. Thus, in the present experiments prostaglandin E_2, a potent pyrogen, was delivered into the cerebral ventricles of endotoxin tolerant rats to assess the possibility of a cross tolerance phenomenon. In addition, a separate group of animals were perfused within the VSA to measure AVP release before and after the development of endotoxin tolerance.

METHODS: Male Sprague-Dawley rats (275-375 g) were used in all experiments. Under pentobarbital anesthesia animals were implanted with a Silastic catheter which was advanced into the right jugular vein and exteriorized at the nape of the neck. The head was then secured in a stereotaxic device and a 23 gauge (TW) guide cannula was positioned above the right or left lateral cerebral ventricle. Body temperature was measured remotely using biotelemetry devices implanted intraperitoneally. Animals for push-pull perfusion were implanted with the jugular catheter and transmitter as well as a unilateral 23 gauge (TW) cannula directed toward the VSA for subsequent push-pull perfusion.

Surgical recovery was 5-10 days. Tolerance was induced by 2 successive daily injections of *E. coli* endotoxin (50 μg/kg iv). Intracerebroventricular (icv) injections of PGE₂ (10 ng/5 μl 0.9% saline) were made 15 min or 180 min following a third or fourth successive endotoxin injection. PGE₂ was also injected icv, in non-tolerant, pyrogen naive animals.

Push-pull perfusion was performed in rats before and after a first (naive) and a third (tolerant) endotoxin injection. The perfusate (artificial CSF) was collected on ice over a 30 min period and stored at -70°C until radioimmunoassay for AVP. A pre-endotoxin sample was collected and 7 subsequent samples were collected following the injection of endotoxin. Data are expressed as pg AVP/30 min sample. All data were subjected to a one way analysis of variance with Newman-Keuls test for multiple comparisons.

RESULTS: Administration of endotoxin typically results in a biphasic fever upon a first exposure to the pyrogen. However, subsequent injections of endotoxin results in a brief monophasic fever. The thermal responses to icv injection of PGE_2 in non-tolerant and tolerant animals are depicted in Table I. Administration of PGE_2 in non-tolerant animals evoked a maximal thermal response of 1.27 ± 0.20°C by 30 min. In contrast, PGE_2 administered in tolerant rats 15 min after endotoxin (a time when body temperature was still stable), had a response of 0.53 ± 0.13°C ($p < 0.05$, compared to PGE_2 alone) 30 min following the central injection. PGE_2 administered 180 min after endotoxin in tolerant animals resulted in a response that was similar to non-tolerant rats 30 min after PGE_2 (1.48 ± 0.09°C).

Analysis of VSA push-pull perfusates (Table II) revealed that AVP concentrations were not significantly altered from pre-endotoxin values in animals receiving their first endotoxin injection. However, in tolerant rats, AVP increased significantly from a pre-injection level of 0.70 ± 0.08 pg/sample to 1.94 ± 0.37 pg/sample ($p < 0.05$), in the 30 min interval following endotoxin. Subsequent samples were not significantly different from baseline.

TABLE I: Mean (± S.E.M.) body tempeature (°C) responses 30 min after icv PGE_2 in endotoxin naive (non-tolerant) or endotoxin tolerant rats

Non-Tolerant	Tolerant (+15 min)	Tolerant (+180 min)
1.27 ± 0.20	0.53 ± 0.13[1]	1.48 ± 0.09
(n, 12)	(n, 7)	(n, 6)

Tolerant animals received iv endotoxin followed 15 or 180 min later by PGE_2.
[1]$p < 0.05$ ANOVA, Newman-Keuls (tolerant versus non-tolerant).

DISCUSSION: It is generally believed that repeated central injections of pyrogenic compounds do not result in the development of tolerance to that pyrogen [7-9]. The results of the present study demonstrate that the response to a centrally administered pyrogen, in this case PGE_2, can indeed be affected by the physiological state of endotoxin tolerance. The demonstration of tolerance in the brain, following peripheral injection of endotoxin, is dependent upon the timing of the central injection of PGE_2. When injected after the tolerant monophasic fever had ended, PGE_2 mediated temperature increases were similar to those observed in non-tolerant rats. This hyperthermia, however, was reduced when PGE_2 was injected prior to the monophasic tolerant response to endotoxin. In addition, analysis of AVP levels from VSA push-pull perfusates provides supportive evidence which suggests that endogenous AVP is released within the first 30 min of a third endotoxin injection and may be

TABLE II: Mean ($\pm$ S.E.M.) AVP concentrations (pg/30 min) in VSA push-pull perfusates from animals receiving a first (naive, n, 6) or third (tolerant, n, 4) endotoxin injection

Time (min)	0	30	60	90	120	150	180
Naive	1.23$\pm$0.22	1.27$\pm$0.15	1.32$\pm$0.45	1.04$\pm$0.24	0.90$\pm$0.20	0.95$\pm$0.32	0.75$\pm$0.23
Tolerant	0.70$\pm$0.08	1.94$\pm$0.34[1]	0.79$\pm$0.25	0.76$\pm$0.27	0.43$\pm$0.13	0.57$\pm$0.06	0.75$\pm$0.30

Endotoxin was injected at time 0 and perfusates collected at 30 min intervals.
[1] $p < 0.05$, ANOVA, Newman-Keuls, compared to time 0 within groups.

responsible for suppressing the thermogenic effect of PGE_2. The fact that exogenous AVP administered into the VSA of the non-tolerant rat brain can also suppress PGE_2-induced fever [10] supports the contention that the endogenous peptide is responsible for the reduced response to PGE_2.

Recently, it was observed that icv delivered endotoxin in the endotoxin tolerant rabbit does not result in a diminished febrile respone [11]. These authors, however, did not precede their central injection with an intravenous 'boost' of endotoxin which is apparently necessary to activate the endogenous antipyretic system. Thus, endogenous activity of AVP is dependent upon an as yet undefined endotoxin induced stimulus.

The present results were somewhat unexpected in that the antipyretic activity of endogenous AVP would be predicted to be during the defervescent phase of the febrile response. In the tolerant rat the refractory phase of endotoxin fever occurs approximately 3-4 hours after iv administration. Because it seems unlikely that the response time for AVP is in excess of 3 h, it is probable that AVP acts as an initiator of a sequence of events, probably central and peripheral, which leads to the diminished febrile reaction to repeated endotoxin challenges. This is supported by studies employing AVP antagonists whereby AVP receptor blockade within the VSA of the tolerant rat results in a resumption of the febrile response to intravenous endotoxin [6].

This study further demonstrates that the endogenous antipyretic, AVP, plays a role in the pyrogenic tolerance to intravenous endotoxin. Furthermore, the results indicate that antipyretic activity, presumably involving AVP, during 'active' endotoxin tolerance can be demonstrated by the suppression of pyresis evoked by centrally administered PGE_2.

ACKNOWLEDGEMENTS: MFW is a Fellow of the Medical Research Council of Canada (MRC). NWK is an MRC and QJP an AHFMR Scientist. This research was supported by MRC grants to NWK and QJP.

REFERENCES

1. Cooper, K.E. & Cranston, W.I.: Clearance of radioactive bacterial pyrogen from the circulation. J. Physiol. (London) **166:**41P (1963).
2. Herring, W.B., Herion, J.C., Walker, R.I. & Palmer, J.G.: Distribution and clearance of circulating endotoxin. J. Clin. Invest. **42:**79-87 (1963).
3. Dinarello, C.A., Bodel, P.T. & Atkins, E.: The role of the liver in the production of fever and in pyrogenic tolerance. Trans. Assoc. Am. Physicians **81:**334-343 (1968).
4. Cooper, K.E., Blähser, S., Malkinson, T.J., Merker, G., Roth, J. & Zeisberger, E.: Changes in body temperature and vasopressin content of brain neurons, in pregnant and non-pregnant guinea pigs, during fevers produced by Poly I:Poly C. Pflügers Arch. **412:**292-296 (1988).
5. Merker, G., Blähser, S. & Zeisberger, E.: Reactivity pattern of vasopressin-containing neurons and its relation to the antipyretic reaction in the pregnant guinea pig. Cell. Tis. Res. **212:**47-61 (1980).
6. Wilkinson, M.F. & Kasting, N.W.: Centrally acting vasopressin contributes to endotoxin tolerance. Am. J. Physiol. **258:** (Regulatory Integrative Comp. Physiol. **27**):R443-R449 (1990).
7. Sheth, U.K. & Borison, H.L.: Central pyrogenic action of *Salmonella Typhosa* lipopolysaccharide injected into the lateral cerebral ventricle in cats. J. Pharmacol. Exp. Ther. **130:**411-417 (1960).
8. Splawinski, J., Górka, Z., Zacny, E. & Kaluza, J.: Fever produced in the rat by intracerebral *E. coli* endotoxin. Pflügers Arch. **368:**117-123 (1977).

9.   Myers, R.D., Rudy, T.A. & Yaksh, T.L.: Fever produced by endotoxin injected into the hypothalamus of the monkey and its antagonism by salicylate. J. Physiol. (London) **243:**167-193 (1974).

10.   Ruwe, W.D., Naylor, A.M. & Veale, W.L.: Perfusion of vasopressin within the rat brain suppresses prostaglandin E-hyperthermia. Brain Res. **338:**219-224 (1985).

11.   Kozak, W., Soszynksi, D., Szewczenko, M. & Bodurka, M.: Lack of pyrogenic tolerance transmission between brain and periphery in the rabbit. Experientia **46:**1010-1011 (1990).

ADDENDUM

Since the submission of our paper, subsequent experiments indicate that PGE$_2$ induced hyperthermia is not modified in the endotoxin tolerant rat. The following table summarizes our new data. PGE$_2$ was administered icv in control (non-tolerant) and then in endotoxin tolerant rats 15 min after iv endotoxin. The values shown are the change in temperature (°C $\pm$ S.E.M.) observed 30 min after the icv injection. There were no statistical differences between control and tolerant groups.

10 ng PGE$_2$		50 ng PGE$_2$	
Control	Tolerant	Control	Tolerant
0.93 $\pm$ 0.16	1.30 $\pm$ 0.24	1.70 $\pm$ 0.09	2.17 $\pm$ 0.17

Lomax, Schönbaum (eds.) **Thermoregulation: The Pathophysiological Basis of Clinical Disorders.**
8th International Symposium Pharmacology of Thermoregulation, Kananaskis, Alberta, Canada 1991, pp. 152-156 (Karger, Basel 1992)

THE PUTATIVE ANTIPYRETIC ARGININE VASOPRESSIN MAY INDUCE MOTOR BEHAVIOR THROUGH MULTIPLE SITES OF ACTION

B.J. WILLCOX, P. POULIN, Q.J. PITTMAN and W.L. VEALE

Neuroscience Research Group, Department of Medical Physiology, Faculty of Medicine, The University of Calgary, 3330 Hospital Drive N.W., Calgary, Alberta, Canada T2N 4N1

There is now considerable evidence that arginine vasopressin (AVP) may act as an endogenous antipyretic in the brain (for review see [1]). The mechanism(s) by which AVP induces antipyresis are unknown, but the reduction of febrile body temperature towards prefebrile levels involves multiple components [2]. These include efferent pathways for increased heat loss and reduced heat production including thermoregulatory behaviors, such as grooming, prostration and intermittent locomotion [3-5]. The observation that AVP induces both antipyresis [2] and motor behavior [8-10] when injected into a lateral cerebral ventricle of the rat brain raises the possibility that AVP may reduce febrile body temperature, at least in part, by activating behavioral heat loss mechanisms. This hypothesis is particularly attractive because AVP perfused into the ventral septal area (VSA; an area extending from the diagonal bands of Broca to the anterior hypothalamus), of the rat basal forebrain, has been found to induce both antipyresis [1,2] and motor behaviors, including prostration [11]. Hence, the VSA provides a potential tissue locus for AVP induced behavioral heat reduction. Recently, the medial amygdala of the rat brain has been found to be another tissue site at which exogenous AVP reduces febrile body temperature [12]. Thus, in this study we investigated the possibility that AVP may also induce motor behaviors when infused into the medial amygdala of the rat brain.

METHODS: Male Sprague Dawley rats (250-300 g) were anaesthetized with sodium pentobarbital (50 mg/kg) and bilateral stainless steel, 23 gauge guide cannulae were implanted stereotaxically directed towards the medial amygdala. Rats were allowed to recover from surgery for 7 to 10 days. AVP (100 pmol in 1.0 μl sterile, pyrogen free, physiological saline) infusions were administered into unrestrained rats through 27 gauge cannulae, over a 60 sec period using an infusion pump. AVP infusions were administered twice, 24 h apart, to examine the initial motor responses to a central AVP infusion (Day 1), and to test for a possible sensitization phenomenon of AVP induced motor effects (Day 2) previously described [8,9]. On each experimental day, the animals were placed in a large plexiglass chamber 1 h prior to infusion. Motor behaviors were scored after infusion, for 10 min at 1 min intervals, on a ranking scale modified from that developed by Kasting et al. [8], that allows for ranking the severity of departure from normal motor behavior. Motor behaviors were scored as follows: 0, no effect; 1, pauses defined by periods (10 sec or longer) of absence of activity; 2, prostration; 3, locomotor difficulties; 4, barrel rotation; 5, myoclonus/myotonus; 6, death. Results are presented as the highest score each animal received throughout the 10-min period. Without knowledge of behavioral scores, the infusion sites were verified histologically upon completion of the experiment. Differences in responses within groups, from Day 1 to Day 2, were analyzed by the Wilcoxon matched pairs signed ranks test and differences in responses between groups were analyzed by the Mann-Whitney U test.

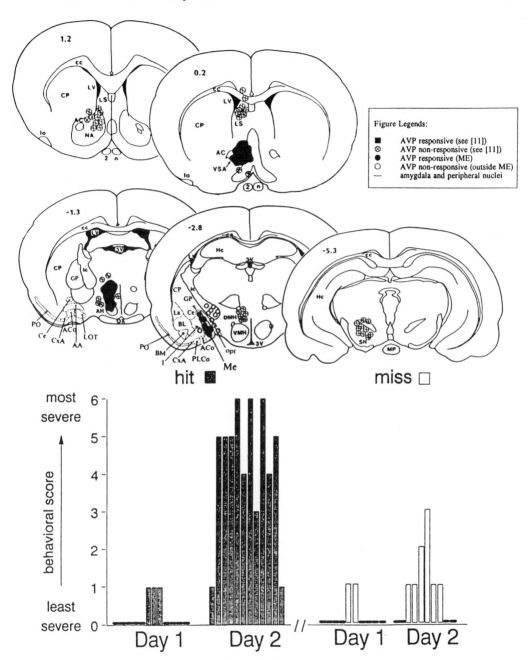

FIGURE 1: Behavioral responses of rats to bilateral infusions of AVP (100 pmol/1.0 μl pyrogen-free, physiological saline) on 2 consecutive days into the medial amygdala compared to behavioral responses of a different group of rats to the same treatment but outside of the medial amygdala. Each bar represents the most severe behavioral score an individual animal (n, 12 hits; n, 10 misses) received during the 10 min observation period following AVP infusion. The data show an increase in magnitude of the motor responses to AVP infusion from Day 1 to Day 2 (p < 0.004; Wilcoxon matched pairs signed ranks test) for the group which received infusions inside the medial amygdala. The data also show a much greater response when the infusions occurred inside the medial amygdala

compared to surrounding areas (p < 0.0004; Mann-Whitney U test). No significant sensitization of responses was seen in the group who received AVP infusions in areas outside of, but surrounding, the medial amygdala (p > 0.05; Wilcoxon matched pairs signed ranks test). Numbers in the coronal sections indicate the distance in mm from bregma (+, rostral; -, caudal). Abbreviations: AA, anterior amygdaloid area; AC, anterior commissure; ACo, anterior cortical amygdaloid nucleus; AH, anterior hypothalamus; BL, basolateral amygdaloid nucleus; BM, basomedial amygdaloid nucleus; cc, corpus callosum; CeL, central amygdaloid nucleus; CP, caudate putamen; CxA, cortex amygdala transition zone; DMH, dorsomedial hypothalamus; En, endopiriform nucleus; GP, globus pallidus; Hc, hippocampus; I, intercalated nuclei amygdala; ic, internal capsule; La, lateral amygdaloid nucleus; lo, olfactory tract; LOT, nucleus of lateral olfactory tract; LS, lateral septum; LV, lateral ventricle; ME, medial amygdaloid nucleus; 2n, optic nerve;NA, nucleus accumbens; opt, optic tract; ox, optic chiasm; PLCo, posterolateral cortical amygdaloid nucleus; PO, primary olfactory cortex; SI, substantia innominata; SN, substantia nigra; 3V, third ventricle; VMH, ventromedial hypothalamus; VSA, ventral septal area.

RESULTS: The behavioral scores of rats following a first (Day 1) and a subsequent (Day 2) AVP (100 pmol) infusion in the medial amygdala are shown in Fig. 1. After the initial exposure to AVP, rats displayed minor behavioral responses consisting of long pauses. Following AVP infusion, animals also engaged in grooming behavior (data not shown). When the animals were retested one day later, the motor responses of the animals infused within the medial amygdala were significantly increased from those of Day 1 (p < 0.004; Wilcoxon matched pairs signed ranks test). Most animals exhibited prostration, which then progressed to more severe departures from normality. The motor responses of animals whose infusions were outside the medial amygdala were not significantly different from Day 1 (p > 0.05; Wilcoxon matched pairs signed ranks test). Although several animals which received AVP infusions outside the medial amygdala exhibited minor motor responses on both days, including pauses, their behavioral scores were significantly lower than in the group of rats who received AVP infusion into the medial amygdala (p < 0.0004; Mann-Whitney U test).

DISCUSSION: In this study, we have shown that AVP infusion into the medial amygdala induces motor responses that may be involved in thermoregulatory behavior. For example, infusion of AVP into the medial amygdala induced prostration, intermittent locomotion and grooming behavior. These behaviors have been reported to play an important role in behavioral heat reduction [3-5]. The recent finding that infusion of AVP into the medial amygdala reduces febrile body temperature [12] is consistent with a postulated role for AVP in antipyresis. The observation that AVP, infused into the medial amygdala, induces both motor responses and antipyresis suggests that AVP may activate different components of complex systems involved in reducing febrile body temperature. A similar response to AVP infusion occurs in the ventral septal area where this neuropeptide induces both motor [11] and an antipyretic responses [1]. Thus, there appear to be multiple sites where infusion of AVP induces both motor behaviors as well as reduction in febrile body temperature.

Numerous studies have shown that the anterior hypothalamic/ preoptic nuclei and lateral hypothalamic nuclei are major central thermoregulatory centers in the brain and may play a role in behavioral thermoregulation [3-7]. Both the ventral septal area and the medial amygdala have been shown to have extensive vasopressinergic connections with these areas [13-16]. In addition, immunocytochemical studies have shown increased AVP reactivity in fibers connecting these areas during fever [14]. Thus, it is possible that AVP acting in the ventral septal area and in the medial amygdala reduces febrile body temperature through interaction with these brain loci perhaps, in part, through activating behavioral heat reduction mechanisms. Similarly, all these sites are indirectly connected through the stria terminalis and the ventral amygdalofugal pathway to motor areas (see [13] for review) and the amygdala itself has recently been shown to have direct reciprocal connections with the motor cortex [17]. These pathways may provide an anatomical substrate for AVP's motor effects, including behavioral heat reduction, and if overstimulated might induce motor disturbances.

The motor effects in response to amygdalar AVP infusion are increased after an initial exposure to AVP, demonstrating a sensitization effect. Sensitization of the motor effects of AVP also occurs after repeated AVP infusion into the ventral septal area [1]. Repeated intracerebroventricular administration of AVP sensitizes both the motor effects of AVP and AVP induced antipyresis [18]. Since the sites of action for the antipyretic and motor effects of AVP are similar, and because both the antipyretic and the motor effects can be sensitized by repeated exposure to AVP, it is possible that the enhanced antipyresis and enhanced motor effects observed following repeated AVP administration may be correlated. This would support a role for AVP in behavioral heat reduction. Because repeated administration of AVP can result in severe motor behaviors such as myoclonic/myotonic convulsions, it is possible that AVP induced sensitization could play a role in pathophysiological thermoregulatory behaviors, such as febrile convulsion (see [1] for review).

This study suggests that AVP can act in a specific region of the brain to initiate motor behaviors that may be of importance in behavioral thermoregulation. Previous studies suggest that the ventral septal area is also an active site for similar motor behaviors. This raises the possibility that these sites are part of a complex neural network that may induce antipyresis, in part through behavioral heat loss mechanisms, and may be involved in the pathogenesis of febrile convulsions.

ACKNOWLEDGEMENTS: Supported by the Medical Research Council of Canada.

REFERENCES

1. Pittman, Q.J., Naylor, A., Poulin, P., Disturnal, J., Veale, W.L., Martin, S.M. & Malkinson, T.J.: The role of vasopressin as an antipyretic in the ventral septal area and its possible involvement in convulsive disorders. Brain Res. Bull. **20:**887-892 (1988).

2. Cooper, K.E.: The neurobiology of fever: thoughts on recent developments. Ann. Rev. Neurosci. **10:**297-324 (1987).

3. Hainsworth, F.R.: Saliva spreading, activity, and body temperature regulation in the rat. Am. J. Physiol. **212:**1288-1292 (1969).

4. Roberts, W.W. & Robinson, T.C.L.: Relaxation and sleep induced by warming of preoptic region and anterior hypothalamus in cats. Exp. Neurol. **25:**282-294 (1969).

5. Roberts, W.W. & Mooney, R.D.: Brain areas controlling thermoregulatory grooming, prone extension, locomotion, and tail vasodilation in rats. J. Comp. Physiol. Psychol. **86:**470-480 (1974).

6. Hainsworth, F.R. & Epstein, A.N.: Severe impairment of heat-induced saliva-spreading in rats recovered from lateral hypothalamic lesions. Science **153:**1255-1257 (1966).

7. Satinoff, E. & Shan, S.Y.Y.: Loss of behavioral thermoregulation after lateral hypothalamic lesions in rats. J. Comp. Physiol. Psychol. **77:**302-312 (1971).

8. Kasting, N.W., Veale, W.L. & Cooper, K.E.: Convulsive and hypothermic effects of vasopressin in the brain of the rat. Can. J. Physiol. Pharmacol. **58:**316-319 (1980).

9. Burnard, D.M., Pittman, Q.J. & Veale, W.L.: Increased motor disturbances in response to arginine vasopressin following hemorrhage or hypertonic saline: evidence for central AVP release in rats. Brain Res. **273:**59-65 (1983).

10. Burnard, D.M., Veale, W.L. & Pittman, Q.J.: Prevention of arginine-vasopressin-induced motor disturbances by a potent vasopressor antagonist. Brain Res. **362:**40-46 (1986).

11. Naylor, A.M., Ruwe, W.D., Burnard, D.M., McNeely, P.D., Turner, S.L., Pittman, Q.J. & Veale, W.L.: Vasopressin-induced motor disturbances: localization of a sensitive forebrain site in the rat. Brain Res. **361:**242-246 (1985).

12. Federico, P., Malkinson, T.J., Cooper, K.E., Pittman, Q.J. & Veale, W.L.: Vasopressin-induced antipyresis in the medial amygdaloid nucleus of the urethan-anaesthetized rat. Soc. Neurosci. Abstr. **16**:1204 (1990).

13. De Olmos, J.S., Alheid, G.F. & Beltramino, C.A.: Amygdala. In Paxinos, *The Rat Nervous System, Vol. 1. Forebrain and Midbrain*, pp. 223-334 (Academic Press, 1985).

14. Zeisberger, E., Merker, G., Blahser, S. & Krannig, M.: Changes in activity of vasopressin neurons during fever in the guinea pig. Neurosci. Lett. (Suppl.) **14**:S414 (1983).

15. Disturnal, J.E., Veale, W.L. & Pittman, Q.J.: Electrophysiological analysis of potential arginine vasopressin projections to the ventral septal area of the rat. Brain Res. **342**:162-167 (1985).

16. Bleier, R. & Byne, W.: Septum and hypothalamus. In Paxinos, *The Rat Nervous System, Vol. 1. Forebrain and Midbrain*, pp. 87-118 (Academic Press, 1985).

17. Kita, H. & Kitai, S.T.: Amygdaloid projections to the frontal cortex and the striatum in the rat. J. Comp. Neurol. **298**:40-49 (1990).

18. Poulin, P.: (unpublished results, 1991).

Lomax, Schönbaum (eds.) **Thermoregulation: The Pathophysiological Basis of Clinical Disorders.**
8th International Symposium Pharmacology of Thermoregulation, Kananaskis, Alberta, Canada 1991, pp. 157-166 (Karger, Basel 1992)

CIRCADIAN BODY TEMPERATURE IN PATIENTS WITH PSYCHOGENIC PROLONGED HYPERTHERMIA

S. YOSHIUE[1], H. YOSHIZAWA[1], H. ITOH[1], T. YAZUMI[1], M. NAKAMURA[1], H. SEKINE[1], H. TAKAHASHI[1], T. KANAMORI[1], H. SUZUKI[1], N. IHASHI[1], R. SAKAKI[1]*, M. ISHIDA and J. OGATA[2]

[1]The First Department of Internal Medicine, St. Marianna University School of Medicine, 2-16-1, Sugao Miyamae-ku, Kawasaki, Japan, Postal Code 213 and [2]Division of Nutritional Physiology, Department of Food and Nutrition, Kyoritsu Women's University, 2-2-1, Hitotsubashi Chiyoda-ku, Tokyo, Postal Code 101 (Japan)

Although there are some reports of animal experiments, there is very limited information [1] dealing with psychogenic prolonged hyperthermia from the clinical point of view, particularly concerning the mechanism by which hyperthermia may occur. In 1988 we investigated [2] the correlation between psychogenic stress and hyperthermia, estimating simultaneously tympanic (T_t), rectal (T_r), oral (T_o), axillary (T_a) and finger (T_f) temperatures. The study was designed to search for any difference between patients and healthy subject in terms of circadian patterns. The following questions were raised:

1. Does the circadian rhythm in patients with psychogenic prolonged hyperthermia differ from that of healthy subjects?

2. Is vasoconstriction in the extremities the major reason for the hyperthermia?

3. Is a set point change the cause of psychogenic hyperthermia?

4. Could the elevation in body temperature in patients with psychogenic hyperthermia be attributable to an endogenous pyrogen?

METHODS: Thirty two healthy young subjects (14 women and 18 men) volunteered for the circadian rhythm study [3]. Seven patients (3 women and 4 men) with prolonged hyperthermia for at least 1 year or more were subjects for recording circadian temperatures at 2 min intervals. One female was found to have an infection.

T_a, T_o, T_r, T_t and T_f were measured in four groups of patients: hyperthyroidism (4); organic disease (4); infectious disease (6); psychogenic hyperthermia (8); healthy subject (98 women and 80 men), under ambient conditions of 24°C and 50% humidity.

RESULTS: The clinical profile of patients with psychogenic prolonged hyperthermia is shown in Table 1.

Comparison of the body temperatures at different sites in the four groups is seen in Table 2.

TABLE I: Clinical profile

No.	Sex Age	T_a (°C)	T_o (°C)	Extremities	Complication	Trait	Duration	Psychological Approach	Occupation	Hyperthermia in Family
1.	M. 39	36.6-37.6	36.7-37.3	cold	--	anxious or nervous	about 6 years	unchanged	secretary	+
2.	M. 19	37.0-37.8	37.0-37.4	"	allergy?	"	over 1 year	"	student	+
3.	M.	36.2-37.4	36.5-37.4	"	--	"	over 4 years	"	public officer	-
4.	M. 56	36.9-37.5	37.6 (Tr)	"	--	" & depressive	over 6 years	"	no	-
5.	F. 19	37.3-38.0	37.5-38.3	not cold	headache	" & distressed	about 5 years	poor	student	-
6.	F. 27	36.5-37.5	36.9-37.4	cold	history of cystitis		over 1 year	?	programmer	?
7.	F. 20	37.0-37.5	37.1-37.4	not cold	history of infection? & iron deficiency		about 1 year	?	nurse	?

TABLE II: Body temperature in four hyperthermic groups

No.	Group	Temperature (°C)				
		T_t	T_r	T_o	T_a	T_f
1	Psychogenic	37.31±0.26	37.50±0.24	37.04±0.19	37.20±0.34	34.12±3.28
2.	Infectious or post-infectious origin	37.48±0.36	37.58±0.27	37.10±0.32	36.92±0.40	32.02±3.93
3	Organic origin	38.28±0.54	38.24±0.64	37.86±0.90	38.25±0.73	33.24±2.78
4	Hyper-thyroidism	37.37±0.12	37.34±0.05	37.04±0.13	37.00±0.41	36.14±0.40
5	Control					
	Male	36.92±0.24	37.23±0.22	36.77±0.24	36.50±0.43	35.11±0.88
	Female	36.99±0.24	37.27±0.26	36.88±0.27	36.53±0.37	32.86±3.56

Representative data from patient number 1 (Table 1) were:

39 year-old man, secretary. Circadian rectal temperature was recorded on different occasions. The initial pattern revealed a "morning elevated type" compared with the normal pattern. However, subsequently the pattern gradually changed. The lowest temperature was at 03:00-04:16 h, and the highest at 17:00-18:00 h (left panel Fig. 1). Circadian rhythm curves on 3 consecutive days demonstrated the mirror-like reciprocal relationship between T_r and T_h (right panel in Figure 1). T_a was always higher than T_o (bottom panel in Figure 1).

Representative data from patient number 5 (Table 1):

Records from a 19 year old girl student are shown in Fig. 2. T_r was 36.4°C at 02:40 h when the curve reached its nadir, then there was a gradual increase and it peaked at 18:00 h (38.1°C).

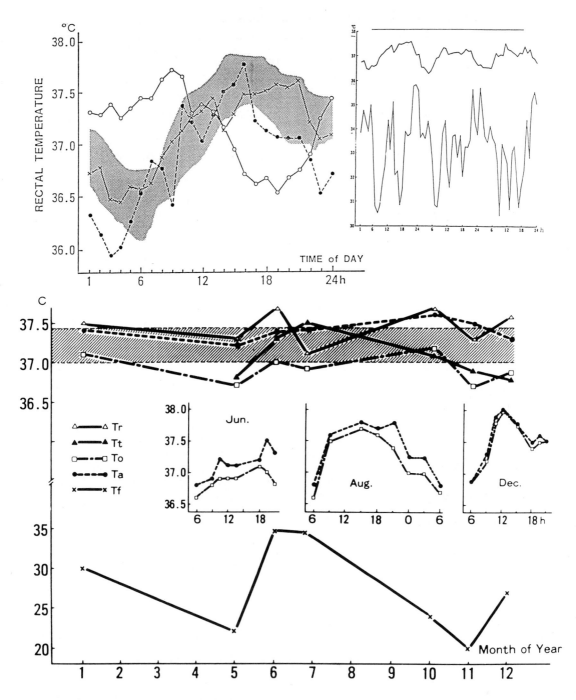

FIGURE 1: Representative patients (number 1).

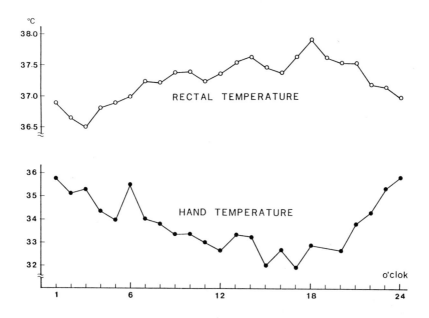

FIGURE 2: Representative patient (number 5).

The highest T_h was 35.8°C at 24:00 h and the lowest (31.9°C) at 17:00 h. Mean values of 1 hourly circadian T_r are seen in Fig. 3. At 03:00 h the minimum T_r was 36.35 ± 0.25°C in females and 36.42 ± 0.46°C in males. T_r gradually rose through the afternoon and evening when the maximum was from 37.37 ± 0.21 to 37.46 ± 0.31°C between 13:00 and 19:00 h in females and 37.23 ± 0.26 to 37.34 ± 0.43°C between 13:00 and 17:00 h in males. In healthy subject at 04:38-05:44 h the minimum T_r was 36.82 ± 0.48°C in females in the luteal phase, 36.46 ± 0.22°C in females in the follicular phase and 36.41 ± 0.30°C in males. At 17:00-18:00 h the maximum T_r was 37.66 ± 0.30°C in the luteal phase, 37.65 ± 0.24°C in follicular phase and 37.61 ± 0.26°C in males.

Mean values of 1 hourly circadian T_h curves are shown in Fig. 4. The maximum T_h was 35.48 ± 0.83°C in females and 34.68 ± 0.90°C in males at 23:00-24:00 h. T_h began to rise from 18:00-19:00 h when it was 32.62 ± 2.28°C in females and 31.69 ± 2.13°C in males, again reaching the previous maximum T_h at 23:00-24:00 h. In healthy subject, the lowest T_h was at 17:00-18:00 h and was 30.18 ± 6.08°C in females and 30.09 ± 4.05°C in males, followed by a gradual increase towards the next morning.

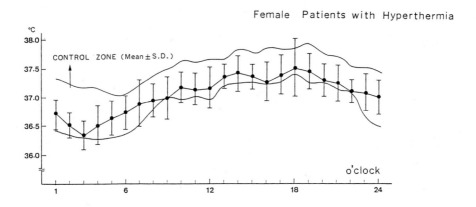

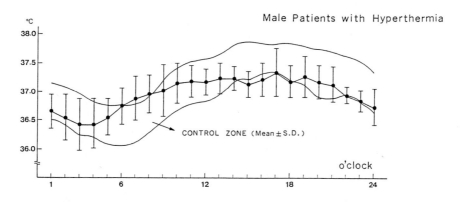

FIGURE 3: Mean values of 1 hourly circadian rhythms of T_r in females and males.

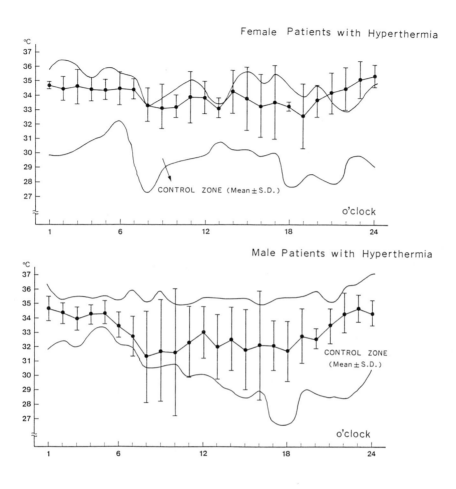

FIGURE 4: Mean values of 1 hourly circadian rhythms of T_h in females and males.

Mean values of 10 minute circadian rhythms of T_r are shown in Fig. 5. Fig. 6 shows the relationship between the circadian rhythms of T_r and T_h, in patients No. 1 and 5 in Table 1. At the turning point, a clear difference exists between controls and patients.

DISCUSSION: The average temperature values were higher on days when the patients were depressed. This can be considered as a desynchronization of circadian rhythm, related to the manic-depressive disorder, suggesting a disturbance of brain centers or a neurological disorder [4-6]. Several studies have confirmed differences in the circadian body temperature, with an approximately 2 h time difference in sleep-wake cycles [7-9].

The initial fall in core temperature that occurs typically during the first 3 h after sleep onset can be curtailed by an increase in ambient temperature [10].

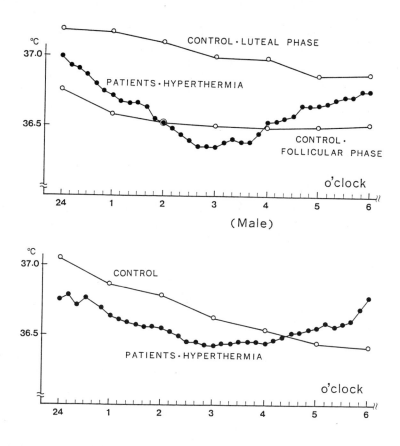

FIGURE 5: Mean values of 10 minute circadian rhythms of T_r in females and 10 males (24:00-06:00 h).

When a subject was active at night time during sleep deprivation, T_r was elevated in comparison to normal. Continuous bedrest caused a normal temperature pattern during the night and reduced temperatures during the day [11].

A major component of the rise in body temperature induced by psychological stress in rats is mediated by prostaglandins released in the central nervous system, and constitutes a fever [12]. Naloxone was able to prevent stress induced hyperthermia in rats, suggesting that endorphinergic mechanisms underlie the effect [13].

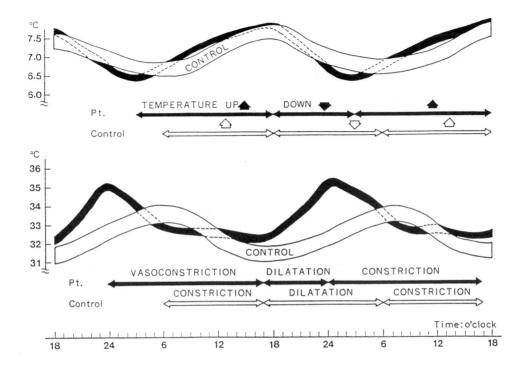

FIGURE 6: Circadian rhythms in patients with psychogenic prolonged hyperthermia.

It is concluded:

1. Circadian rhythms in patients with psychogenic prolonged hyperthermia have a different pattern compared with healthy subjects. The lowest morning temperature was around 03:00 h, 2-3 h earlier than in healthy subjects. Then rectal temperature rose gradually towards noon and peaked between 13:00 and 17:00 h, though there were differences between males and females.

    Circadian hand temperature peaked at 23:00-24:00 h, then gradually fell to 08:00-10:00 h.

    Patients tended to have a longer period of peripheral vasoconstriction than did healthy subjects.

2. The duration of peripheral vasoconstriction was approximately 17 h which was about 6 h longer than in healthy subjects.

    One of the major factors responsible for the rise in body temperature is the peripheral vasoconstriction and decreased heat dissipation.

3. The reciprocal relationship between circadian rectal temperature and peripheral temperatures suggest that a change in set-point may occur during psychogenic hyperthermia.

ACKNOWLEDGEMENTS: The authors wish to express their appreciation to Dr. K. Uchino of Department of Student Health Center, Yokohama National University and Dr. M. Iriki of Department of Physiology, Yamanashi Medical College for evaluation of the data and Dr. Y. Kawashima of Yokohama National University for technical help.

REFERENCES

1. Renbourn, E.T.: Body temperature and pulse rate in boys and young men prior to sporting contests. A study of emotional hyperthermia: with a review of the literature. Psychosom. Res. **4:**147-175 (1960).

2. Yoshiue, S., Yoshizawa, H., Itoh, H., Sekine, H., Nakamura, M., Kanamori, T., Yazumi, T., Suzuki, H., Ogata, J. & Ishida, M.: Analysis of body temperature at different sites in patients having slight fever caused by psychogenic stress. In Lomax & Schönbaum, *Thermoregulatory Mechanisms and Their Therapeutic Implications*, pp. 169-170 (Karger, Basel 1979).

3. Yazumi, T.: Thermal circadian rhythm in healthy subjects. The St. Marianna Medical J. **13:**632-641 (1985).

4. Pflug, B., Erikson, R. & Johnsson, A.: Depression and daily temperature. A long study. Acta Psychiat. Scand. **54:**254-266 (1976).

5. Nikitopoulou, G. & Grammer, J.L.: Endogenous anxiety and circadian rhythms. Brit. Med. J. **1:**1311 (1979).

6. Kripke, D.F., Mullaney, D.J., Atkinson, M. & Wolf, S.: Circadian rhythm disorders in manic-depressives. Biol. Psychiat. **13:**335-351 (1978).

7. Horne, J.A. & Oesterberg, O.: Individual differences in human circadian rhythms. Biol. Psychiat. **5:**179-190 (1987).

8. Horne, J.A., Brass, C.G. & Pettitt, A.N.: Circadian performance differences between morning and evening 'types'. Ergonomics **23:**29-36 (1980).

9. Stephan, K. & Dorow, R.: Circadian core temperature, psychomotor performance and subjective ratings of fatigue in morning and evening 'types'. In Redfern, Campbell, Davis & Martin, *Circadian Rhythms in the Central Nervous System*, pp. 233-236 (VCH Publishers, London 1985).

10. Bonegio, R.G.B., Driver, H.S., King, L.A., Laburn, H.P. & Shapiro, C.M.: Circadian temperature rhythm blunting and sleep composition. Acta Physiol. Scand. **133(Suppl. 574):**44-47 (1988).

11. Wever, R.A.: Internal interactions within the human circadian system: the masking effect. Experientia **41:**332-342 (1985).

12. Kluger, M.J., O'Reilly, B., Shope, T.R. & Vander, A.J.: Further evidence that stress hyperthermia is a fever. Physiology and Behavior **39:**763-766 (1987).

13. Blaesig, J., Hoellt, V., Baeuerle, U. & Herz, A.: Involvement of endorphins in emotional hyperthermia of rats. Life Sci. **23:**2525-2532 (1978).

Lomax, Schönbaum (eds.) **Thermoregulation: The Pathophysiological Basis of Clinical Disorders.**
8th International Symposium Pharmacology of Thermoregulation, Kananaskis, Alberta, Canada 1991, pp. 167-171 (Karger, Basel 1992)

THE LAMINA TERMINALIS CONTRIBUTES TO THE PATHOLOGY OF FEVER

EUGEN ZEISBERGER and GESA MERKER

Physiologisches Institut, Klinikum der Justus-Liebig-Universität, Aulweg 129, D-6300 Giessen (Germany)

The interconnections between the immune and central nervous systems have been reviewed recently [1]. It has been shown that hypothalamic structures respond to certain mediators of the immune system (some lymphokines, e.g., interleukins, interferons and tumor necrosis factor) by increasing the set point temperature and causing fever [2]. The increase in body temperature may be beneficial because it accelerates and facilitates the activation of the immune defense system. To prevent an excessive, harmful rise in body temperature, the febrile response is controlled and limited by endogenous antipyretics [3-5]. These are neuropeptides released at distinct sites in the limbic system. A known effective site is the ventral septal area (VSA) [6,7], located frontal to the anterior commisure, between the lateral septum and the dorsal band of Broca (DBB). This area is closely connected to structures along the lamina terminalis which play a role in the control of the water balance [8]. The febrile responses to pyrogens could also be modified by changes in water balance [7,9].

The purpose of this study was to re-evaluate our earlier experiments in which we influenced the febrile responses to bacterial endotoxin (LPS from *E. coli*, 20 μg/kg) by microinfusions of arginine vasopressin (AVP) or its V_1 and V_2 agonists into the VSA with respect to their possible action on structures along the lamina terminalis.

METHODS: The methods have been described previously [10,11]. A cannula was implanted into the VSA. The microinfusions (bilaterally, speed 0.1 μl/min) of AVP (9 μg/6 h) or its V_1 and V_2 agonists (14 μg/6 h) started 1 h before injection of bacterial pyrogen and lasted 6 h. The tests were repeated at weekly intervals in each animal; thus each guinea pig served as its own control. The columns of the inserted graph of Fig. 1 follow the sequence of the experiments. For details on methods for febrile tests and intraseptal microinfusions, see reference [10] and for immunocytochemical techniques [11].

RESULTS: Fig. 1 shows a schematic sagittal section through the brain of a guinea pig, together with a diagram showing the febrile responses.

The first test with bacterial endotoxin (control) preceded the stereotaxic operation for the microinfusions. The second test/column shows that AVP microinfusion into the VSA prevented fever, in contrast to solvent infusion (third test). In the fourth test, no pyrogen was given to the guinea pigs. AVP was then microinfused into the VSA and did not influence colonic temperature. Tests 5 and 6 indicate that intraseptal infusions of V_1 and V_2 receptor specific AVP agonists were less effective than AVP, but adding the effects of V_1 and V_2 agonists would likely have resulted in fever suppression similar to the effect of AVP.

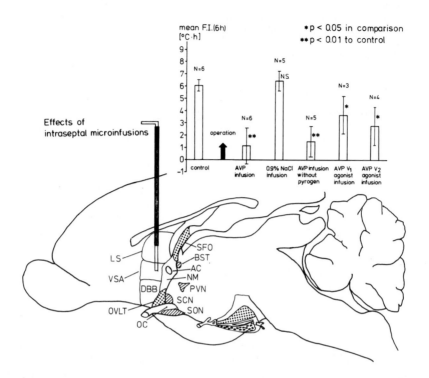

FIGURE 1: Sagittal section of the guinea pig's brain showing the areas of the lamina terminalis (OVLT, NM, SFO) and a cannula in the VSA through which solutions containing AVP or V_1 and V_2 receptor agonists were microinfused. The diagram summarizes the effects of intraseptal microinfusions on the febrile responses to bacterial endotoxin in a group of 6 guinea pigs. For details see text.

The immunocytochemical investigations of the areas of the lamina terminals revealed numerous AVP reactive terminals and also disseminated perikarya, particularly within the organum vasculosum laminae terminalis (OVLT). Characteristic for these disseminated AVP neurons was that they had close contacts to blood vessels. Fig. 2 gives an example of these connections.

Some of these neurons (indicated by arrows) either invade or send their axons directly to the neighbouring blood vessels. Double staining techniques showed that some of these perivascular AVP neurons in the OVLT also receive afferents from the VSA.

DISCUSSION: Anatomically the VSA is close to the preoptic region (which is thermosensitive) and to structures along the lamina terminalis. Three areas of the lamina terminals are depicted in Fig. 1.

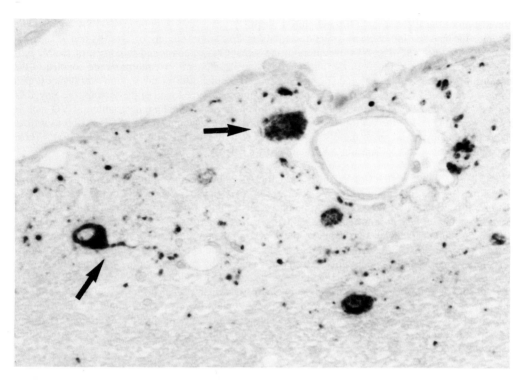

FIGURE 2: Frontal section through the guinea pig's brain showing the immunoreactive staining of AVP structures in the OVLT. The arrows indicate AVP neurons invading the perivascular space or sending their axons to the blood vessels in a close proximity. Enlargement: 960x.

Two of them, the subfornical organ (SFO) and OVLT, are circumventricular oragns (CVO) and possess fenestrated capillaries, allowing an exchange of large molecules between the blood and glial and neuronal processes in the perivascular space. Both these CVO are connected to the nucleus medianus (NM), also known as the median preoptic nucleus. This nucleus is, however, situated within the blood brain barrier. Supposedly, the OVLT senses blood plasma osmolality [12] as well as signals from the peripheral immune system, e.g., endogenous pyrogens [13], whereas the SFO has receptors for angiotensin II [14]. The NM receives inputs from both OVLT and SFO and also from peripheral cardiovascular receptors via the solitary tract. Neural tracing studies have established that all these areas send projections to the hypothalamic nuclei containing AVP neurons, such as the paraventricular (PVN), supraoptic (SON), suprachiasmatic (SCN) nuclei and the bed nucleus of stria terminalis (BST) indicated in Fig. 1 by shaded areas. From these nuclei different AVP pathways originate. In addition to the projections of magnocellular AVP neurons of PVN and SON to the neural lobe of the pituitary, other pools of magnocellular neurons project to the lower brain stem and spinal cord [15]. The parvocellular neurons of PVN, BST and SCN on the other hand project predominantly to the median eminence and to different areas of the limbic system. Some projections are distributed in the amygdala and hippocampus, others pass the OVLT and ascend through the DBB to different septal areas [16,17]. The VSA receives AVP afferents originating from the BST in the rat [18] and from the PVN in the guinea pig [16]. These studies support our findings of a change in the immunoreactivity to AVP antiserum in a parvocellular neuronal pool of the PVN in animals with suppressed fever [19]. Increased release of AVP in VSA has been demonstrated during electrical stimulation of the PVN in rats [20] and guinea pigs [21]. The AVP actions in the VSA appear to be receptor mediated as indicated by structure-activity studies with a variety of agonists and antagonists of the AVP molecule. The AVP receptors in the septum have been found to consist of the V_1 subtype, i.e., receptors coupled to the phosphatidyl inositol system. V_2 receptors are coupled to the adenylate cyclase system. The specific binding to the receptor sites in the septum was demonstrated autoradiographically in rats [22] and V_1 specific binding sites were found in the septum, the amygdala and the hippocampus [23]. Surprisingly, V_1 specific binding sites were not detectable in CVO such as OVLT and SFO and in the AVP producing nuclei of the hypothalamus (PVN, SON, SCN) as well as the neurohypophysis, although these structures were densely labelled with tritiated AVP [23]. These hypothalamic sites bear V_2 specific AVP binding sites [24].

The antipyretic effects of V_1 and V_2 specific AVP agonists shown in our microinfusion experiments may be due to binding to the V_1 receptors in VSA and to V_2 receptors in the nearby OVLT. The AVP neurons with close contacts to blood vessels could influence local permeability, or at least the accessibility of receptors for endogenous pyrogens in the perivascular space of the OVLT. Double staining techniques showed that some of these perivascular AVP neurons in the OVLT receive afferents from the VSA [25]. Thus AVP has a dual antipyretic action: First, it could activate, via V_1 receptors, septal neurons which block the changes induced by pyrogens in the hypothalamic centers (Possibly, other neuropeptides participate in this function and modulate the action of AVP [10,26]). Second, the release of AVP from the disseminated perivascular system of the OVLT could influence the permeability or the binding of pyrogens to their receptors by a V_2 specific mechanism. This effect could also be modulated by other neuropeptides. For instance, modulation by various neuropeptides of interleukin 1β induced production of prostaglandin E_2 was reported recently in cultured astrocytes [27].

It seems that various peptides modulate the activation of the antipyretic neuronal system in the VSA as well as the binding of endogenous pyrogens to the astroglial receptors in the OVLT and other areas of the lamina terminalis.

ACKNOWLEDGEMENTS: This study was supported by the "Deutsche Forschungsgemeinschaft, Project Ze 183/4-1. The technical assistance of Miss B. Störr and Mrs. A. Kaps is gratefully acknowledged.

REFERENCES

1. Blatteis, C.M.: The neurobiology of endogenous pyrogens. In Bligh & Voigt, *Thermoreception and Temperature Regulation*, pp. 257-272 (Springer, Berlin 1990).
2. Kluger, M.J.: Endogenous pyrogens and fever. In Mercer, *Thermal Physiology 1989*, pp. 35-44 (Elsevier, Amsterdam 1989).
3. Cooper, K.E.: The neurobiology of fever: Thoughts on recent developments. Ann. Rev. Neurosci. **10**:297-324 (1987).
4. Pittman, Q.J. & Landgraf, R.: Vasopressin in thermoregulation and blood pressure control. In Lord & Jamison, *Vasopressin Vasopressine*, pp. 177-184 (Collogue INSERM Vol. 208 (John Libbey Eurotext 1991).
5. Zeisberger, E.: Peptides and amines as putative factors in endogenous antipyresis. In *Proceedings of the XXth International Congress of Neurovegetative Research in Tokyo 1990, Excerpta Medica International Congress* (Elsevier, Amsterdam 1991) (in press).
6. Naylor, A.M., Cooper, K.E. & Veale, W.L.: Vasopressin and fever: evidence supporting the existence of an endogenous antipyretic system in the brain. Can. J. Physiol. Pharmacol. **65**:1333-1338 (1987).
7. Kasting, N.W.: Criteria for establishing a physiological role for brain peptides. A case in point: The role of vasopressin in thermoregulation during fever and antipyresis. Brain Res. Rev. **14**:143-153 (1989).

8. Thrasher, T.N.: Role of forebrain circumventricular organs in body fluid balance. Acta Physiol. Scand. **136(Suppl. 583)**:141-150 (1989).

9. Roth, J., Schulze, K., Merker, G., Simon, E. & Zeisberger, E.: Influence of osmotic stimulation on release of arginine-vasopressin and fever in the guinea pig. Neuroendocrinology **52(Suppl. 1)**:114 (1990).

10. Zeisberger, E.: Antipyretic action of vasopressin in the ventral septal area of the guinea-pig's brain. In Lomax & Schönbaum, *Thermoregulation: Research and Clinical Applications*, pp. 65-68 (Karger, Basel 1989).

11. Merker, G., Blähser, S. & Zeisberger, E.: Reactivity pattern of vasopressin-containing neurons and its relation to the antipyretic reaction in the pregnant guinea pig. Cell Tissue Res. **212**:47-61 (1980).

12. Thrasher, T.N. & Keil, L.C.: Regulation of drinking and vasopressin secretion: Role of organum vasculosum laminae terminalis. Am. J. Physiol. **253**:R108-R120 (1987).

13. Stitt, J.T. & Shimada, S.G.: Immunoadjuvants enhance the febrile responses of rats to endogenous pyrogen. J. Appl. Physiol. **67**:1734-1739 (1989).

14. Phillips, M.I.: Functions of angiotensin in the central nervous system. Ann. Rev. Physiol. **49**:413-435 (1987).

15. Kiss, J.Z.: Dynamism of chemoarchitecture in the hypothalamic paraventricular nucleus. Brain Res. Bull. **20**:699-708 (1988).

16. Staiger, J.F. & Nürnberger, F.: Pattern of afferents to the lateral septum in the guinea pig. Cell Tissue Res. **257**:471-490 (1989).

17. Dubois-Dauphin, M., Tribollet, E. & Dreifuss, J.J.: Distribution of neurohypophysial peptides in the guinea pig brain. I. An immunocytochemical study of the vasopressin-related glycopeptide. Brain Res. **496**:45-65 (1989).

18. De Vries, G.J., Buijs, R.M., Van Leeuwen, F.W., Caffé, A.R. & Swaab, D.F.: The vasopressinergic innervation of the brain of normal and castrated rats. J. Comp. Neurol. **233**:236-254 (1985).

19. Merker, G., Roth, J. & Zeisberger, E.: Thermoadaptive influence on reactivity pattern of vasopressinergic neurons in the guinea pig. Experientia **45**:722-726 (1989).

20. Neumann, I., Schwarzberg, H. & Landgraf, R.: Measurement of septal release of vasopressin and oxytocin by the push-pull technique following electrical stimulation of the paraventricular nucleus of rats. Brain Res. **462**:181-184 (1988).

21. Unger, M., Merker, G., Roth, J. & Zeisberger, E.: Influence of noradrenergic input into the hypothalamic paraventricular nucleus on fever in the guinea pig. Pflügers Arch. (in press 1991).

22. Poulin, P., Lederis, K. & Pittman, Q.J.: Subcellular localization and characterization of vasopressin binding sites in the ventral septal area, lateral septum, and hippocampus of the rat brain. J. Neurochem. **50**:889-898 (1988).

23. Gerstberger, R. & Fahrenholz, F.: Autoradiographic localization of V_1 vasopressin binding sites in rat brain and kidney. Eur. J. Pharmacol. **167**:105-116 (1989).

24. Cheng, S.W.T. & North, W.G.: Vasopressin reduces release from vasopressin-neurons and oxytocin-neurons by acting on V_2-like receptors. Brain Res. **479**:35-39 (1989).

25. Staiger, J.F. & Wouterlood, F.G.: Efferent projections from the lateral septal nucleus to the anterior hypothalamus in the rat: A study combining Phaseolus vulgaris-leucoagglutinin tracing with vasopressin immunocytochemistry. Cell Tissue Res. **261**:17-23 (1990).

26. Zeisberger, E.: Comparison of antipyretic actions of different neuropeptides in the same site of brain septum in the guinea pig. In Mercer, *Thermal Physiology 1989*, pp. 117-122 (Elsevier, Amsterdam 1989).

27. Katsuura, G., Gottschall, P.E., Dahl, R.R. & Arimura, A.: Interleukin-1β increases prostaglandin E_2 in rat astrocyte cultures: Modulatory effect of neuropeptides. Endocrinology **124**:3125-3127 (1989).

CUMULATIVE BIBLIOGRAPHY

Aarden, L.A., DeGroot, E.R., Schaap, O.L. & Landsdorp, P.M.: Production of hybridoma growth factors by human monocytes. Eur. J. Immunol. **17**:1411-1416 (1987).

Akins, C.W.: Noncardioplegic myocardial preservation for coronary revascularization. J. Thorac Cardiovas. Surg. **88**:174-181 (1984).

Akira, S., Hirando, T., Taga, T. & Kishimoto, T.: Biology of multifunctional cytokines: IL-6 and related molecules (IL 1 and TNF). FASEB J. **4**:2860-2867 (1990).

Aksel, S., Schomberg, D.W., Tyrey, L. & Hammond, C.B.: Vasomotor symptoms, serum estrogens, and gonadotropin levels in surgical menopause. Am. J. Obstet. Gynecol. **126**:165-169 (1976).

Albano, E., Tomasi, A., Mannuzzu, L. & Arese, P.: Detection of a free radical intermediate from divicine of Vicia faba. Biochem. Pharmacol. **33**:1701-1704 (1984).

Aman, J., Berne, C., Ewald, U. & Tuvemo, T.: Lack of cutaneous hyperaemia in response to insulin-induced hypoglycaemia in IDDM. Diabetes Care **13**:1029-1033 (1990).

Arbid, M.S. & Bashandy, M.A.: A study of the antimetabolites (Divicine) isolated from faba beans (Vicia faba L.) on some physiological responses with special references to its thermoregulatory effects. 7th International Symposium on the Pharmacology of Thermoregulation, Odense, pp. 149-152, 1988 (Karger, Basel 1989).

Arbid, M.S.S. & Marquardt, R.R.: Effect of intraperitoneally injected vicine and convicine on the rats: induction of favism-like signs. J. Sci. Food Agric. **37**:539-547 (1986).

Arbid, M.S.S. & Marquardt, R.R.: Favism-like effects of divicine and isouramil in the rat: Acute and chronic effects on animal health, mortalities, blood parameters and ability to exchange respiratory gases. J. Sci. Food Agric. **43**:75-90 (1988).

Arbid, M.S., Marquardt, R.R. & El-Habbak, M.M.: A study of the toxic effects of high levels of dehulled faba beans (Vicia faba L.) in the diets of laying hens. Egyptian Poultry Science, Faculty of Agriculture, 5 (1985).

Arch, J.R.S.: The brown adipocyte β-adrenoceptor. Proc. Nutr. Soc. **48**:215-223 (1989).

Arese, P.: Rev. Pure Appl. Pharmacol. Sci. **3**:123 (1982).

Arese, P., Bosia, A., Naitana, A., Gaetani, S., D'Aquino,M. & Gaetan, G.P.: In Brewer, *The Red Cell*, p. 725 (Alan R. Liss, New York 1981).

Asch, R.H. & Greenblatt, R.B.: Steroidogenesis in the postmenopausal ovary. Clin. Obstet. Gynaecol. **4**:85-106 (1977)Aschoff, J.: Circadian rhythms in man: a self-sustained oscillator with an inerent frequency underlies human 24-hour periodicity. Science **148**:1427-1432 (1965).

Aschoff, J.: Circadian rhythms in man: a self-sustained oscillator with an inherent frequency underlies human 24-hour periodicity. Science **148**:1427-1432 (1965).

Baeyens, J.M., Esposito, E., Ossowska, G. & Samanin, R.: Effects of peripheral and central administration of calcium channel blockers in the naloxone-precipitated abstinence in morphine-dependent rats. Eur. J. Pharmacol. **137**:9-13 (1987).

Balaban, C.D., Starcevic, V.P. & Severs, W.B.: Neuropeptide modulation of central vestibular circuits. Pharm. Rev. **41**:53-90 (1989).

Balderman, S.C.: The most appropriate temperature for myocardial preservation. In Roberts, *Myocardial Protection in Cardiac Surgery*, Cardiothoracic Surgery, Series Z, pp. 303-359 (Marcel Dekker, NY 1987).

Bansinath, M., Ramabadran, K., Turndorf, H. & Puig, M.M.: Effect of κ and μ selective agonists on colonic temperature in normoglycemic and streptozotocin-treated hyperglycemic mice. Pharmacol. Toxicol. **66**:324-328 (1990).

Bansinath, M., Turndorf, H. & Puig, M.M.: Influence of hypo- and hyperthermia on disposition of morphine. J. Clin. Pharmacol. **28**:860-864 (1988).

Barcroft, H. & Swan, H.J.C.: *Sympathetic Control of Human Blood Vessels* (Edward Arnold, London 1953).

Barlow, D.H., Brockie, J.A., Rees, C.M.P. & Oxford General Practitioners Menopause Study Group: Study of general practice consultations and menopausal problems. Br. Med. J. **302:**274-276 (1991).

Beavis, A.D.: The mitochondrial inner-membrane anion channel possesses two mercurial-reactive regulatory sites. Eur. J. Biochem. **185:**511-519 (1989).

Beckman, A.L. & Carlisle, H.J.: Effect of intrahypothalamic infusion of acetylcholine on behavioral and physiological thermoregulation in the rat. Nature **221:**561-562 (1969).

Beleslin, D.B., Jovanovic-Micic, D. & Samardzic, R.: Nature of hypo- and hyperthermia induced by the calcium antagonist nicardipine. Arch. Int. Physiol. Biochim. **95:**347-353 (1987).

Benedek, G. & Szikszay, M.: Potentiation of thermoregulatory and analgesic effects of morphine by calcium antagonists. Pharmac. Res. Comm. **16:**1009-1018 (1984).

Berger, R.J., Palca, J.W., Walker, J.M. & Phillips, N.H.: Correlations between body temperatures, metabolic rate and slow wave sleep in humans. Neurosci. Lett. **86:**230-234 (1988).

Berger, R.L., Davis, K.B., Kaiser, G.C., Foster, E.D., Hammond, G.L., Tong, T.G.L., Kennedy, J.W., Sheffield, T., Ringqvist, I., Wiens, R.D., Chaitman, B.R. & Mock, M.: Preservation of the myocardium during coronary artery bypass grafting. Circulation **64(Suppl. II):**61-66 (1981).

Bernardini, G.L., Richards, D.B. & Lipton, J.M. Antipyretic effects of centrally administered CRF. Peptides **5:**57-59 (1984).

Berne, C. & Fagius, J.: Skin nerve sympathetic activity during insulin-induced hypoglycaemia. Diabetologia **29:**855-860 (1986).

Bers, D.M.: Ca influx and sarcoplasmic reticulum Ca release in cardiac muscle activation during postrest recovery. Am. J. Physiol. **248:**H336-H381 (1985).

Beyersdorf, F., Krause, E., Sarai, K., Sieber, B., Deutschlander, N., Zimmer, G., Mainka, L., Probst, S., Zegelman, M., Schneider, W. & Satter, P.: Clinical evaluation of hypothermic ventricular fibrillation, multi-dose blood cardioplegia and single-dose Bretschneider cardioplegia in coronary surgery. Thorac Cardiovasc. Surg. **38:**20-29 (1990).

Bianco, A.C., Sheng, X. & Silva, J.E.: Triiodothyronine amplifies norepinephrine stimulation of uncoupling protein gene transcription by a mechanism not requiring protein synthesis. J. Biol. Chem. **263:**18168-18175 (1988).

Bider, D., Ben-Rafael, Z., Shalev, J., Mashiach, S., Serr, D.M. & Blankstein, J.: Hot flushes during Gn-RH analogue administration despite normal serum oestradiol levels. Maturitas **11:**223-228 (1989).

Binkley, S., Kluth, E.& Menaker, M.: Pineal function in sparrows: Circadian rhythms and body temperature. Science **174:**311-314 (1971).

Biswas, S. & Poddar, M.K.: Does GABA act through dopaminergic/cholinergic interaction in the regulation of higher environmental tempreature-induced change in body temperature? Meth. Find. Exp. Clin. Pharmacol. **12:**303-307 (1990).

Biswas, S. & Poddar, M.K.: Effect of short- and long-term exposures to low environmental temperature on brain regional GABA metabolism. Neurochem. Res. **15:**821-826 (1990).

Blaesig, J., Hoellt, V., Baeuerle, U. & Herz, A.: Involvement of endorphins in emotional hyperthermia of rats. Life Sci. **23:**2525-2532 (1978).

Blatteis, C.M.: Functional anatomy of the hypothalamus from the point of view of temperature regulation. In Szelenyi & Szekely, *Advances in Physiological Science, Vol. 32, Contributions to Thermal Physiology*, pp. 3-12 (Pergamon, Oxford 1981).

Blatteis, C.M.: Hypothalamic substances in the control of body temperature: general characteristics. Fed. Proc. **40:**2731-2740 (1981).

Blatteis, C.M.: The neurobiology of endogenous pyrogens. In Bligh & Voigt, *Thermoreception and Temperature Regulation*, pp. 257-272 (Springer, Berlin 1990).

Bleier, R. & Byne, W.: Septum and hypothalamus. In Paxinos, *The Rat Nervous System, Vol. 1. Forebrain and Midbrain*, pp. 87-118 (Academic Press, 1985).

Bligh, J.: Aminoacids as central synaptic transmitters or modulators in mammalian thermoregulation. Fed. Proc. **40**:2746-2749 (1981).

Blight, J. & Cottle, W.H.: The influence of ambient temperature on thermoregulatory responses to 5-hydroxytryptamine, noradrenaline and acetylcholine injected into the lateral cerebral ventricles of sheep, goats and rabbits. J. Physiol. Lond. **212**:377-392 (1969).

Bonchek, L.I. & Burlingame, M.W.: Coronary artery bypass without cardioplegia. J. Thorac Cardiovasc. Surg. **93**:261-267 (1987).

Bonegio, R.G.B., Driver, H.S., King, L.A., Laburn, H.P. & Shapiro, C.M.: Circadian temperature rhythm blunting and sleep composition. Acta Physiol. Scand. **133(Suppl. 574)**:44-47 (1988).

Bongianni, F., Carla, V., Moroni, F. & Pellegrini-Giampietro, D.E.: Calcium channel inhibitors suppress the morphine-withdrawal syndrome in rats. Br. J. Pharmac. **88**:561-567 (1986).

Boschi, G. & Launay, N.: Differential effects of neuroleptic and serotonergic drugs on amphetamine-induced hypothermia in mice. Neuropharmacology **24**:117-122 (1985).

Boschi, G. & Rips, R.: Forebrain sites for the hypothermic effect of dexamphetamine in mice. Neurosci. Lett. **31**:153-158 (1982).

Boschi, G. & Rips, R.: Tyrotropin releasing hormone (TRH) induced hyperthermia and its potentiation in the mouse: peripheral or central origin. IRCS Med. Sci. **9**:200-201 (1981).

Bristow, G.K.: Clinical aspects of accidental hypothermia. In Heller, Musacchia & Wang, *Living in the Cold*, pp. 513-521 (Elsevier, New York 1986).

Buijs, R.M. & Swaab, D.F.: Immuno-electron microscopical demonstration of vasopressin and oxytocin synapses in the limbic system of the rat. Cell Tissue Res. **204**:355-365 (1979).

Bunnell, D.E. & Horvath, S.M.: Effects of body heating during sleep interruption. Sleep **8(3)**:274-282 (1985).

Bunting, S., Gryglewski, R., Moncada, S. & Vane, J.R.: Arterial walls generate from prostaglandin endoperoxides a substance (Prostaglandin X) which relaxes strips of mesenteric and coeliac arteries and inhibits platelet aggregation. Prostaglandins **12**:897-913 (1976).

Burcher, E., Atterhög, J-H., Pernow, B. & Rosell, S.: Cardiovascular effects of substance P: Effects on the heart and regional blood flow in the dog. In Euler and Pernow, *Substance P*, pp. 261-268 (Raven Press, New York 1977).

Burnard, D.M., Pittman, Q.J. & Veale, W.L.: Increased motor disturbances in response to arginine vasopressin following hemorrhage or hypertonic saline: evidence for central AVP release in rats. Brain Res. **273**:59-65 (1983).

Burnard, D.M., Veale, W.L. & Pittman, Q.J.: Arginine vasopressin: its possible involvement in febrile convulsions. In Cooper, Lomax, Schönbaum & Veale, *Homeostasis and Thermal Stress. 6th Int. Symp. Pharmacol. Thermoregulation*, pp. 57-61 (Karger, Basel 1986).

Burnard, D.M., Veale, W.L. & Pittman, Q.J.: Prevention of arginine-vasopressin-induced motor disturbances by a potent vasopressor antagonist. Brain Res. **362**:40-46 (1986).

Busbridge, N.J., Dascombe, M.J., Tilders, F.J.H., van Oers, J.W.A.M., Linton, E.A. & Rothwell, N.J.: Central activation of thermogenesis and fever by interleukin-1β and interleukin-1α involves different mechanisms. Biochem. Biophys. Res. Comm. **162**:591-596 (1989).

Caffé, A.R., van Leeuwen, F.W. & Luiten, P.G.M.: Vasopressin cells in the medial amygdala of the rat project to the lateral septum and ventral hippocampus. J. Comp. Neurol. **261**:237-252 (1987).

Cagnacci, A., Bonuccelli, U., Melis, G.B., Soldani, R., Piccini, P., Napolitano, Muratorio, A. & Fioretta, P.: Effect of naloxone on body temperature in postmenopausal women with Parkinson's disease. Life Sci. **46**:1241-1247 (1990).

Cagnacci, A., Melis, G.B., Paoleti, A.M., Soldani, R. & Fioretti, P.: Thermoregulatory and endocrine effects of a low dose of danazol in postmenopausal women: Interaction with the effect of naloxone. Life Sci. **48**:1051-1058 (1991).

Cannon, B. & Johansson, B.W.: Nonshivering thermogenesis in the newborn. Mol. Aspects Med. **3**:119-223 (1980).

Cannon, B. & Nedergaard, J.: Adipocytes, preadipocytes, and mitochondria from brown adipose tissue. In Hausman & Martin, *Biology of the Adipocyte: Research Approaches*, pp. 21-51 (Van Nostrand Reinhold, New York 1987).

Carpentier, S., Murawsky, M. & Carpentier, A.: Cytotoxicity of cardioplegic solutions: evaluation by tissue culture. Circulation **64(Suppl. II)**:90-95 (1981).

Casper, R.F., Yen, S.S.C. & Wilkes, M.M.: Menopausal flushes: A neuroendocrine link with pulsatile luteinizing hormone secretion. Science **205**:823-825 (1979).

Cenarruzabeitia, M.N., Santidrian, S., Bello, J. & Larralde, J.: Effect of raw field bean (vicia faba) on amino-acid-degrading enzymes in rats and chicks. Nutr. Metb. **23(3)**:203-210 (1979).

Challis, R.A.J., Leighton, B., Lozeman, F.J. & Newsholme, E.A.: The hormone-modulatory effects of adenosine in skeletal muscle. In Gerlach & Becker, *Topics and Perspectives in Adenosine Research*, pp. 275-285 (Springer-Verlag, Berlin 1987).

Charney, D.S., Heninger, G.R. & Sternberg, D.E.: Assessment of α_2 adrenergic autoreceptor function in humans: Effects of oral yohimbine. Life Sci. **30**:2033-2041 (1982).

Cheng, S.W.T. & North, W.G.: Vasopressin reduces release from vasopressin-neurons and oxytocin-neurons by acting on V_2-like receptors. Brain Res. **479**:35-39 (1989).

Chevion, M., Navok, T., Glaser, G. & Mager, J.: The chemistry of favism-inducing compounds. The properties of isouramil and divicine and their reaction with glutathione. Eur. J. Biochem. **12**:405-409 (1982).

Chipkin, R.E.: Effects of D1 and D2 antagonists on basal and apomorphine decreased body temperature in mice and rats. Pharmacol. Biochem. Behav. **30**:683-686 (1988).

Clark, W.G. & Lipton, J.M.: Brain and pituitary peptides in thermoregulation. Pharmac. Ther. **22**:249-297 (1983).

Clark, W.G. & Lipton, J.M.: Changes in body temperature after administration of adrenergic agents and related drugs including antidepressants. Neurosci. Behav. **10**:153-220 (1986).

Clayden, J.R., Bell, J.W. & Pollard, P.: Menopausal flushing: Double blind trial of a non-hormonal medication. Br. Med. J. **1**:409-412 (1974).

Colditz, G.A., Stampfer, M.J., Willett, W.C., Hennekens, C.H., Rosner, B. & Speizer, F.E.: Prospective study of estrogen replacement therapy and risk of breast cancer in postmenopausal women. **264**:2648-2653 (1990).

Collins, M.G., Hunter, W.S. & Blatteis, C.M.: Factors producing elevated core temperature in spontaneously hypertensive rats. J. Appl. Physiol. **63**:740-745 (1987).

Conrad, L.C.A. & Pfaff, D.W.: Efferents from medial basal forebrain and hypothalamus in the rat. I. An autoradiographic study of the medial preoptic area. J. Comp. Neurol. **169**:185-220 (1976).

Conrad, L.C.A. & Pfaff, D.W.: Efferents from medial basal forebrain and hypothalamus in the rat. II. An autoradiographic study of the anterior hypothalamus. J. Comp. Neurol. **169**:221-262 (1976).

Consolo, S., Dolfini, E., Garattini, S. & Valzelli, L.: Desipramine and amphetamine metabolism. J. Pharm. Pharmacol. **19**:253-256 (1967).

Cooper, K.E.: The neurobiology of fever: Thoughts on re cent developments. Ann. Rev. Neurosci. **10**:297-324 (1987).

Cooper, K.E., Blähser, S., Malkinson, T.J., Merker, G., Roth, J. & Zeisberger, E.: Changes in body temperature and vasopressin content of brain neurons, in pregnant and non-pregnant guinea pigs, during fevers produced by Poly I:Poly C. Pflügers Arch. **412**:292-296 (1988).

Cooper, K.E. & Cranston, W.I.: Clearance of radioactive bacterial pyrogen from the circulation. J. Physiol. (London) **166**:41P (1963).

Cooper, K.E., Cranston, W.J. & Snell, E.S.: Observation on the site and mode of action of pyrogens in the rabbit brain. J. Physiol. **191**:325-337 (1967).

Corbett, D., Evans, S., Thomas, C., Wang, D. & Jonas, R.A.: MK-801 reduced cerebral ischemic injury by inducing hypothermia. Brain Res. **514**:300-304 (1990).

Cox, B.: Dopamine. In Lomax & Schönbaum, *Body Temperature*, pp. 231-255 (Dekker, New York 1979).

Cox, B., Ary, M. & Lomax, P.: Dopaminergic involvement in withdrawal hypothermia and thermoregulatory behavior in morphine dependents rat. Pharmacol. Biochem. Behav. **4**:259-262 (1976).

Cox, B. & Lomax, P.: Pharmacologic control of temperature regulation. Ann. Rev. Pharmacol. Toxicol. **17**:341-353 (1977).

Crawshaw, L.I.: Temperature regulation in vertebrates. Ann. Rev. Physiol. **42**:473-491 (1980).

Danon, A., Leibson, V. & Assouline, J.: Effects of aspirin, indomethacin, flufenamic acid and paracetamol on prostaglandin output from rat stomach and renal papilla in-vitro and ex-vivo. J. Pharm. Pharmacol. **35**:576-579 (1983).

D'Amico, J.F., Greendale, G.A., Lu, J.K.H. & Judd, H.L.: Induction of hypothalamic opioid activity with transdermal estradiol administration in postmenopausal women. Fertil. Steril. **55**:754-758 (1991).

D'Aquino, M., Gaetani, S. & Spadoni, M.A.: Effect of factors of favism on the protein and lipid components of rat erythrocyte membrane. Biochem. Biophys. Acta **731**:161-167 (1983).

Dascombe, M.J.: Cyclic nucleotides and fever. In Milton, *Pyretics and Antipyretics*, pp. 219-255 (Springer-Verlag, Berlin 1982).

Dascombe, M.J.: Evidence against adenosine 3',5'-monophosphate as a mediator of fever in the brain. Neuropharmacology **25**:309-313 (1986).

Dascombe, M.J.: The pharmacology of fever. Prog. Neurobiol. **25**:327-373 (1985).

Dascombe, M.J. & Milton, A.S.: Cyclic adenosine 3',5'-monophosphate in cerebrospinal fluid during thermoregulation and fever. J. Physiol. (Lond.) **263**:441-463 (1976).

Dascombe, M.J. & Milton, A.S.: The effects of cyclic adenosine 3',5'-monophosphate and other adenine nucleotides on body temperature. J. Physiol. (Lond.) **250**:143-160 (1975).

Davatelis, G., Wolpe, S.D., Sherry, B., Dayer, J.-M., Chicheportiche, R. & Cerami, A.: Macrophage inflammatory protein-1: a prostaglandin-independent endogenous pyrogen. Science **243**:1066-1068 (1989).

Davoren, P.R. & Sutherland, E.W.: The effect of l-epinephrine and other agents on the synthesis and release of adenosine 3',5'-phosphate by whole pigeon erythrocytes. J. Biol. Chem. **238**:3009-3015 (1963).

Dawson, R. Jr. & Lordon, J.F.: Behavioral and neurochemical effects of neonatal administration of monosodium L-glutamate in mice. J. Comp. Physiol. Psychol. **95**:71-84 (1981).

De Aloysio, D., Fabiani, A.G., Mauloni & Bottiglioni, F.: Analysis of the climacteric syndrome. Maturitas **11**:43-53 (1989).

DeFronzo, R.A., Jordan, D., Tobin, J.D. & Andres, R.: Glucose clamp technique: a method for quantifying insulin secretion and resistance. Am. J. Physiol. **237**:E214-223 (1979).

de Jong, J.W.: Cardioplegia and calcium antagonists: a review. Ann. Thorac. Surg. **42**:593-598 (1986).

de Olmos, J.S., Alheid, G.F. & Beltramino, C.A.: Amygdala. In Paxinos, *The Rat Nervous System (Vol. 1): Forebrain and Midbrain*, pp. 223-334 (Academic Press, Toronto 1985).

De Vries, G.J., Buijs, R.M., van Leeuwen, F.W., Caffé, A.R. & Swaab, D.F.: The vasopressinergic innervation of the brain in normal and castrated rats. J. Comp. Neurol. **233**:236-254 (1985).

Dhumal, V.R., Gulati, O.D. & Nandkumar, S.S.: Effects on rectal temperature in rats of γ-aminobutyric acid: Possible mediation through putative transmitters. Eur. J. Pharmacol. **35**:341-347 (1976).

Dicker, A., Raasmaja, A., Cannon, B. & Nedergaard, J.: Effects of hypothyroidism on adrenergic receptors in brown adipose tissue. (Submitted 1991).

Dinarello, C.A.: Interleukin-1. Rev. Infect. Dis. **6**:51-95 (1984).

Dinarello, C.A., Bernheim, H.A. & Duff, G.W.: Mechanisms of fever induced by recombinant human interferon. J. Clin. Invest. **74**:906-913 (1984). J. Clin. Invest. **74**:906-913 (1984).

Dinarello, C.A., Bodel, P.T. & Atkins, E.: The role of the liver in the production of fever and in pyrogenic tolerance. Trans. Assoc. Am. Physicians **81**:334-343 (1968).

Dinarello, C.A., Cannon, S.M., Wolff, H.A., Bernheim, B., Beutler, A., Cerami, I.S., Figari, M.A., Palladino, Jr. & O'Connor, J.V.: Tumor necrosis factor (cachectin) is an endogenous pyrogen and induces production of interleukin 1. J. Exp. Med. **163**:1433-1450 (1986).

Disturnal, J.E., Veale, W.L. & Pittman, Q.J.: Electrophysiological analysis of potential arginine vasopressin projections to the ventral septal area of the rat. Brain Res. **342**:162-167 (1985).

Dorsa, D.M., Petracca, F.M., Baskin, D.G. & Cornett, L.E.: Localization and characterization of vasopressin-binding sites in the amygdala of the rat brain. J. Neurosci. **4:**1764-1770 (1984).

Drummond, P.D. & Edis, R.H.: Loss of facial sweating and flushing in Holmes-Adie syndrome. Neurology **40:**847-849 (1990).

Dubois-Dauphin, M., Tribollet, E. & Dreifuss, J.J.: Distribution of neurohypophysial peptides in the guinea pig brain. I. An immunocytochemical study of the vasopressin-related glycopeptide. Brain Res. **496:**45-65 (1989).

Duloo, A.G. & Miller, D.S.: Unimpaired thermogenic response to noradrenaline in genetic (ob/ob) and hypothalamic (MSG) obese mice. Bioscience Reports **4:**343-349 (1984).

Duncombe, W.G.: The colorimetric micro-determination of long-chain fatty acids. Biochem. J. **88:**7-10 (1963).

Dunn, A.J. & Berridge, C.W.: Physiological and behavioural responses to corticotropin releasing factor administration: is CRF a mediator of anxiety or stress responses? Brain Res. Rev. **15:**71-100 (1990).

Erlik, Y., Tataryn, I.V., Meldrum, D.R., Lomax, P., Bajorek, J.G. & Judd, H.L.: Association of waking episodes with menopausal hot flushes. JAMA **245(17):**1741-1744 (1981).

Espevic, T. & Nissen-Meyer, J.: A highly sensitive cell line, WEHI 164 clone 13, for measuring cytotoxic factor/tumor necrosis factor from human monocytes. J. Immunol. Meth. **95:**99-105 (1986).

Euler, U.S. von and Pernow, B. (Eds.): *Substance P* (Raven Press, New York 1977).

Farrar, W., Kilian, P.L., Ruff, M.R., Hill, J.M. & Pert, C.B.: Visualization and characterization of interleukin 1 receptors in brain. J. Immunol. **139:**459-463 (1987).

Federico, P., Malkinson, T.J., Cooper, K.E., Pittman, Q.J. & Veale, W.L.: Vasopressin-induced antipyresis in the medial amygdaloid nucleus of the urethan-anesthetized rat. Soc. Neurosci. Abstr. **16:**1204 (1990).

Fisher, S., Raskin A. & Uhlenhuth, E.H. (eds): *Cocaine: Clinical and Biobehavioral Aspects* (Oxford University Press, New York 1987).

Flameng, W., Van-der-Vusse, J.G., DeMeyere, R., Borgers, M., Sergeant, P., Meersch, E.V., Geboers, J. & Suy, R.: Intermittent aortic cross-clamping versus St. Thomas' hospital cardioplegia in extensive aorta-coronary bypass grafting. J. Thorac Cardiovasc. Surg. **88:**164-173 (1984).

Fleming, J.A., Byck, R. & Barash, P.G.: Pharmacology and therapeutic applications of cocaine. Anesthesiology **73:**518-531 (1990).

Flint, M., Kronenberg, F. & Utian, W. (eds): Multidisciplinary Persectives on Menopause. Ann. N.Y. Acad. Sci. 592 (1990).

Folin (1950): (Cited from Hawk's physiological chemistry, 14th edition, 1965).

Foster, D.O.: Quantitative role of brown adipose tissue in thermogenesis. In Trayhurn & Nicholls, *Brown Adipose Tissue*, pp. 31-51 (Edward Arnold, London 1986).

Foster, D.O. & Frydman, M.L.: Nonshivering thermogenesis in the rat. I. Measurements of blood flow with microspheres point to brown adipose tissue as the dominant site of calorigenesis induced by noradrenaline. Can. J. Physiol. Pharmacol. **56:**110-122 (1978).

France, C.P., Winger, G.D. & Woods, J.H.: Analgesic, anesthetic and respiratory effects of the competitive N-methyl-D-aspartate (NMDA) antagonist CGS 19755 in rhesus monkeys. Brain Res. **526:**355-358 (1990).

Fredholm, B.B. & Dunwiddle, T.V.: How does adenosine inhibit transmitter release? Trends Pharmac. Sci. **9:**130-134 (1988).

Freedman, R.R.: Laboratory and ambulatory monitoring of menopausal hot flushes. Psychophysiology **26:**573-579 (1989).

Freedman, R.R., Woodward, S. & Sabharwal, S.C.: α_2-Adrenergic mechanism in menopausal hot flushes. Obstet. Gynecol. **76:**573-578 (1990).

Freeman, J.J. & Sulser, F.: Iprindole-amphetamine interactions in the rat: the role of aromatic hydroxylation of amphetamine in its mode of action. J. Pharmacol. Exp. Ther. **183:**307-315 (1972).

Fregly, M.J.: A simple and accurate feeding device for rats. J. Appl. Physiol. **15:**539 (1960).

Fregly, M.J., Nelson, E.L., Jr. & Tyler, P.E.: Water exchange in rats exposed to cold, hypoxia, and both combined. Aviat. Space Environ. Med. **47:**600-607 (1976).

French, E.B. & Kilpatrick, R.: The role of adrenaline in hypoglycaemic reactions in man. Clin. Sci. **14:**639-651 (1955).

Freund-Mercier, M.J., Stoeckel, M.E., Dietl, M.M., Palacios, J.M. & Richard, P.: Quantitative autoradiographic mapping of neurohypophyseal hormone binding sites in the rat forebrain and pituitary gland-I. Characterization of different binding sites and their distribution in the Long-Evans strain. Neurosci. **26:**261-272 (1988).

Fromme, G.A., White, R.D. & Housmans, P.R.: Myocardial preservation. In Roberts, *Myocardial Protection in Cardiac Surgery*, pp. 395-408 (Marcel Dekker, NY 1987).

Fuxe, K., Hökfelt, T., Ljungdahl, A., Agnati, L., Johansson, O. & Perez de la Mora, M.: Evidence for an inhibitory gabaergic control of the mesolimbic dopamine neurons: Possibility of improving treatment of schizophrenia by combined treatment with neuroleptics and gabaergic drugs. Med. Biol. **53:**177-183 (1975).

Gambone, J., Meldrum, D.R., Laufer, L., Chang, R.J., Lu, J.K.H. & Judd, H.L.: Further delineation of hypothalamic dysfunction responsible for menopausal hot flashes. J. Clin. Endocrinol. Metab. **59:**1097-1102 (1984).

Gaykema, R.P.A., Van Weeghel, R., Hersh, L.B. & Luiten, P.G.M.: Prefrontal cortical projections to the cholinergic neurons in the basal forebrain. J. Compl. Neurol. **303:**563-583 (1991).

Gearing, M. & Terasawa, E.: The α-1-adrenergic neuronal system is involved in the pulsatile release of luteinizing hormone-releasing hormone in the ovariectomized female rhesus monkey. Neuroendocrinology **53:**373-381 (1991).

Gebhard, M.M.: Myocardial protection and ischemia tolerance of the globally ischemic heart. Thorac Cardiovasc. Surg. **38:**55-59 (1990).

Gerlier, D. & Thomasset, N.: Use of MTT colorimetric assay to measure cell activation. J. Immunol. Meth. **94:**57-63 (1986).

Gerstberger, R. & Fahrenholz, F.: Autoradiographic localization of V_1 vasopressin binding sites in rat brain and kidney. Eur. J. Pharmacol. **167:**105-116 (1989).

Gill, D.M.: Mechanism of action of cholera toxin. Adv. Cyclic Nucleotide Res. **8:**85-118 (1977).

Gillis, B.J. & Cain, D.P.: Amygdala and pyriform cortex kindling in vasopressin deficient rats (Brattleboro strain). Brain Res. **271:**375-378 (1983).

Girardier, L. & Seydoux, J.: Neural control of brown adipose tissue. In Trayhurn & Nicholls, *Brown Adipose Tissue*, pp. 122-151 (Edward Arnold, London 1986).

Goldstein, D.S., McCarty, R., Polinsky, R.J. & Kopin, I.J.: Relationship between plasma norepinephrine and sympathetic neural activity. Hypertension **5:**552-559 (1983).

Hadas, H., Sod-Moriah, U.A. & Kaplanski, J.: The effect of lipopolysaccharide on fever and thermoregulation in rats. In Mercer, *Thermal Physiology*, pp. 395-400 (Elsevier, Amsterdam 1989).

Hagazy, M.I. & Marquardt, R.R.: Metabolism of vicine and convicine in rat tissues: Absorption and excretion patterns and sites of hydrolysis. J. Sci. Food Agric. **35:**139-146 (1984).

Hainsworth, F.R.: Saliva spreading, activity, and body temperature regulation in the rat. Am. J. Physiol. **212:**1288-1292 (1969).

Hainsworth, F.R. & Epstein, A.N.: Severe impairment of heat-induced saliva-spreading in rats recovered from lateral hypothalamic lesions. Science **153:**1255-1257 (1966).

Hales, J.R.S., Foldes, A., Fawcett, A.A. & King, R.B.: The role of adrenergic mechanisms in thermoregulatory control of blood flow through capillaries and arteriovenous anastomoses in the sheep hind limb. Pflügers Arch. **395:**93-98 (1982).

Hales, J.R.S. & Molyneux, G.S.: Control of cutaneous arteriovenous anastomoses. In Vanhoutte, *Vasodilatation: Vascular Smooth Muscle, Peptides, Autonomic Nerves and Endothelium*, pp. 321-332 (Raven Press, New York 1988).

Hales, J.R.S., Stephens, F.R.N., Fawcett, A.A., Daniel, K., Sheahan, J., Westerman, R.A. & James, S.B.: Observations on a new non-invasive monitor of skin blood flow. Clin. Exp. Pharm. Physiol. **16:**403-415 (1989).

Hamill, O.P., Marty, A., Neher, E., Sakmann, B. & Sigworth, F.J.: Improved patch-clamp techniques for high resolution current recording from cells and cell-free membrane patches. Pflügers Arch. **391**:85-100 (1981).

Harris *et al.* (1951): (Cited from Hawk's physiological chemistry, 14th edition, 1965).

Harris, R.B.S.: Role of set-point theory in regulation of body weight. FASEB J. **4**:33110-33118 (1990).

Hashimoto, M., Bando, T., Iriki, M. & Hashimoto, K.: Effect of indomethacin on febrile response to recombinant human interleukin 1- in rabbits. Am. J. Physiol. **255**:R527-R533 (1988).

Haskell, E.H., Palca, J.W., Walker, J.M., Berger, R.J. & Heller, H.C.: The effects of high and low ambient temperatures on human sleep stages. Electroecephalogr. Clin. Neurophysiol. **51**:494-501 (1981).

Hearse, D.J., Yamamoto, F. & Shattock, M.J.: Calcium antagonists and hypothermia: the temperature dependency of the negative inotropic and anti-ischemic properties of verapamil in the isolated rat heart. Circulation **70**:154-164 (1984).

Hedqvist, P.: Actions of prostacyclin (PGI$_2$) on adrenergic neuroeffector transmission in the rabbit kidney. Prostaglandins **17**:249-258.

Heldmaier, G. & Steinlechner, S.: Seasonal control of energy requirements for thermoregulation in the Djungarian hamster (Phodopus sungorus), living in natural photoperiod. J. Comp. Physiol. **142**:429-437 (1981).

Helperin, B.N., Beezi, G., Mene, G. & Benaceroff, B.: Etude quantitative de l'activate granulo plexyue Due systeme reteculo-ends lial por l'injection intraveneus d'encre de chin chez les diverses especes animals. Anr. Inst. Pastuer **80**:582-604 (1951).

Heritage, A.S., Stumpf, W.E., Sar, M. & Grant, L.D.: Brainstem catecholamine neurons are target sites for sex steroid hormones. Science **207**:1377-1379 (1980).

Herring, W.B., Herion, J.C., Walker, R.I. & Palmer, J.G.: Distribution and clearance of circulating endotoxin. J. Clin. Invest. **42**:79-87 (1963).

Hess, M.L., Krause, S.M., Robbins, A.D. & Greenfield, L.J.: Excitation-contraction coupling in hypothermic ischemic myocardium. Am. J. Physiol. **240**:H336-H341 (1981).

Hissa, R. & Hirsimäki, P.: Calorigenic effects of noradrenaline and inderal in the temperature-acclimated golden hamster. Comp. Gen. Pharmac. **2**:217-224 (1971).Hjelms, E. & Steiness, E.:Myocardial protection in coronary artery bypass surgery. A study comparing cold cardioplegia and intermittent aortic cross clamping. J. Cardiovasc. Surg. **23**:403-406 (1982).

Hökfelt, T., Skirboll, L., Rehfeld, J.F., Goldstein, H., Markey, K. & Dann, O.: A subpopulation of mesencephalic dopamine neurons projecting to limbic areas containing a cholecystokinin-like peptide: evidence from immunohistochemistry combined with retrograde tracing. Neuroscience **5**:2093-2124 (1980).

Holte, A. & Mikkelsen, A.: Climacteric complaints as a major health problem in the ageing population year 2000: Prognoses based on the distribution of climacteric complaints in a Scandinavian normal population. In Cortes-Prieto, Alvarez de los Heros, Neves-E-Castro & Vasquez-Benitez *Medicina de la Reproduccion Año 2000. Revista de la universidad de Alcala, No. 1*, pp. 233-243 (1990).

Holzbauer, T.R. & Vogt, M.: The concentration of adrenaline in the peripheral blood during insulin hypoglycaemia. Brit. J. Pharmacol. **9**:249 (1954).

Hoo-Paris, R., Jourdan, M.L., Moreau-Hamsany, C. & Wang, L.C.H.: Plasma glucagon, glucose, and free fatty acid concentrations and secretion during prolonged hypothermia in the rat. Am. J. Physiol. **260**:R480-R485 (1991).

Hoo-Paris, R., Jourdan, M.L., Wang, L.C.H. & Rajotte, R.V.: Insulin secretion and substrate homeostasis in prolonged hypothermia in rats. Am. J. Physiol. **255**:R1035-R1040 (1988).

Horita, A., Carino, M.A. & Lai, H.: Pharmacology of thyrotropin-releasing hormone. Ann. Rev. Pharmacol. Toxicol. **26**:311-332 (1986).

Horne, J.A., Brass, C.G. & Pettitt, A.N.: Circadian performance differences between morning and evening 'types'. Ergonomics **23**:29-36 (1980).

Horne, J.A. & Oesterberg, O.: Individual differences in human circadian rhythms. Biol. Psychiat. **5**:179-190 (1987).

Horne, J.A. & Reid, A.J.: Night-time sleep EEG changes following body heating in a warm bath. Electroencephalogr. Clin. Neurophysiol. **60:**154-157 (1985).

Horne, J.A. & Shackell, B.S.: Slow wave sleep elevations after body heating: Proximity to sleep and effects of aspirin. Sleep **10(4):**383-392 (1987).

Horne, J.A. & Staff, L.H.E.: Exercise and sleep: Body-heating effects. Sleep **6:**36-46 (1983).

Hsieh, A.C.L., Carlson, L.D. and Gray, G.: Role of the sympathetic nervous system in the control of chemical regulation of heat production. Am. J. Physiol. **190:**247-251 (1957).

Inokuchi, K. & Malik, K.U.: Attenuation by prostaglandins of adrenergically induced renal vasoconstriction in anesthetized rats. Am. J. Physiol. **246:**R228-R235 (1984).

Iriki, M. & Simon, E.: Regional differentiation of sympathetic efferents. In Ito, *Integrative Control Function of the Brain*, pp. 221-238 (Kodansha, Tokyo 1978).

Jacocks, M.A., Fowler, B.N., Chaffin, J.S., Lowenstein, E., Lappas, D.G., Pohost, G.M., Boucher, C.A., Okada, R.D., Hanna, N., Daggett, W.M., Butler, J., Balkas, C.: Hypothermic ischemic arrest versus hypothermic potassium cardioplegia in human beings. Ann. Thorac Surg. **34:**157-165 (1982).

Janis, R.A., Silver, P. & Triggle, D.J.: Drug action and cellular regulation. Adv. Drug Res. **16:**309-591 (1987).

Janský, L., Bartunkova, R., Kockova, J., Mejsnar, J. & Zeisberger, E.: Interspecies differences in cold adaptation and nonshivering thermogenesis. Fed. Proc. **28:**1053-1058 (1969).

Jepson, M.M., Millward, D.J., Rothwell, N.J. & Stock, M.J.: Involvement of sympathetic nervous system and brown fat in endotoxin-induced fever in rats. Am. J. Physiol. **255:**E617-E620 (1988).

Johansson, B.W.: Biologiska rytmer. Observanda Medica **4:**27-32 and 57-60 (1977).

Johnson, J.M., Brengelmann, G.L., Hales, J.R.S., Vanhoutte, P.M. & Wenger, C.B.: Regulation of the cutaneous circulation. Fed. Proc. **45:**2841-2850 (1986).

Jones, S.B. & Romano, F.D.: Functional characteristics and responses to adrenergic stimulation of isolated heart preparations from hypothermic and hibernating subjects. Cryobiology **21:**615-626 (1984).

Jourdan, M.L., Hoo-Paris, R. & Wang, L.C.H.: Characterization of hypothermia in nonhibernator: the rat. In Malan & Canguilhem, *Living in the Cold II*, pp. 289-296 (John Libbey Eurotext, Ltd., Montrouge, France 1989).

Jourdan, M.L., Lee, T.F. & Wang, L.C.H.: Survival and resuscitation from hypothermia: what natural hibernation can tell us about mammalian response to hypothermia. In Groat & Fuller, *Clinical Applications of Cryobiology* (CRC Press 1991) (in press).

Jourdan, M.L. & Wang, L.C.H.: An improved technique for the study of hypothermia physiology. J. Therm. Biol. **12:**175-178 (1987).

Kafka, M.S., Benedito, M.A., Roth, R.H., Steele, L.K., Wolfe, W.W. & Castravas, G.N.: Circadian rhythms in catecholamine metabolites and cyclic nucleotide production. Chronobiol. Int. **3:**101-115 (1986).

Kalra, P.S., Sahu, A. & Kalra, S.P.: Interleukin-1 inhibits the ovarian steroid-induced luteinizing hormone surge and release of hypothalamic luteinizing hormone-releasing hormone in rats. Endocrinology **126:**2145-2152 (1990).

Kaplanski, J., Hadas, H. & Sod-Moriah, U.A.: Effect of dexamethasone on fever and thermoregulation in acutely heat exposed rats. In Mercer, *Thermal Physiology*, pp. 407-412 (Elsevier, Amsterdam 1989).

Kaplanski, J., Hadas, H. & Sod-Moriah, U.A.: Effect of indomethacin on hyperthermia induced by lipopolysaccharides on high ambient temperature in rats. In Lomax & Schönbaum, *Thermoregulation: Research and Clinical Application*, pp. 176-178 (Karger, Basel 1989).

Karande, V.C., Scott, R.T. & Archer, D.F.: The relationship between serum estradiol-17β concentrations and induced pituitary luteinizing hormone surges in postmenopausal women. Fertil. Steril. **54:**217-221 (1990).

Kasting, N.W.: Criteria for establishing a physiological role for brain peptides. A case in point: The role of vasopressin in thermoregulation during fever and antipyresis. Brain Res. Rev. **14:**143-153 (1989).

Kasting, N.W., Veale, W.L. & Cooper, K.E.: Convulsive and hypothermic effects of vasopressin in the brain of the rat. Can. J. Physiol. Pharmacol. **58**:316-319 (1980).

Kasting, N.W., Veale, W.L., Cooper, K.E. & Lederis, K.: Vasopressin may mediate febrile convulsions. Brain Res. **213**:327-333 (1981).

Katovich, M.J. & O'Meara, J.: Effect of chronic estrogen on the skin temperature response to naloxone in morphine-dependent rats. Can. J. Physiol. Pharmacol. **65**:563-567 (1987).

Katovich, M.J., Pitman, D.L. & Barney, C.C.: Mechanisms mediating the thermal response to morphine withdrawal in rats. Proc. Soc. Exp. Biol. Med. **193**:129-135 (1990).

Katovich, M.J. & Simpkins, J.W.: Adrenergic modulation of the LHRH flush response in rats. Physiologist **33**:A105 (1990).

Katovich, M.J. & Simpkins, J.W.: Further evidence for an animal model for the hot flush. In Lomax & Schönbaum, *Thermoregulation: Research and Clinical Applications*, pp. 101-106 (Karger, Basel 1989).

Katovich, M.J., Simpkins, J.W. & Barney, C.C.: Alpha-Adrenergic mediation of the tail skin temperature response to naloxone in morphine-dependent rats. Brain Res. **426**:55-61 (1987).

Katovich, M.J., Simpkins, J.W. & O'Meara, J.: Effects of acute central LHRH administration on the skin temperature response in morphine dependent rats. Brain Res. **494**:85-94 (1989).

Katsuura, G., Gottschall, P.E., Dahl, R.R. & Arimura, A.: Interleukin-1β increases prostaglandin E$_2$ in rat astrocyte cultures: Modulatory effect of neuropeptides. Endocrinology **124**:3125-3127 (1989).

Kelly, P.H. & Moore, K.E.: Dopamine concentrations in the rat brain following injections into the substantia nigra of baclofen, γ-aminobutyric acid, γ-hydroxybutyric acid, apomorphine and amphetamine. Neuropharmacology **17**:169-174 (1978).

Kinnally, K.W., Campo, M.L. & Tedeschi, H.: Mitochondrial channel activity studied by patch-clamping mitoplasts. J. Bioenergetics Biomembranes **21**:497-506 (1989).

Kiss, J.Z.: Dynamism of chemoarchitecture in the hypothalamic paraventricular nucleus. Brain Res. Bull. **20**:699-708 (1988).

Kita, H. & Kitai, S.T.: Amygdaloid projections to the frontal cortex and the striatum in the rat. J. Comp. Neurol. **298**:40-49 (1990).

Klitsch, T. & Siemen, D.: The inner mitochondrial membrane anion channel is present in brown adipocytes but is not identical with the uncoupling protein. J Membrane Biol. **122**:69-75 (1991).

Kluger, M.J.: Endogenous pyrogens and fever. In Mercer, *Thermal Physiology 1989*, pp. 35-44 (Elsevier, Amsterdam 1989).

Kluger, M.J.: The febrile response. In *Stress Proteins in Biology and Medicine*, pp. 61-78 (Cold Spring Harbor Laboratory Press 1990).

Kluger, M.J., O'Reilly, B., Shope, T.R. & Vander, A.J.: Further evidence that stress hyperthermia is a fever. Physiology and Behavior **39**:763-766 (1987).

Kluger, M.J., Ringler, D.H. & Anver, M.R.: Fever and survival. Science **188**:166-168 (1975).

Kozak, W., Soszynksi, D., Szewczenko, M. & Bodurka, M.: Lack of pyrogenic tolerance transmission between brain and periphery in the rabbit. Experientia **46**:1010-1011 (1990).

Kripke, D.F., Mullaney, D.J., Atkinson, M. & Wolf, S.: Circadian rhythm disorders in manic-depressives. Biol. Psychiat. **13**:335-351 (1978).

Kronenberg, F., Carraway, R., Cote, L.J., Crawshaw, L.I. & Downey, J.A.: Changes in thermoregulation, immunoreactive neurotensin, catecholamines and LH during menopausal hot flashes. Maturitas **6**:31-43 (1984).

Ladinsky, H., Consolo, S., Bianchi, S. & Jori, A.: Increase in striatal acetylcholine by picrotoxin in the rat: Evidence for a GABAergic-dopaminergic-cholinergic link. Brain Res. **108**:351-361 (1976).

Langub, M.C., Jr., Maley, B.E. & Watson, R.E., Jr.: Ultrastructural evidence for luteinizing hormone-releasing hormone neuronal control of estrogen responsive neurons in the preoptic area. Endocrinology **128**:27-36 (1991).

Laufer, L.R., Erlik, Y., Meldrum, D.R. & Judd, H.L.: Effect of clonidine on hot flushes in postmenopausal women. Obstet. Gynecol. **60**:583-589 (1982).

Lauter, S. & Baumann, H.: Kreislauf und Atmung im hypoglykamischen Zustand. Dtsch. Arch. klin. Med. **163**:161-175 (1929).

Lavoinne, A., Buc, H.A., Claeyssens, S., Pinosa, M. & Matray, F.: The mechanism by which adenosine decreases gluconeogenesis from lactate in isolated rat hepatocytes. Biochem. J. **246**:449-454 (1987).

Lazarow, A.: Methods for quantitative measurement of water intake. Meth. Med. Res. **6**:225-229 (1954).

Leckman, J.F., Maas, J.W., Redmond, D.E. & Heninger, G.E.: Effects of oral clonidine on plasma MHPG in man. Life Sci. **26**:2179-2185 (1980).

Lee, K.S. & Reddington, M.: Autoradiographic evidence for multiple CNS binding sites for adenosine derivatives. Neuroscience **19**:535-549 (1986).

Lee, T.F., Li, D.J., Jacobson, K.A. & Wang, L.C.H.: Improvement of cold tolerance by selective A_1 adenosine receptor antagonists in rats. Pharmac. Biochem. Behav. **37**:107-112 (1990).

Leibowitz, S.F.: Brain monoamines and peptides: role in the control of eating behavior. Fed. Proc. **45**:1396-1403 (1986).

LeMay, D.R., LeMay, L.G., Kluger, M.J. & D'Alecy, L.G.: Plasma profiles of IL-6 and TNF with fever-inducing doses of lipopolysaccharide in dogs. Am. J. Physiol. **259**:R126-R132 (1990).

LeMay, L.G., Vander, A.J. & Kluger, M.J.: Role of interleukin 6 in fever in rats. Am. J. Physiol. **258**:R798-R803 (1990).

L'Hermite, M. (ed.): *Update on Hormonal Treatment in the Menopause. Progr. Reprod. Biol. Med.* 13 (Karger, Basel 1989).

Lin, C.S. & Klingenberg, M.: Characteristics of the isolated purine nucleotide binding protein from brown fat mitochondria. Biochem. (Wash.) **21**:2950-2956 (1982).

Lin, J.Y. & Ling, K.H.: Favism 2. Studies on physiological activities of vicine in vivo. J. Formosan Med. Assoc. **62**:490-494 (1962).

Lin, M.T., Chandra, A. & Liu, G.G.: The effects of theophylline and caffeine on thermoregulatory functions of rats at different ambient temperatures. J. Pharm. Pharmac. **32**:204-208 (1980).

Lin, M.T., Wang, P.S., Chuang, J., Fan, L.J. & Won, S.J.: Cold stress or a pyrogenic substance elevates thyrotropin releasing hormone levels in the rat hypothalamus and induces thermogenic reactions. Neuroendocrinology **50**:177-181 (1989).

Lipton, J.M. & Clark, W.G.: Neurotransmitters in temperature control. Ann. Rev. Physiol. **48**:a613-623 (1986).

Liu, B., Wohlfart, B.& Johansson, B.W.: Mechanical restitution at different temperatures in papillary msucles from rabbit, rat and hedgehog. Cryobiology **27**:596-604 (1990).

Lock, M.: Hot flushes in cultural context: The Japanese case as a cautionary tale for the West. In Schönbaum *The Climacteric Hot Flush. Progr. Basic Clin. Pharmacol. Vol. 6*, pp. 40-60 (Karger, Basel 1991).

Lock, M., Kaufert, P. & Gilbert, P.: Cultural construction of the menopausal syndrome: the Japanese case. Maturitas **10**:317-332 (1988).

Löfström, E., Pernow, B. & Wahren, J.: Vasodilating action of substance P in the human forearm. Acta Physiol. Scand. **63**:311-324 (1965).

Lomax, P.: Drugs and body temperaure. Int. Rev. Neurobiol. **12**:1-43 (1970).

Lomax, P.: The pathophysiology of postmenopausal hot flushes. In Schönbaum *The Climacteric Hot Flush. Progr. Basic Clin. Pharmacol. Vol. 6*, pp. 61-82 (Karger, Basel 1991).

Lomax, P. Bajorek, J.G., Chesarek, W. & Tataryn, I.V.: Thermoregulatory effects of luteinizing hormone releasing hormone in the rat. In Cox, Lomax, Milton & Schönbaum *Thermoregulatory Mechanisms and Their Therapeutic Implications*, pp. 208-211 (Karger, Basel 1980).

Lomax, P. & Daniel, K.A.: Body temperature changes induced by cocaine in the rat. In Mercer, *Thermal Physiology 1989*, pp. 265-271 (Excerpta Medica, Amsterdam 1989).

Lomax, P. & Daniel, K.A.: Cocaine and body temperature in the rat: effect of exercise. Pharmacol. Biochem. Behav. **36**:889-892 (1990).

Lomax, P. & Daniel, K.A.: Cocaine and body temperature in the rat: effects of ambient temperature. Pharmacol. **40**:103-109 (1990).

Lomax, P. & Schönbaum, E.: Neuroendocrine mechanisms in postmenopausal hot flushes. Submitted to: Life Sci. Adv.

Long, N.C., Kunkel, S.L., Vander, A.J. & Kluger, M.J.: Antiserum against tumor necrosis factor enhances lipopolysaccharide fever in rats. Am. J. Physiol. **258**:R332-R337 (1990).

Lopaschuk, G.D., Hansen, C.A. & Neely, J.R.: Fatty acid metabolism in hearts containing elevated levels of CoA. Am. J. Physiol. **250**:H351-H359 (1986).

Macdonald, I.A., Bennett, T., Gale, E.A.M., Green, J.H. & Walford, S.: The effect of propranolol on thermoregulation during insulin-induced hypoglycaemia in man. Clin. Sci. **63**:301-310 (1982).

Macdonald, I.A. & Lake, D.M.: An improved technique for extracting catecholamines from body fluids. J. Neurosci. Methods **13**:239-248 (1985).

Mager, J., Chevion, M. & Glaser, G.: In Liener, *Toxic Constituents of Plant Foods*, p. 266 (Academic Press, New York 1980).

Mager, J., Glaser, G., Razin, A., Izak, G., Bien, S. & Noam, M.: Metabolic effects of pyrimidines derived from faba bean glycosides on human erythrocytes deficient in glucose-6-phosphate dehydrogenase. Biochem. Biophys. Res. Comm. **20**:235-240 (1965).

Malan, A. & Mioskowski, E.: pH-temperature interactions on protein function and hibernation: GDP binding to brown adipose tissue mitochondria. J. Comp. Physiol. B **158**:487-493 (1988).

March, C.J., Mosley, B., Larsen, A., Cerretti, D.P., Braedt, G., Price, V., Gillis, S., Henney, C.S., Kronheim, S.R., Grabstein, K., Conlon, P.J., Hopp, T.P. & Cosman, D.: Cloning, sequence and expression of two distinct human interleukin-1 complementary DNAs. Nature **315**:641-647 (1985).

Mathieson, W.B., Federico, P., Veale, W.L. & Pittman, Q.J.: Single-unit activity in the bed nucleus of the stria terminalis during fever. Brain Res. **486**:49-55 (1989).

Matsuda, L.A., Hanson, G.R. & Gibb, J.W.: Neurochemical effects of amphetamine metabolites on central dopaminergic and serotonergic systems. J. Pharmacol. Exp. Ther. **251**:901-908 (1989).

McArthur, M.D., Jourdan, M.L. & Wang, L.C.H.: Effects of hypothermia and rewarming on plasma metabolites in rats. In Lomax & Schönbaum, *Thermoregulation: The Pathophysiological Basis of Clinical Disorders*, 8th International Symposium Pharmacology of Thermoregulation, Kananaskis, Canada 1991, pp. 119-123 (Karger, Basel 1992).

McArthur, M.D., Jourdan, M.L. & Wang, L.C.H.: Prolonged stable hypothermia: effects on blood gases and pH in rats and ground squirrels. Am. J. Physiol. (submitted 1990).

McEwan, J.R., Benjamin, N., Larkin, S., Fuller, R.W., Dollery, C.T., MacIntyre, I. & Path, F.R.C.: Vasodilation by calcitonin gene-related peptide and by substance P: A comparison of their effects on resistance and capacitance vessels of human forearms. Circulation **77**:1072-1080 (1988).

McGinty, D., Szymusiak, R.: The basal forebrain and slow wave sleep: Mechanistic and functional aspects. In Wauquier, Dugovic & Radulovacki, *Slow Wave Sleep: Physiological, Pathophysiological, and Functional Aspects*, pp. 61-71 (Raven Press, Ltd., New York 1989).

McGoon, D.C.: The ongoing quest for ideal myocardial protection. A catalog of the recent English literature. J. Thorac Cardiovasc. Surg. **89**:639-653 (1985).

Mefford, I.N., Ward, M.M., Miles, L., Taylor, B., Chesney, M.A., Keegan, D.L. & Barchas, J.D.: Determination fo plasma catecholamines and free 3,4-dihydroxyphenylacetic acid in continuously collected human plasma by high performance liquid chromatography with electrochemical detection. Life Sci. **20**:477-483 (1981).

Melis, G.H., Gambacciani, M., Cagnacci, A., Paoletti, A.M., Mais, V. & Fiorett, P.: Effects of the dopamine antagonist veralipride on hot flushes and luteinizing hormone secretion in postmenopausal women. Obstet. Gynecol. **72**:688-692 (1988).

Menon, R.K., Okonofua, F.E., Agnew, J.E., Thomas, M., Bell, J., O'Brien, P.M.S. & Dandona, P.: Endocrine and metabolic effects of simple hysterectomy. Int. J. Gynaecol. Obstet. **25**:459-463 (1987).

Menzel, W.: *Menschliche Tag-Nacht-Rhytmik und Schichtarbeit.* (Benno Schwabe & Co. Verlag, Basel 1962).

Merker, G., Blähser, S. & Zeisberger, E.: Reactivity pattern of vasopressin-containing neurons and its relation to the antipyretic reaction in the pregnant guinea pig. Cell Tissue Res. **212**:47-61 (1980).

Merker, G., Roth, J. & Zeisberger, E.: Thermoadaptive influence on reactivity pattern of vasopressinergic neurons in the guinea pig. Experientia **45**:722-726 (1989).

Milton, A.S.: Antipyretics and antipyretics. In Milton, *Handbook of Experimental Pharmacology, Vol. 60,* pp. 257-303 (Springer Verlag, Berlin 1982).

Milton, A.S.: Thermoregulatory actions of eicosanoids in the central nervous system with particular regard to the pathogenesis of fever. Ann. N.Y. Acad. Sci. **559**:392-410 (1989).

Milton, N.G.N., Hillhouse, E.W., Nicholson, S.A., Self, C.H. & McGregor, A.M.: Production and utilisation of monoclonal antibodies to human/rat corticotrophin-releasing factor-41. J. Mol. Endocrinol. **5**:159-166 (1990).

Minano, F.J., Sancibrian, M. & Serrano, J.S.: Hypothermic effect of GABA in conscious stressed rats: Its modification by cholinergic agonists and antagonists. J. Pharm. Pharmacol. **39**:721-726 (1987).

Mohell, N. & Dicker, A.: The β-adrenergic radioligand [^{3}H]CGP-12177, generally classified as an antagonist, is a thermogenic agonist in brown adipose tissue. Biochem. J. **261**:401-405 (1989).

Mohell, N., Nedergaard, J. & Cannon, B.: Quantitative differentiation of α- and β-adrenergic respiratory responses in isolated hamster brown fat cells: evidence for the presence of an α_1-adrenergic component. Eur. J. Pharmacol. **93**:183-193 (1983).

Molnar, G.W.: Body temperatures during menopausal hot flashes. J. Appl. Physiol. **38(3)**:499-503 (1975).

Moncada, S., Gryglewski, R., Bunting, S. & Vane, J.R.: An enzyme isolated from arteries transforms prostaglandin endoperoxides to an unstable substance that inhibits platelet aggregation. Nature **263**:663-665 (1976).

Moore-Ede, M.C., Czeisler, C.A. & Richardson, G.S.: Circadian timekeeping in health and disease. New Engl. J. Med. **309**:469-476 and 530-536 (1983).

Morray, J.P. & Pavlin, E.G.: Oxygen delivery and consumption during hypothermia and rewarming in the dog. Anesthesiology **72**:510-516 (1990).

Moss, D., Ma, A. & Cameron, D.P.: Defective thermoregulatory thermogenesis in monosodium glutamate-induced obesity in mice. Metabolism **34**:626-630 (1985).

Muduuli, D., Marquardt, R. & Guenter, W.: Effect of dietary vicine on the productive performance of laying chickens. Can. J. Anim. Sci. **61**:757-761 (1981).

Muduuli, D.S., Marquardt, R.R. & Guenter, W.: Effect of dietary vicine and vitamine E supplementation on the productive performance of growing and laying chickens. Br. J. Nutr. 47-53 (1982).

Musacchia, X.J.: Comparative physiological and biochemical aspects of hypothermia as a model for hibernation. Cryobiology **21**:583-592 (1984).

Myers, R.D.: The role of ions in thermoregulation and fever. In Milton, *Handbook of Experimental Pharmacology, Vol. 60. Pyretics and Antipyretics,* pp. 151-186 (Springer, Berlin 1982).

Myers, R.D., Rudy, T.A. & Yaksh, T.L.: Fever produced by endotoxin injected into the hypothalamus of the monkey and its antagonism by salicylate. J. Physiol. (London) **243**:167-193 (1974).

Nakajima, M. & Toda, N.: Prejunctional and postjunctional actions of prostaglandins $F_{2\alpha}$ and I_2 and carbocyclic thromboxane A_2 in isolated dog mesenteric arteries. Europ. J. Pharmacol. **120**:309-318 (1986).

Nakamura, H., Mizushima, Y., Seto, Y., Motoyoshi, S. & Kadokawa, T.: Dexamethasone fails to produce antipyretic and analgesic actions in experimental animals. Agents & Actions **16**:542-547 (1985).

Nakashima, T., Hori, T. & Kiyohara, T.: Intracellular recording analysis of septal thermosensitive neurons in the rat. In Mercer, *Thermal Physiology,* pp. 69-72 (Elsevier, New York 1989).

Nakashima, T., Hori, T., Kuriyama, K. & Matsuda, T.: Effects of interferon-alpha on the activity of preoptic thermosensitive neurons in tissue slices. Brain Res. **454**:361-367 (1988).

Nakashima, T., Hori, T., Kuriyama, K. & Kiyohara, T.: Naloxone blocks the interferon-alpha induced changes in hypothalamic neuronal activity. Neurosci. Lett. **82**:332-336 (1987).

Naylor, A.M., Cooper, K.E. & Veale, W.L.: Vasopressin and fever: evidence supporting the existence of an endogenous antipyretic system in the brain. Can. J. Physiol. Pharmacol. **65**:1333-1338 (1987).

Naylor, A.M., Ruwe, W.D., Burnard, D.M., McNeely, P.D., Turner, S.L., Pittman, Q.J. & Veale, W.L.: Vasopressin-induced motor disturbances: localization of a sensitive forebrain site in the rat. Brain Res. **361**:242-246 (1985).

Nedergaard, J. & Cannon, B.: Apparent unmasking of [^{3}H]GDP binding in rat brown-fat mitochondria is due to mitochondrial swelling. Eur. J. Biochem. **164**:681-686 (1986).

Nehls, D.G., Park, C.K., MacCormack, A.G. & McCulloch, J.: The effects of N-methyl-D-aspartate receptor blockade with MK-801 upon the relationship between cerebral blood flow and glucose utilization. Brain Res. **511**:271-279 (1990).

Neri Serneri, G.G., Castellani, S., Scart, L., Trotta, F., Chen, J.L., Carnovali M., Poggesi, L. & Masotti, G: Repeated sympathetic stimuli elicit the decline and disappearance of prostaglandin modulation and an increase of vascular resistance in humans. Circulation Res. **67**:580-588 (1990).

Nesbakken, R.: Aspects of free fatty acid metabolism during induced hypothermia. Scand. J. Clin. Lab. Invest. **31**(131):5-72 (1973).

Neumann, I., Schwarzberg, H. & Landgraf, R.: Measurement of septal release of vasopressin and oxytocin by the push-pull technique following electrical stimulation of the paraventricular nucleus of rats. Brain Res. **462**:181-184 (1988).

Nicholls, D.G., Cunningham, S.A. & Rial, E.: The bioenergetic mechanism of brown adipose tissue thermogenesis. In Trayhurn & Nicholls *Brown Adipose Tissue*, pp. 52-85 (Edward Arnolds, London 1986).

Nicholls, D.G. & Locke, R.M.: Thermogenic mechanisms in brown fat. Physiol. Rev. **64**:1-65 (1984).

Nicholls, D.G., Snelling, R. & Rial, E.: Proton and calcium circuits across the mitochondrial inner membrane. Biochem. Soc. Trans. **12**:388-390 (1984).

Nieuwenhuys, R.: *Chemoarchitecture of the Brain.* (Springer-Verlag, Berlin 1985).

Nijsten, M.W.N., DeGroot, H.J., Klasen, H.J., Hack, C.E. & Aarden, L.A.: Serum levels of interleukin-6 and acute phase response. Lancet II:921 (1987).

Nikitopoulou, G. & Grammer, J.L.: Endogenous anxiety and circadian rhythms. Brit. Med. J. **1**:1311 (1979).

Nikolaishvili, L.S. & Devdariani, M.I.: Dynamics of local blood flow in different regions of the hypothalamus in the sleep-wakefulness cycle. Neurosci. Behav. Physiol. **18**(4):310-315 (1988).

Nomoto, T., Uchida, Y. Boschi, G. & Rips, R.: Thyroid hormone involvement in TRH induced hyperthermia in mice with various thyroid states. In Lomax & Schönbaum, *Thermoregulation: Research adn Clinical Applications*, pp. 152-155 (Karger, Basel 1986).

Norizzano, O.C., Karora, A., Rettori, V., Ponzio, R. & McCann, S.M.: GABAergic control of TSH secretion: Effect of bicuculline injected in the median preoptic area and the arcuate nucleus on the release of TSH in the rat. Commun. Biol. **6**:383-392 (1988).

Norman, D.C., Grahn, D. & Yoshikawa, T.T.: Fever and aging. J. Am. Geriatr. Soc. **33**:859-863 (1985).

Ohisalo, J.J.: Regulatory function of adenosine. Med. Biol. **65**:181-191 (1987).

Okonofua, F.E., Lawal, A. & Bamgbose, J.K.: Features of menopause and menopausal age in Nigerian women. Int. J. Gynecol. Obstet. **31**:341-345 (1990).

Oldenhave, A. & Jaszmann, L.J.B.: The climacteric: Absence or presence of hot flushes and their relation to other complaints. In Schönbaum *The Climacteric Hot Flush. Progr. Basic Clin. Pharmacol. Vol. 6*, pp. 6-39 (Karger, Basel 1991).

Olinger, G.N.: Intermittent ischemic arrest. In Roberts, *Myocardial Protection in Cardiac Surgery*, pp. 207-219 (Marcel Dekker, NY 1987).

Opp, M., Obál Jr., F. & Krueger, J.M.: Corticotropin-releasing factor attenuates interleukin 1-induced sleep and fever in rabbits. Am. J. Physiol. **257**:R528-R535 (1989).

Otero Losada, M.E.: Changes in central GABAergic function following acute and repeated stress. Brit. J. Pharmacol. **93**:483-490 (1988).

Owman, C., Hanko, J., Hardebo, J.E. & Kåhrström, J.: Neuropeptides and classical autonomic transmitters in the cardiovascular system: Existence, coexistence, action, interaction. In Christensen, Henriksen & Lassen, *The Sympatho-adrenal System*, Alfred Benzon Symposium 23, pp. 340-383 (Munksgaard, Copenhagen 1986).

Palmi, M. & Sgaragli, G.: Hyperthermia induced in rabbits by organic calcium antagonists. Pharmac. Biochem. Behav. **34**:325-330 (1989).

Parmeggiani, P.L.: Thermoregulation during sleep in mammals. NIPS **5**:208-212 (1990).

Paton, B.C.: Accidental hypothermia. Pharmac. Ther. **22**:331-377 (1983).

Pau, K-Y.F., Gliessman, P.M., Hess, D.L., Ronnekleiv, O.K., Levine, J.E. & Spies, H.G.: Acute administration of estrogen suppresses LH secretion without altering GnRH release in ovariectomized rhesus macaques. Brain Res. **517**:229-235 (1990).

Pellegrini-Giampietro, D.E., Bacciottini, L., Carla, V. & Moroni, F.: Morphine withdrawal in cortical slices: suppression by Ca^{2+}-channel inhibitors of abstinence-induced [^{3}H] noradrenaline release. Br. J. Pharmac. **93**:535-540 (1988).

Pellegrino, L.J., Pellegrino, A.S. & Cushman, A.J.: *A Stereotaxic Atlas of the Rat Brain*, (Plenum Press, New York 1979).

Pepper, J.R., Lockey, E., Cankovic-Darracott, S. & Braimbridge, M.V.: Cardioplegia versus intermittent ischaemic arrest in coronary bypass surgery. Thorax **37**:887-892 (1982).

Pflug, B., Erikson, R. & Johnsson, A.: Depression and daily temperature. A long study. Acta Psychiat. Scand. **54**:254-266 (1976).

Philipp-Dormston, W.K. & Siegert, R.: Adenosine 3',5'-cyclic monophosphate in rabbit cerebrospinal fluid during fever induced by *E. coli*-endotoxin. Med. Microbiol. Immun. **161**:11-13 (1975).

Phillips, M.I.: Functions of angiotensin in the central nervous system. Ann. Rev. Physiol. **49**:413-435 (1987).

Pittman, Q.J. & Landgraf, R.: Vasopressin in thermoregulation and blood pressure control. In Lord & Jamison, *Vasopressin Vasopressine*, INSERM Vol. 208, pp. 177-184 (John Libbey Eurotext, Collogue 1991).

Pittman, Q.J., Naylor, A., Poulin, P., Disturnal, J., Veale, W.L., Martin, S.M. & Malkinson, T.J.: The role of vasopressin as an antipyretic in the ventral septal area and its possible involvement in convulsive disorders. Brain Res. Bull. **20**:887-892 (1988).

Popovic, V.P. & Kent, K.M.: Cardiovascular responses in prolonged hypothermia. Am. J. Physiol. **209**:1069-1074 (1965)

Poulin, P.: (unpublished results, 1991).

Poulin, P., Lederis, K. & Pittman, Q.J.: Subcellular localization and characterization of vasopressin binding sites in the ventral septal area, lateral septum, and hippocampus of the rat brain. J. Neurochem. **50**:889-898 (1988).

Prokocimer, P.G., Maze, M., Vickery, R.G., Kraemer, F.B., Gandjei, R. & Hoffman, B.B.: Mechanism of halothane-induced inhibition of isoproterenol-stimulated lipolysis in isolated rat adipocytes. Mol. Pharmacol. **33**:338-343 (1988).

Quan, N. & Blatteis, C.M.: Intrapreoptically microdialyzed and microinjected norepinephrine evoke different thermal responses. Am. J. Physiol. **257**:R816-R821 (1989).

Quan, N. & Blatteis, C.M.: Microdialysis: a system for localized drug delivery into the brain. Brain Res. Bull. **22**:621-625 (1989).

Ramabadran, K., Bansinath, M., Turndorf, H. & Puig, M.M.: A pharmacological analysis of the interaction of ketamine with kappa opiates. In Domino, *Status of Ketamine in Anesthesiology*, pp. 211-227 (NPP Books, Ann Arbor 1990).

Rance, N.E., McMullen, N.T., Smialek, J.E., Price, D.L. & Young, III, W.S.: Postmenopausal hypertrophy of neurons expressing the estrogen receptor gene in the human hypothalamus. J. Clin. Endocrinol. Metab. **71**:79-85 (1990).

Ravnikar, V.: Physiology and treatment of hot flushes. Obstet. Gynecol. **75**:3s-8s (1990).

Raz, A., Isakson, P.C., Minkes, M.S. & Needleman, P.: Characterization of a novel metabolic pathway of arachidonate in coronary arteries which generates a potent endogenous coronary vasodilator. J. Biol. Chem. **252**;1123-1126 (1977).

Rechtschaffen, A. & Kales, A. (eds.): *A Manual of Standardized Terminology, Techniques, and Scoring Systems for Sleep Stages of Human Subjects*. (U.S. Government Printing Office, Washington, D.C. 1968).

Redford, E.J. & Dascombe, M.J.: Interleukin 1β and lipopolysaccharide effects on prostaglandin E_2 release from rat brain slices. Br. J. Pharmacol. **98**:708P (1989).

Reinberg, A., Gervais, P., Pollak, E., Abulker, Ch. & Dupont, J.: Circadian rhythms during drug induced coma. Intern. J. Chronobiol. **1**:157-162 (1973).

Renbourn, E.T.: Body temperature and pulse rate in boys and young men prior to sporting contests. A study of emotional hyperthermia: with a review of the literature. Psychosom. Res. **4**:147-175 (1960).

Resch, G.E. & Musacchia, X.J.: A role of glucose in hypothermic hamsters. Am. J. Physiol. **231**:1729-1734 (1976).

Reyes, A., Luckhause, J. & Ferin, M.: Unexpected inhibitory action of N-methyl-D,L-aspartate on luteinizing hormone release in adult ovariectomized rhesus monkeys: A role of the hypothalamic-adrenal axis. Endocrinology **127**:724-729 (1990).

Richter, C.P.: *Biological Clocks in Medicine and Psychiatry*. (Charles C. Thomas, Springfield 1965).

Riedel, W., Kozawa, E. & Iriki, M.: Renal and cutaneous vasomotor and respiratory rate adjustments to peripheral cold and warm stimuli and to bacterial endotoxin in conscious rabbits. J. Autonom. Nerv. Syst. **5**:177-194 (1982).

Rivier, J., Rivier, C. & Vale, W.: Synthetic competitive antagonists of corticotrophin releasing factor: effects on ACTH secretion in the rat. Science **224**:889-891 (1984).

Roberts, A.J., Sanders Jr., J.H., Moran, J.M., Kaplan, K.J., Lichtenthal, P.R., Spies, S.M. & Michaelis, L.L.: Nonrandomized matched pair analysis of intermittent ischemic arrest versus potassium crystalloid cardioplegia during myocardial revascularization. Ann. Thorac Surg. **31**:502-511 (1981).

Roberts, P.J., Gupta, H.K. & Shargill, N.S.: The interaction of baclofen (β-(4-chlorophenyl) GABA) with GABA systems in the rat brain: evidence for a releasing action. Brain Res. **155**:209-212 (1978).

Roberts, W.W. & Mooney, R.D.: Brain areas controlling thermoregulatory grooming, prone extension, locomotion, and tail vasodilation in rats. J. Comp. Physiol. Psychol. **86**:470-480 (1974).

Roberts, W.W. & Robinson, T.C.L.: Relaxation and sleep induced by warming of preoptic region and anterior hypothalamus in cats. Exp. Neurol. **25**:282-294 (1969).

Roselli, C.E. & Resko, J.A.: Regulation of hypothalamic luteinizing hormone-releasing hormone levels by testosterone and estradiol in male rhesus moneys. Brain Res. **509**:343-346 (1990).

Roth, J., Schulze, K., Merker, G., Simon, E. & Zeisberger, E.: Influence of osmotic stimulation on release of arginine-vasopressin and fever in the guinea pig. Neuroendocrinology **52**(**Suppl. 1**):114 (1990).

Roth, R.H.: Neuronal activity, impulse flow and MHPG production. In Mass, *MHPG: Basic Mechanisms and Psychopathology*, pp. 19-33 (Academic Press, New York 1983).

Roth, R.H., Walters, J.R. & Aghajanian, G.K.: Effect of impulse flow on the release and synthesis of dopamine in the rat striatum. In Snyder & Costa, *Frontiers in Catecholamine Research*, pp. 567-574 (Pergamon Press, New York 1973).

Rothwell, N.J.: CRF is involved in the pyrogenic and thermogenic effects of interleukin 1β in the rat. Am. J. Physiol. **256**:E111-E115 (1989).

Rothwell, N.J. & Stock, M.J.: Influence of noradrenaline on blood flow to brown adipose tissue in rats exhibiting diet-induced thermogenesis. Pflügers Arch. **389**:237-242 (1981).

Rothwell, N.J. & Stock, M.J.: A role for brown adipose tissue in diet-induced thermogenesis. Nature **281**:31-35 (1979).

Rotondo, D., Abul, H.T., Milton, A.S. & Davidson, J.: Pyrogenic immunomodulators increase the level of prostaglandin E_2 in the blood simultaneously with the onset of fever. Eur. J. Pharmacol. **154**:145-152 (1988).

Ruwe, W.D., Naylor, A.M. & Veale, W.L.: Perfusion of vasopressin within the rat brain suppresses prostaglandin E-hyperthermia. Brain Res. **338**:219-224 (1985).

Russchen, F.T. & Price, J.L.: Amygdalostriatal projections in the rat. Topographical organization and fiber morphology shown using the lectin PHA-L as an anterograde tracer. Neurosci. Lett. **47**:15-22 (1984).

Saigusa, T. & Iriki, M.: Regional differentiation of sympathetic nerve activity during fever caused by intracerebroventricular injection of PGE_2. Pflügers Arch. **411**:121-125 (1988).

Saigusa, T.: Participation of interleukin-1 and tumor necrosis factor in the responses of the sympathetic nervous system during lipopolysaccharide-induced fever. Pflügers Arch. **416**:225-229 (1990).

Sánchez, C: The effects of dopamine D-1 and D-2 receptor agonists on body temperature in male mice. Eur. J. Pharmacol. **171**:201-206 (1989).

Santiago, J.V., White, N.H., Skor, D.A., Levandoski, L.A., Bier, D.M. & Cryer, P.E.: Defective glucose counterregulation, limits intensive therapy of diabetes mellitus. Am. J. Physiol. **247**:E215-E220 (1984).

Satinoff, E. & Shan, S.Y.Y.: Loss of behavioral thermoregulation after lateral hypothalamic lesions in rats. J. Comp. Physiol. Psychol. **77**:302-312 (1971).

Sawyer, C.H., Everett, J.M. & Green, J.D.: The rabbit diencephalon in stereotaxic coordinates. J. Com. Neurol. **101**:801-824 (1954).

Scarpace, P.J., Bender, B.S. & Borst, S.E.: *E. coli* peritonitis activates thermogenesis in brown adipose tissue: Relationship to fever. Can. J. Physiol. Pharmacol. (June 1991).

Scarpace, P.J., Bender, B.S. & Borst, S.E.: The febrile response to *E. coli* peritonitis is impaired in senescent rats. Gerontologist **30(special issue)**:215A (1990).

Scarpace, P.J. & Matheny, M.: Adenylate cyclase agonist properties of CGP-12177A in brown fat: Evidence for atypical β-adrenergic receptors. Am. J. Physiol. **260**:E226-E231 (1991).

Scarpace, P.J., Matheny, M. & Borst, S.E.: Thermogenesis induced by a unique brown adipose tissue agonist is decreased with age. FASEB J. **5**:A1654 (1991).

Scarpace, P.J., Mooradian, A.D. & Morley, J.E.: Age-associated decrease in beta-adrenergic receptors and adenylate cyclase activity in rat brown adipose tissue. J. Gerontol. **43**:B65-B70 (1988).

Schindler, A.E., Muller, D., Keller, E., Goser, R. & Runkel, F.: Studies with clonidine (Dixarit) in menopausal women. Arch. Gynecol. **227**:341-347 (1979).

Schmidt, Th.H.: *Thermoregulatorische Grössen in Abhängigkeit von Tageszeit und Menstruationszyklus.* Thesis, München 1972.

Schmitt, H.: The pharmacology of clonidine and related products. In Gross, *Antihypertensive agents*, pp. 299-396 (Springer-Verlag, New York 1977).

Schönbaum, E. (ed). *The Climacteric Hot Flush. Progr. Basic Clin. Pharmacol. vol. 6* (Karger, Basel 1991).

Schönbaum, E. & Lomax, P. (eds): *Thermoregulation. Physiology and Biochemistry. Int. Encycl. Pharmacol. Ther. Section 131* (Pergamon Press, New York 1990); *Thermoregulation. Pathology, Pharmacology and Therapy. Int. Encycl. Pharmacol. Ther. Section 132* (Pergamon Press, New York 1991).

Sealy, W.C.: Hypothermia: its possible role in cardiac surgery. Ann. Thorac. Surg. **47**:788-791 (1989).

Sellers, E.A. & You, S.S.: Role of the thyroid in metabolic responses to a cold environment. Am. J. Physiol. **163**:81-91 (1950).

Sherwin, B.B. & Gelfand, M.M.: Effects of parenteral administration of estrogen and androgen on plasma hormone levels and hot flushes in the surgical menopause. Am. J. Obstet. Gynecol. **148:**552-557 (1984).

Sheth, U.K. & Borison, H.L.: Central pyrogenic action of Salmonella Typhosa lipopolysaccaride injected into the lateral cerebral ventricle in cats. J. Pharmacol. Exp. Ther. **130:**411-417 (1960).

Shohami, E. & Gross, J.: An ex-vivo method for evaluating prostaglandin synthetase activity in cortical slices of mouse brain. J. Neurochem. **45:**132-136 (1985).

Sibley, D.R. & Lefkowitz, R.J.: Molecular mechanism of receptor desensitization using the β-adrenergic receptor coupled adenylate cyclase system as a model. Nature Lond. **317:**124-129 (1985).

Siesjo, B.K.: Hypothermia and hyperthermia. In Siesjo, *Brain Energy Metabolism*, pp. 324-344 (Wiley and Sons, New York 1978).

Silva, J.E.: Full expression of uncoupling protein gene requires the concurrence of norepinephrine and triiodothyronine. Mol. Endocrinol. **2:**706-713 (1988).

Silverman, R.W., Bajorek, J.G.,Lomax, P. & Tataryn, I.V.: Monitoring the pathophysiological correlates of postmenopausal hot flushes. Maturitas **3:**39-46 (1981).

Simpkins, J.W., Andreadis, D.K., Millard, W.J. & Katovich, M.J.: The effects of celular glucoprivation on skin temperature regulation in the rat. Life Sci. **47:**107-115 (1990).

Simpkins, J.W., Katovich, M.J. & Millard, W.J.: Glucose modulation of skin temperature responses during morphine withdrawal in the rat. Psychopharmacol. **102:**213-220 (1990).

Simpkins, J.W., Katovich, M.J. & Song, I-C.: Similarities between morphine withdrawal in the rat and the menopausal hot flush. Life Sci. **32:**1957-1966 (1983).

Snedecor, G.W. & Cochran, W.G.: Statistical methods. Iowa State University Press, Ames 7th Edition (1980).

Sokoloff, P., Giros, B., Martres, M.-P., Bouthenet, M.-L. & Schwartz, J.-C.: Molecular cloning and characterization of a novel dopamine receptor (D_3) as a target for neuroleptics. Nature (Lond.) **347:**146-151 (1990).

Sorgato, M.C., Keller, B.U. & Stühmer, W.: Patch-clamping of the inner mitochondrial membrane reveals a voltage-dependent ion channel. Nature **330:**498-496 (1987).

Sorgato, M.C., Moran, O., de Pinto, V., Keller, B.U. & Stühmer, W.: Further investigation on the high conductive ion channel of the inner membrane of mitochondria. J. Bioenergetics Biomembranes **21:**485-506 (1989).

Squires, R.D.: Thermoregulatory effects of injections of γ-aminobutyric acid (GABA) and picrotoxin into medial preoptic region of cats. Fed. Proc. **26:**555 (abstr.) (1967).

Spangelo, B.L., Judd, A.M., MacLeod, R.M., Goodman, D.W. & Isakson, P.C.: Endotoxin induced release of interleukin-6 from rat medial basal hypothalami. Endocrinology **127:**1779-1785 (1990).

Spence, R.J., Rhodes, B.A. & Wagner, H.N., Jr.: Regulation of arteriovenous anastomotic and capillary blood flow in the dog leg. Am. J. Physiol. **222:**326-332 (1972).

Splawinski, J., Górka, Z., Zacny, E. & Kaluza, J.: Fever produced in the rat by intracerebral E. coli endotoxin. Pflügers Arch. **368:**117-123 (1977).

Staiger, J.F. & Nürnberger, F.: Pattern of afferents to the lateral septum in the guinea pig. Cell Tissue Res. **257:**471-490 (1989).

Staiger, J.F. & Wouterlood, F.G.: Efferent projections from the lateral septal nucleus to the anterior hypothalamus in the rat: A study combining Phaseolus vulgaris-leucoagglutinin tracing with vasopressin immunocytochemistry. Cell Tissue Res. **261:**17-23 (1990).

Stanley, B.G., Kyrkouli, S.E., Lampert, S. & Leibowitz, S.F.: Neuropeptide Y chronically injected into the hypothalamus: a powerful neurochemical inducer of hyperphagia and obesity. Peptides **7:**1189-1192 (1986).

Starke, K., Gothert, M. & Kilbringer, H.: Modulation of neurotransmitter release by presynaptic autoreceptors. Physiol. Rev. **69:**864-989 (1989).

Steffen, J.M.: Glucose, glycogen, and insulin responses in the hypothermic rat. Cryobiology **25:**94-101 (1988).

Stephan, K. & Dorow, R.: Circadian core temperature, psychomotor performance and subjective ratings of fatigue in morning and evening 'types'. In Redfern, Campbell, Davis & Martin, *Circadian Rhythms in the Central Nervous System*, pp. 233-236 (VCH Publishers, London 1985).

Stitt, J.T.: Prostaglandin E as the neural mediator of the febrile response. Yale J. Biol. Med. **59**:137-149 (1986).

Stitt, J.T.: Prostaglandin E_1 fever induced in rabbits. J. Physiol. **232**:163-179 (1973).

Stitt, J.T. & Shimada, S.G.: Immunoadjuvants enhance the febrile responses of rats to endogenous pyrogen. J. Appl. Physiol. **67**:1734-1739 (1989).

Stojilkovic, S.S., Merell, F., Iida, T., Krsmanovic, L.Z. & Catt, K.J.: Endothelin stimulation of cytosolic calcium and gonadotropin secretion in anterior pituitary cells. Science **248**:1663-1666 (1990).

Stolwijk, J.J. & Hardy, J.D.: Control of body temperature. In Lee, *Handbook of Physiology, Section 9. Reactions to Environmental Agents* (Am. Physiol. Soc., Bethesda, Maryland 1977).

Stone, S.C., Mickal, A. & Rye, P.H.: Postmenopausal symptomatology, maturation index, and plasma estrogen levels. Obstet. Gynecol. **45**:625-627 (1975).

Studd, J.W.W. & Whitehead, M.I. (eds): *The Menopause* (Blackwell, Oxford 1988).

Studler, J.M., Reibaud, M., Tramu, G., Blanc, G., Glowinski, J. & Tassin, J.P.: Distinct properties of cholecystokinin-8 and mixed dopamine-cholecystokinin-8 neurons innervating the nucleus accumbens. In Vanderkalghen & Crawley, *Cholecystokinin*, pp. 306-314 (Academic Science, New York 1985).

Susic, H. & Malik, K.U.: Prostacyclin and prostaglandin E_2 effects on adrenergic transmission in the kidney of anesthetized dog. J. Pharmacol. Exp. Ther. **218**:588-592 (1981).

Swartzman, L.C., Edelberg, R. & Kemmann, E. Impact of stress on objectively recorded menopausal hot flushes and on flush report bias. Health Psychology **9**:529-545 (1990).

Tataryn, I.V., Lomax, P., Bajorek, J.G., Chesarek, W., Meldrum, D.R. & Judd, H.L.: Postmenopausal hot flushes: a disorder of thermoregulation. Maturitas **2**:101-107 (1980).

Tataryn, I.V. Meldrum, D.R., Frumar, A.M., Lu, K.H., Judd, H.L., Bajorek, J.G., Chesarek, W. & Lomax, P.: The hormonal and thermoregulatory changes in postmenopausal hot flushes. In Cox, Lomax, Milton & Schönbaum *Thermoregulatory Mechanisms and Their Therapeutic Implications*, pp. 202-207 (Karger, Basel 1980).

Tax, L.: Hormone replacement therapy? Livial® (Org OD 14), a new possibility. In Schönbaum *The Climacteric Hot Flush. Progr. Basic Clin. Pharmacol. Vol. 6*, pp. 143-159 (Karger, Basel 1991).

The DCCT Research Group: Diabetes Control and Complications Trial (DCCT): results of feasibility study. Diabetes Care **10**:1-19 (1987).

Thompson, C.J., Thow, J., Jones, I.R. & Baylis, P.H.: Vasopressin secretion during insulin-induced hypoglycaemia: exaggerated response in people with type I diabetes. Diab. Med. **6**:158-163 (1989).

Thomson, J. & Oswald, I.: Effect of oestrogen on the sleep, mood, and anxiety of menopausal women. Br. Med. J. **2**:1317-1319 (1977).

Thrasher, T.N.: Role of forebrain circumventricular organs in body fluid balance. Acta Physiol. Scand. **136(Suppl. 583)**:141-150 (1989).

Thrasher, T.N. & Keil, L.C.: Regulation of drinking and vasopressin secretion: Role of organum vasculosum laminae terminalis. Am. J. Physiol. **253**:R108-R120 (1987).

Tovey, K.C., Oldham, K.G. & Whelan, J.A.M.: A simple direct assay for cyclic AMP in plasma and other biological samples using an improved competitive protein binding technique. Clinica chim. Acta **56**:221-234 (1974).

Trovati, M., Massucco, P., Mularoni, E., Cavalot, F., Anfossi, G., Mattiello, L. & Emanuelli, G.: Insulin-induced hypoglycaemia increases plasma concentrations of angiotensin II and does not modify atrial natriuretic polypeptide secretion in man. Diabetologia **31**:816-820 (1988).

Tulandi, T., Samarthji, L. & Kinch, R.A.: Effect of intravenous clonidine on menopausal flushing and luteinizing hormone secretion. Brit. J. Obstet. Gynec. **990**:854-857 (1983).

Unger, M., Merker, G., Roth, J. & Zeisberger, E.: Influence of noradrenergic input into the hypothalamic paraventricular nucleus on fever in the guinea pig. Pflügers Arch. (in press 1991).

Vanderwende, C., Spoerlein, M.T. & Lapollo, J.: Cocaine potentiates ketamine-induced loss of the righting reflex and sleeping time in mice. Role of catecholamines. J. Pharmacol. Exp. Ther. 222:122-125 (1982).

Van Meel, J.A.C., Qian, J., Timmermans, P.B.M.W.M. & Van Zwieten, P.A.: Differential inhibition of α_2-adrenoceptor mediated pressor response by (+) and (-) verapamil in pithed rats. J. Pharm. Pharmacol. 35:500-504 (1983).

Vasse, M., Chagraoui, A., Henry, J.-P. & Protais, P: The rise of body temperature induced by stimulation of dopamine D_1 receptors is increased in acutely reserpinized mice. Eur. J. Pharmacol. 181:23-33 (1990).

Wallace, J.M. & Harlan, W.R.: Significance of epinephrine in insulin hypoglycaemia in man. Am. J. Med. 38:531-539 (1965).

Wang, L.C.H.: Effects of feeding on aminophylline induced supra-maximal thermogenesis. Life Sci. 29:2459-2466 (1981).

Wang, L.C.H.: Factors limiting maximum cold-induced heat production. Life Sci. 23:2089-2098 (1978).

Wang, L.C.H. & Anholt, E.C.: Elicitation of supramaximal thermogenesis by aminophylline in the rat. J. Appl. Physiol. 53:16-20 (1982).

Wang, L.C.H., Jourdan, M.L. & Lee, T.F.: Mechanisms underlying the supramaximal thermogenesis elicited by aminophylline in rats. Life Sci. 44:927-934 (1989).

Wang, L.C.H. & Lee, T.F.: Enhancement of maximal thermogenesis by reducing endogenous adenosine activity in the rat. J. Appl. Physiol. 68:580-585 (1990).

Wang, L.C.H., Man, S.F.P. & Belcastro, A.N.: Metabolic and hormonal responses in theophylline-increased cold resistance in males. J. Appl. Physiol. 63:589-596 (1987).

Wang, L.C.H., McArthur, M.D., Jourdan, M.L. & Lee, T.F.: Depressed metabolic rates in hibernation and hypothermia: can these be compared meaningfully? In Sutton, Coates & Remmers, Hypoxia: The Adaptations, pp. 78-83 (B.C. Decker, Toronto 1990).

Wang, X.L., Lee, T.F. & Wang, L.C.H.: Do adenosine antagonists improve cold tolerance by reducing hypothalamic adenosine activity in rats? Brain Res. Bull. 24:389-393 (1990).

Watanabe, M., Hashimoto, M., Iriki, M. & Shimada, Y.: Arachidonate metabolites related to TNF-induced fever. Jpn. J. Physiol. 39(Suppl. 781): (1989).

Weber, A. & Siemen, D.: Permeability of the nonselective channel in brown adipocytes to small cations. Pflügers Arch. 414:564-570 (1989).

Weihe, W.H.: The effect of temperature on the action of drugs. Ann. Rev. Pharmacol. 13:409-425 (1973).

West J.B.: Visceral control mechanism. In Best & Taylor, Physiological Basis of Medical Practice, pp. 1211-1234 (Williams and Wilkins, London 1985).

Wever, R.A.: The Circadian System of Man: Results of Experiments Under Temporal Isolation. (Springer Verlag, New York 1979).

Wever, R.A.: Internal interactions within the human circadian system: the masking effect. Experientia 41:332-342 (1985).

Wilkinson, M.F. & Kasting, N.W.: Centrally acting vasopressin contributes to endotoxin tolerance. Am. J. Physiol. 258: (Regulatory Integrative Comp. Physiol. 27):R443-R449 (1990).

Wilkinson, M.F. & Kasting, N.W.: Centrally acting vasopressin contributes to endotoxin tolerance. Am. J. Physiol. 258: (Regulatory Integrative Comp. Physiol. 27):R443-R449 (1990).

Winterbourn, C.C., Benatti, U. & DeFlora, A.: Contributions of superoxide, hydrogen peroxide, and transition metal ions to auto-oxidation of the favism-inducing pyrimidine aglycone, divicine, and its reactions with haemoglobin. Biochem. Pharmacolgoy 23(12):2009-2015 (1986).

Witkin, J.M., Goldberg, S.R. & Katz, J.L.: Lethal effects of cocaine are reduced by the dopamine-1 receptor antagonist SCH 23390 but not by haloperidol. Life Sci. 44:1285-1291 (1989).

Wohlfart, B. & Noble, M.I.M.: The cardiac excitation-contraction cycle. Pharmacol. Ther. 16:1-43 (1982).

Woodward, S. & Freedman, R.R.: Increased menopausal hot flashes in slow wave sleep. Ann. NY Acad. Sci. **592**:479-480 (1990).

Yanagisawa, M., Inoue, A., Ishikawa, T., Kasuya, Y., Kimura, S., Kumagaye, S., Nakajima, K., Watanabe, T.X., Sakakibara, S., Goto, K. & Masaki, T.: Primary structure, synthesis, and biological activity of rat endothelin, an endothelium-derived vasoconstrictor peptide. Proc. Natl. Acad. Sci. USA **85**:6964-6967 (1988).

Yannai, S. & Marquardt, R.R.: Induction of favism-like symptoms in the rat: effects of vicine and divicine in normal and buthionine sulfoximine-treated rats. J. Sci. Food Agric. **36**:1161-1168 (1985).

Yarbrough, G.G. & McGuffin-Clineschimidt, J.C.: In vivo behavioral assessment of central nervous system purinergic receptors. Eur. J. Pharmacol. **76**:137-144 (1981).

Yazumi, T.: Thermal circadian rhythm in healthy subjects. The St. Marianna Medical J. **13**:632-641 (1985).

Yoshida, T., Nishioka, H., Nakamura, Y. & Kondo, M.: Reduced norepinephrine turnover in mice with monosodium glutamate-induced obesity. Metabolism **33**:1060-1063 (1984).

Yoshiue, S., Yoshizawa, H., Itoh, H., Sekine, H., Nakamura, M., Kanamori, T., Yazumi, T., Suzuki, H., Ogata, J. & Ishida, M.: Analysis of body temperature at different sites in patients having slight fever caused by psychogenic stress. In Lomax & Schönbaum, *Thermoregulatory Mechanisms and Their Therapeutic Implications*, pp. 169-170 (Karger, Basel 1979).

Young, A. & Dawson, N.J.: Effect of environmental temperature on the development of a noradrenergic thermoregulatory mechanism in the rat. Pflu. Arch. Eur. J. **412**:141-146 (1988).

Zataman, M.L.: Renal and cardiovascular effects of hibernation and hypothermia. Cryobiology **21**:593-614 (1984).

Zeisberger, E.: Antipyretic action of vasopressin in the ventral septal area of the guinea-pig's brain. In Lomax & Schönbaum, *Thermoregulation: Research and Clinical Applications*, pp. 65-68 (Karger, Basel 1989).

Zeisberger, E.: Comparison of antipyretic actions of different neuropeptides in the same site of brain septum in the guinea pig. In Mercer, *Thermal Physiology 1989*, pp. 117-122 (Elsevier, Amsterdam 1989).

Zeisberger, E.: Peptides and amines as putative factors in endogenous antipyresis. In *Proceedings of the XXth International Congress of Neurovegetative Research in Tokyo 1990, Excerpta Medica International Congress* (Elsevier, Smsterdam 1991) (in press).

Zeisberger, E.: The role of septal peptides in thermoregulation and fever. In Bligh & Voight, *Thermoreception and Temperature Regulation*, pp. 274-283 (Springer, Berlin, Heidelberg 1990).

Zeisberger, E., Merker, G., Blahser, S. & Krannig, M.: Changes in activity of vasopressin neurons during fever in the guinea pig. Neurosci. Lett. (Suppl.) **14**:S414 (1983).

Zsigmond, E.K. & Domino, E.F.: Clinical pharmacology of ketamine. In ino, *Status of Ketamine in Anesthesiology*, pp. 27-67 (NPP Books, Ann Arbor 1990).

AUTHOR INDEX

Subject Index